Endocrine Diseases

ATLAS OF NONTUMOR PATHOLOGY

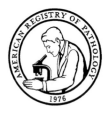
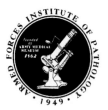

Endocrine Diseases

Ricardo V. Lloyd, MD, PhD
Bruce R. Douglas, MD
William F. Young, Jr, MD

Published by the
American Registry of Pathology
and the
Armed Forces Institute of Pathology
Washington, DC

In Collaboration with
Universities Associated for Research
and Education in Pathology, Inc.
Bethesda, Maryland

2002

ATLAS OF NONTUMOR PATHOLOGY

EDITOR
Donald West King, MD

ASSOCIATE EDITORS
Leslie H. Sobin, MD
J. Thomas Stocker, MD
Bernard Wagner, MD

EDITORIAL ADVISORY BOARD
Ivan Damjanov, MD
Cecilia M. Fenoglio-Preiser, MD
Fred Gorstein, MD
Daniel Knowles, MD
Virginia A. LiVolsi, MD
Florabel G. Mullick, MD
Juan Rosai, MD
Fred Silva, MD
Steven G. Silverberg, MD

Manuscript Reviewed by:
Ronald A. DeLellis, MD
Virginia A. LiVolsi, MD

Accepted for Publication
2001

Available from the American Registry of Pathology
Armed Forces Institute of Pathology
Washington, DC 20306-6000
www.afip.org
ISBN: 1-881041-73.5

INTRODUCTION TO SERIES

This volume introduces the Atlas of Nontumor Pathology, a complementary series to the Armed Forces Institute of Pathology (AFIP) Atlas of Tumor Pathology, first published in 1949.

For several years, various individuals in the pathology community have suggested the formation of a new series of monographs concentrating on this particular area. In 1998, an Editorial Board was appointed and outstanding authors chosen shortly thereafter.

The purpose of the Atlas is to provide surgical pathologists with ready expert reference material most helpful in their daily practice. The lesions described relate principally to medical non-neoplastic conditions as exemplified by our first three Fascicles on endocrine, pulmonary, and skin diseases. Many of these lesions represent complex entities and when appropriate, we have included contributions from internists, radiologists, and surgeons. This has led to some increase in the size of the monographs but the emphasis remains on diagnosis by the surgical pathologist.

Previously, the Fascicles have been available on CD-ROM format as well as in print. In order to provide the widest possible advantages of both modalities, we have formatted the print Fascicle on the World Wide Web. Use of the Internet allows cross-indexing within the Fascicles as well as linkage to MedLine.

Our goal is to continue to provide expert information at the lowest possible cost. Therefore, marked reductions in pricing are available to residents and fellows as well as to staff purchasing on a subscription basis.

We believe that the Atlas of Nontumor Pathology will serve as an outstanding reference for surgical pathologists as well as an important contribution to the literature of other medical specialties.

Donald West King, MD
Leslie H. Sobin, MD
J. Thomas Stocker, MD
Bernard Wagner, MD

PREFACE AND ACKNOWLEDGMENTS

Participating in the inception of a new series of Fascicles is a very exciting and challenging event. This first Fascicle on nontumor endocrine diseases presents a broad overview of the wide spectrum of endocrine disorders. The general themes of hypoplastic, inflammatory, autoimmune, and hyperplastic lesions are maintained in each chapter. Basic concepts, such as feedback mechanisms, which are important for understanding many endocrine disorders are emphasized throughout the book.

We are indebted to many individuals for their contributions to the preparation of this Fascicle. Many of our colleagues at the Mayo Clinic provided illustrations and stimulating conversations during the development of this work. We also acknowledge the contributions of many authors of previous Fascicles whose works on neoplastic as well as non-neoplastic endocrine disorders preceded this one. Several illustrations that have been used in the text are specifically acknowledged in the corresponding legends. We thank Drs. A. M. Neville and M. J. O'Hare who allowed us to publish figures from their previously published work, *The Human Adrenal Cortex*. We also thank the editor, Dr. Donald West King, and the associate editors, Drs. Leslie H. Sobin, J. Thomas Stocker, and Bernard Wagner, for inviting us to participate in this innovative and challenging project.

Ricardo V. Lloyd, MD, PhD
Department of Laboratory Medicine
and Pathology, Mayo Clinic

Bruce R. Douglas, MD
Department of Diagnostic Radiology,
Mayo Clinic

William F. Young, Jr, MD
Department of Internal Medicine/
Endocrinology and Metabolism,
Mayo Clinic

Permission to use copyrighted illustrations has been granted by:

Springer-Verlag:

The Human Adrenal Cortex, 1982. For figure 4-41.

W.B. Saunders Company:

Williams Textbook of Endocrinology, 9th ed., 1998. For figures 1-5, 2-6, 3-1, 4-7, and 5-7.

Contents

Abbreviations

ACTH	adrenocorticotropic hormone
AMP	adenosine monophosphate
APUD	amine precursor uptake and decarboxylase
ß-HSD	beta-hydroxysteroid dehydrogenase
CCK	cholecystokinin
Cg	chromogranin
CRH	corticotropin-releasing hormone
CYP	cytochrome P450
DIT	diiodotyrosine
DNES	diffuse or dispersed neuroendocrine system
EC	enterochromaffin
ECL	enterochromaffin-like
FSH	follicle-stimulating hormone
G cell	gastrin-producing cell
GDNF	glial-derived neurotropic factor
GH	growth hormone
GHRH	growth hormone–releasing hormone
GIP	gastrin inhibitory polypeptide
GnRH	gonadotropin (FSH/LH)-releasing hormone
HLA	histocompatability locus antigen
IDDM	insulin-dependent diabetes mellitus
LH	luteinizing hormone
MEN	multiple endocrine neoplasia
MHC	major histocompatability complex
MIT	monoiodotyrosine
MODY	maternity onset diabetes of the young
MTC	medullary thyroid carcinoma
NCAM	neural cell adhesion molecule

NIDDM	noninsulin-dependent diabetes mellitus
NSP	neuroendocrine-specific protein
$(OH_2)D$	dihydroxy vitamin D
PGA	polyglandular autoimmune syndrome
POMC	pro-opiomelanocortin
PPNAD	primary pigmented nodular adrenocortical disease
PRL	prolactin
PTH	parathyroid hormone
PTHrP	parathyroid hormone–related peptide
RAIU	radioactive iodine uptake
Rb	retinoblastoma
SCN	solid cell nests
SRIF	somatotroph release-inhibitory factor (somatostatin)
T_3	triiodothyronine
T_4	thyroxine
Tg	thyroglobulin
TGI	thyroid growth immunoglobulin
TPO	thyroid peroxidase
TRH	thyrotropin-releasing hormone
TSH	thyroid-stimulating hormone
TSI	thyroid-stimulating immunoglobulin
ZES	Zollinger-Ellison syndrome

ENDOCRINE DISEASES

1
PITUITARY GLAND

NORMAL PITUITARY GLAND

Embryology

The human pituitary gland consists of the adenohypophysis and neurohypophysis, and can be recognized grossly by the third month of fetal development (1,4,6,10,11,17). The adenohypophysis develops from Rathke's pouch, which starts to form around the fourth and fifth fetal weeks from an evagination of the stomateal ectoderm. This ectoderm grows upward, detaches from the buccal cavity, and comes to lie in a depression of the sphenoid bone, the anlage of the sella turcica. The neurohypophysis is formed by the merging of the infundibular process of the primitive diencephalon with Rathke's pouch. The three parts of the neurohypophysis include the infundibulum, the infundibular stem, and the posterior lobe. The anterior lobe is formed by the proliferation of cells in the anterior part of Rathke's pouch. Although an intermediate lobe does not develop in humans, the posterior wall of Rathke's pouch forming the neurohypophysis gives rise to the pars tuberalis, which is an upward extension around the stalk.

The pharyngeal pituitary is formed by nests of adenohypophyseal cells trapped in the pharyngeal mucosa. The most common location of the pharyngeal pituitary is in the sphenoid bone, although various other locations have been reported (3). Ectopic pituitary adenomas may arise from these pharyngeal pituitary nests (14).

The hormone-producing cells of the anterior pituitary can be recognized fairly early in development (2,16). Corticotropin (ACTH) cells can be recognized by 5 weeks, growth hormone (GH) cells by 8 weeks, and the alpha subunit of glycoprotein hormone by 9 weeks of gestation. Thyroid-stimulating hormone (TSH), follicle-stimulating hormone (FSH), and luteinizing hormone (LH) cells can be detected by 12 weeks of gestation. Prolactin (PRL) cells are detected starting around 12 weeks and increase in number to term.

Recent advances in molecular biology have isolated and characterized various transcription factors, which are proteins that regulate cell differentiation and proliferation by binding to DNA in the cell nucleus (Table 1-1). These transcription factors are important for the normal development and function of the anterior pituitary (18). Molecular and other defects in the expression of transcription factors can lead to specific endocrine disorders.

Gross Anatomy

The pituitary gland in adults weighs between 400 and 600 mg and measures about 13 x 9 x 6 mm. During pregnancy the gland can double in weight, and it is consistently heavier

Table 1-1

TRANSCRIPTION FACTORS IMPORTANT FOR PITUITARY DEVELOPMENT

Factor	Target Cells
Pit-1/GHF1	GH/PRL/TSH
Thyrotroph embryonic factor (TEF)	TSH
Corticotroph upstream transcription element-binding (CUTE) protein	ACTH
Steroidogenic factor Ad4BP/SF-1	LH/FSH
Estrogen receptor	PRL/Gonadotroph
Glucocorticoid receptor	ACTH

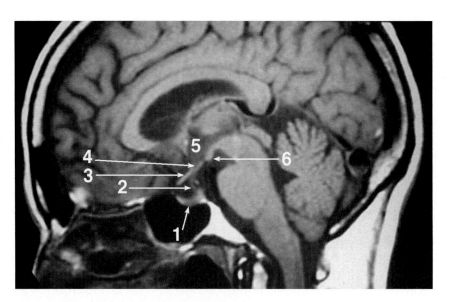

Figure 1-1

NORMAL ANATOMY
OF PITUITARY GLAND

Sagittal T1-weighted image of the normal pituitary demonstrating: 1) pituitary gland, 2) infundibular stalk, 3) optic chiasm, 4) optic nerve, 5) third ventricle, and 6) mammillary body.

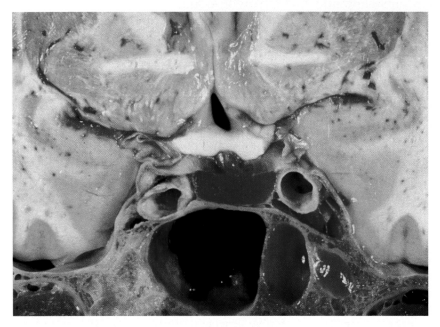

Figure 1-2

GROSS NORMAL ANATOMY
OF PITUITARY GLAND

Gross photograph showing the relationship of the pituitary gland to various structures. The optic chiasm is present on top, the internal carotid arteries laterally, and the sphenoid air sinus. (Courtesy of B. Scheithauer, Rochester, MN.)

in multiparous women (1,11). The pituitary is surrounded by the dura mater which forms the roof of the sella turcica in which the pituitary lies. The pituitary lies adjacent to many important structures including the internal carotid arteries, lateral in the cavernous sinuses, the optic chiasm and optic tracts in front and above, the base of the diencephalon above, and the sphenoid air sinus in front and below (figs. 1-1, 1-2). The sellar diaphragm is also present on the roof of the sella turcica and is made up of a fold of dura mater extending transversely across the sella. Its center is perforated for the passage of the infundibulum.

The adenohypophysis or anterior pituitary constitutes about 70 to 80 percent of the gland. It is composed of: 1) the pars distalis, which contains all of the hormone-producing cells; 2) remnants of the pars intermedia represented by a few colloid-filled cavities lined by epithelial cells; and 3) the pars tuberalis composed of squamous cell nests and a few anterior pituitary cells, especially glycoprotein-producing hormone cells (fig. 1-3).

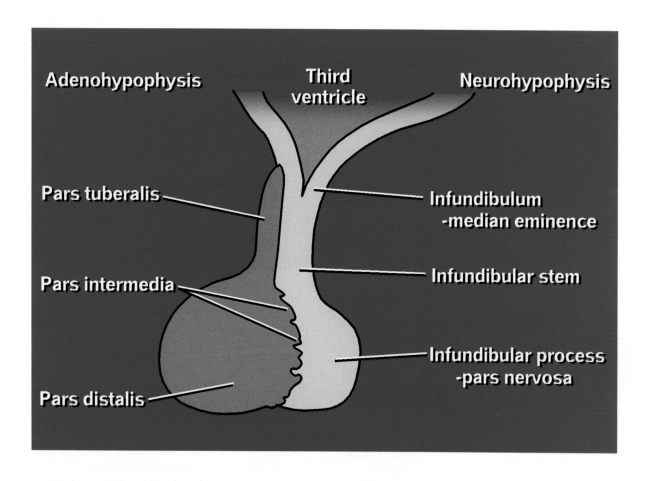

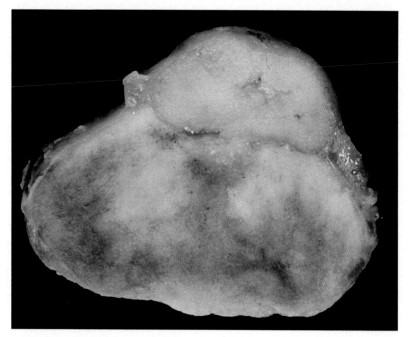

Figure 1-3

NORMAL ANATOMY
OF PITUITARY GLAND

Above: Diagram illustrating the parts of the adenohypophysis and neurohypophysis.

Left: Horizontal cross section showing the anterior (lower) and posterior (upper) lobes. (Figure 1-5 from Fascicle 22, 3rd Series.)

The neurohypophysis or posterior pituitary constitutes the remaining 20 to 30 percent of the gland (fig. 1-3). It is composed of: 1) the infundibulum or median eminence, which is attached to the hypothalamus and receives the hypothalamic peptidergic neurons with releasing and inhibiting hormones that regulate anterior pituitary cell function; 2) the pituitary stalk or infundibular stem composed of unmyelinated nerve fiber tracts which originate in the hypothalamus and portal vessels. These fibers transport hypothalamic peptides to the anterior pituitary; and 3) the posterior lobe, composed of the infundibular process and pars nervosa, which stores vasopressin and oxytocin hormones.

The pituitary gland is located strategically within the sphenoid bone and is adjacent to the internal carotid arteries and lateral to several cranial nerves. The internal carotid arteries give rise to the paired superior, middle, and inferior hypophyseal arteries (7). The external plexus is formed by the superior hypophyseal arteries entering the medial eminence. They terminate in gomitoli or long central arteries with muscle layers and a dense capillary plexus. Parallel veins are formed from the capillaries that travel down the pituitary stalk and end in the fenestrated capillaries of the anterior pituitary lobe. The inferior hypophyseal arteries supply blood to the posterior lobe while the middle hypophyseal arteries enter the anterior lobe and supply some of the adenohypophyseal cells at the periphery of the gland. The short portal vessels which originate in the posterior lobe and distal portions of the stalk supply about 10 to 20 percent of the blood flow to the anterior lobe (7). Venous blood from the pituitary returns via the cavernous sinuses, inferior petrosal sinuses, and internal jugular veins.

The pars distalis has no direct nerve supply, except for a few sympathetic fibers that penetrate the anterior lobe along the capillaries. These pericapillary nerve fibers do not regulate anterior pituitary hormone secretion, but may affect blood flow to the pituitary.

The posterior pituitary lobe is composed of nerve fibers and axon terminals, pituicytes, and dense core granules of stored neurosecretory proteins: oxytocin, vasopressin, and neurophysin. The hypothalamic tracts from the su-

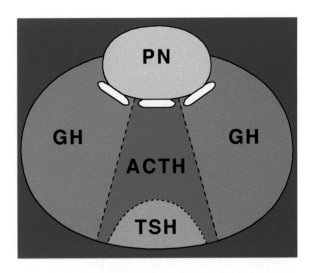

Figure 1-4

NORMAL HISTOLOGY OF PITUITARY GLAND

Diagram illustrating the topographic distribution of various pituitary cell types in the adenohypophysis and the adjacent pars nervosa (PN) of the neurohypophysis.

praoptic and paraventricular nuclei travel from the hypothalamus to the stalk of the posterior lobe as tracts of the supraopticohypophyseal and tuberohypophyseal fibers. Neural connections influence posterior pituitary secretion of oxytocin and vasopressin, as evidenced by the severe atrophy of the neurohypophysis after stalk sectioning or with injury to the axons originating in the supraoptic and paraventricular nuclei.

Microscopic Anatomy and Physiology

A horizontal section across the anterior pituitary reveals fibrous trabeculae in the midcentral portion with lateral wings and a central mucoid wedge (fig. 1-4). Hematoxylin and eosin (H&E)–stained sections show acidophil, basophil, and chromophobe cells. The acidophil cells are present mainly in the lateral wings, the basophil cells are in the mucoid wedge, while the chromophobe cells are widely dispersed (fig. 1-5). Each anterior pituitary cell has a basement membrane, and groups of cells form reticulin-positive clusters with adjacent capillaries (fig. 1-5). Unlike the anterior pituitary which has an indirect arterial blood supply, the posterior pituitary has a direct blood supply from branches of the inferior branches of the internal carotid arteries. Immunohistochemical staining is the method of choice for identifying individual anterior pituitary cells

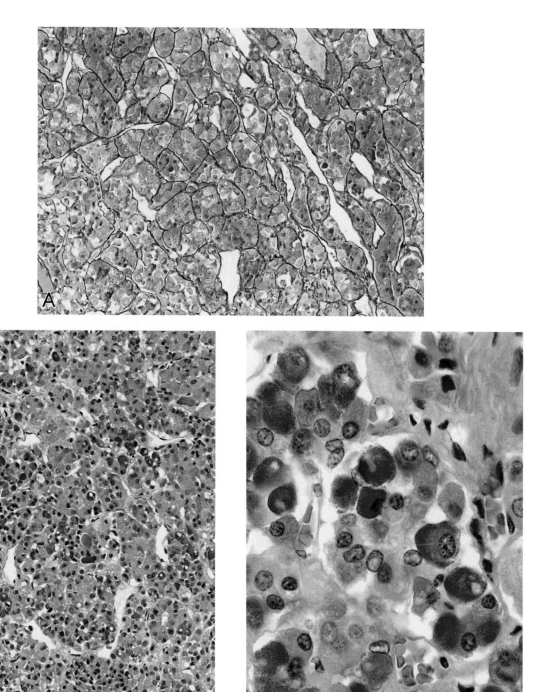

Figure 1-5

NORMAL HISTOLOGY OF ANTERIOR PITUITARY GLAND

Clusters of various cell types are present.

A: Reticulin stain highlights the acinar clusters.

B: The H&E-stained section shows a mixture of various cell types in the acinar clusters.

C: Higher magnification illustrates acidophils with pink cytoplasm, basophils with red cytoplasm, and chromophobes with amphophilic cytoplasm.

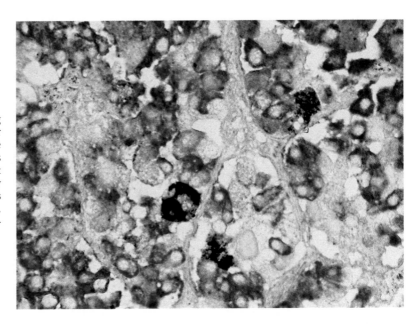

Figure 1-6

IMMUNOHISTOCHEMISTRY
OF PITUITARY GLAND

Immunohistochemical staining shows various cell types in the anterior pituitary. The PRL cells stain brown, the GH cells stain blue, and the LH cells stain gray-black. GH cells are the most abundant type in the anterior pituitary (immunohistochemistry chromogens include: diaminobenzidine [brown], NBT-BCIP [blue], and 4-chloro-1-napthol [gray-black]).

Table 1-2

HYPOTHALAMIC HORMONES REGULATING PITUITARY SECRETION AND TARGET TISSUES

Peptide/Amine	Pituitary Hormone	Target Tissues
Stimulating		
Corticotropin-releasing hormone	ACTH	Adrenal cortex
Gonadotropin-releasing hormone	FSH/LH	Ovaries, testes
Growth hormone–releasing hormone	GH	Many tissues
Thyrotropin-releasing hormone	TSH/PRL	Thyroid, breast, many other tissues
Vasoactive intestinal polypeptide	PRL	Breast, many other tissues
Inhibitory		
Somatostatin	GH	Many tissues
Dopamine	PRL	Breast, many other tissues
Others		
Vasopressin (ADH)	(Posterior pituitary)	Kidney
Oxytocin	(Posterior pituitary)	Uterus, breast

(fig. 1-6). Electron microscopic examination also allows the characterization of unique features of different cell types (fig. 1-7) (9,11).

The hypothalmic-releasing and -inhibiting hormones are important in regulating anterior pituitary function (Table 1-2, fig. 1-8). A negative feedback mechanism operates between specific target organs, the pituitary, and the hypothalamus. For example, thyroid hormone exerts a negative feedback effect on the pituitary and hypothalamus to regulate the secretion of thyrotropin-releasing hormone from hypothalamic neurons and thyroid-stimulating hormone from the pituitary gland.

Somatotroph (GH) Cells

These cells are usually acidophilic on H&E staining. They constitute approximately 40 to 50 percent of the secretory cells in the adult pituitary gland (fig. 1-9). Most GH cells are present in the lateral wings of the anterior pituitary. Ultrastructural analysis show cells with dense secretory granules ranging from 350 to 500 nm in diameter.

The GH gene, located on chromosome 17, is 2.5 kb long and directs the synthesis of a 191 amino acid single-chain peptide with two interchain disulfide bands. At the ultrastructural level, GH secretory granules are present throughout the

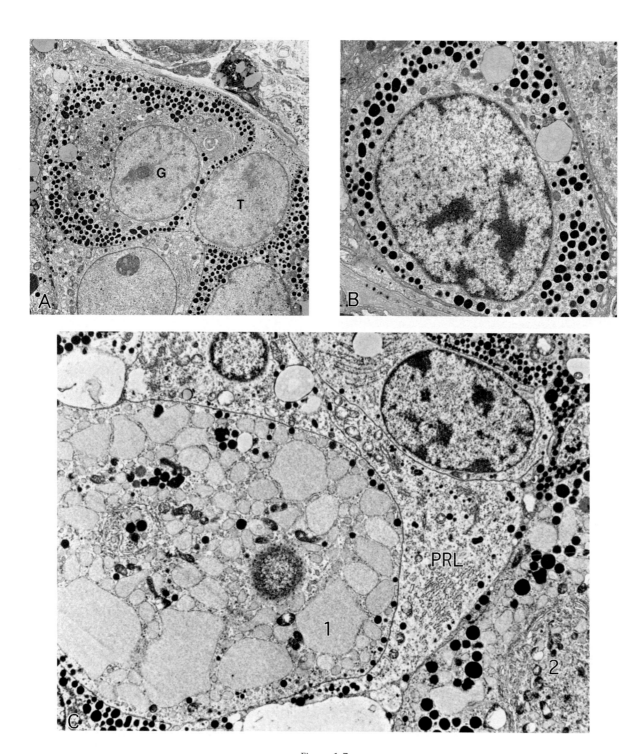

Figure 1-7

ULTRASTRUCTURE OF ANTERIOR PITUITARY GLAND

A: Ultrastructural features of anterior pituitary hormones show a mixture of various cell types with secretory granules of specific size. G, growth hormone cell; T, thyrotroph (X3,000).

B: Higher magnification of a growth hormone cell showing abundant secretory granules 350 to 500 nm in diameter (X7,000).

C: Two stimulated gonadotrophs (1,2) show marked dilation of the rough endoplasmic reticulum and prominent Golgi complex. Secretory granules are sparse and relatively large. A PRL cell (PRL) is between the two gonadectomy cells. (Figure 30 from Fascicle 21, 2nd Series.)

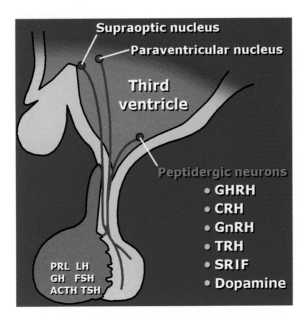

Figure 1-8

HYPOTHALAMIC HORMONES

Schematic diagram showing the hypothalamic neurons producing the various stimulatory and inhibitory substances that regulate anterior pituitary function. The supraoptic and paraventricular nuclei produce oxytocin and vasopressin which are stored in the posterior pituitary. GHRH - growth hormone-releasing hormone; CRH - corticotropin-releasing hormone; GnRH - gonadotropin-releasing hormone; TRH - thyrotropin-releasing hormone; SRIF - somatostatin. Unlike the other peptides, dopamine is an amine that inhibits PRL secretion.

Table 1-3

ANTERIOR PITUITARY HORMONES:
CELL TYPE, DISTRIBUTION, AND FUNCTION

Cell Type	Cell Percentage in Pituitary (Approximately)	Function
GH	40–50	Stimulates linear growth
PRL	10–30	Stimulates breast milk production
ACTH	10–20	Stimulates cortisol synthesis
FSH/LH	10	Stimulates estrogen and testosterone synthesis
TSH	5	Stimulates thyroid hormone synthesis

cytoplasm. GH secretion is regulated by growth hormone-releasing hormone (GHRH) and somatostatin release-inhibiting factor (SRIF). The latter peptide inhibits growth hormone secretion. Insulin-like growth factor 1 (IGH-1) or somatonectin C, which is produced by the liver, mediates many of the effects of GH. IGH-1 exerts a negative feedback effect on GH secretion at the hypothalamic and pituitary levels.

Lactotroph (PRL) Cells

Lactotrophs may be acidophilic or chromophobic and are present in the highest density in the posterolateral wings, but are located throughout the anterior pituitary (fig. 1-10). PRL cells account for 10 to 30 percent of anterior pituitary cells (Table 1-3) (1). The exact percentage varies with age, sex, parity, and hormonal status. Electron microscopy shows that PRL cells are usually sparsely granulated, with secretory granules of up to 650 nm in diameter. The cells usually have well-developed rough endoplasmic reticulum and Golgi complexes.

The PRL gene, located on chromosome 6, is greater than 10 kb long, and the mRNA is about 1 kb long. The protein is a 198 amino acid peptide which has a common evolutionary origin with GH. At the ultrastructural level, PRL cells have secretory granules 200 to 300 nm in diameter. PRL cells have a unique way of extruding granules by "misplaced" exocytosis in which the granule content is secreted into the extracellular space away from the capillaries (fig. 1-11).

One of the functions of PRL hormone is to stimulate lactation. Receptors for PRL are widely distributed in many cells, although the function of the hormone in many tissues remains unknown. Stimulation of pituitary PRL secretion is by thyrotropin-releasing hormone (TRH) and vasoactive intestinal polypeptide (VIP), while dopamine inhibits PRL secretion.

Mammosomatotroph (PRL/GH) Cells

These uncommon cells are present in the normal pituitary gland and increase in number during pregnancy. The regulation of this cell type is unknown, but tumor cells with features of mammosomatotrophs are not uncommon in large series of pituitary adenomas examined ultrastructurally (9,11,12).

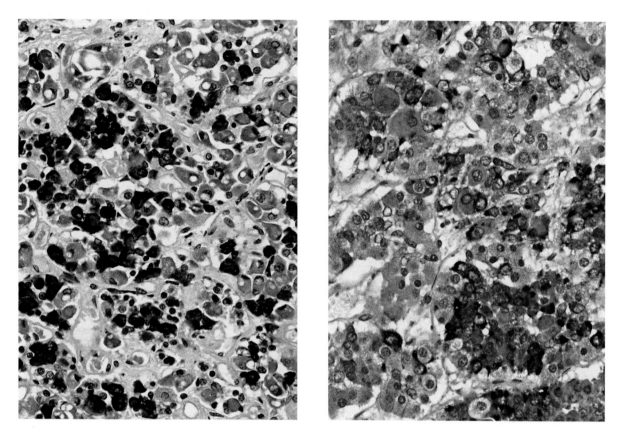

Figure 1-9

IMMUNOHISTOCHEMISTRY OF GH CELLS

Left: Immunohistochemical staining for GH shows many positive cells with brown cytoplasmic staining.

Right: In situ hybridization for GH messenger RNA shows many positive cells with blue cytoplasmic staining using alkaline phosphatase with NBT/BCIF. GH cells constitute about 40 to 50 percent of anterior pituitary cells.

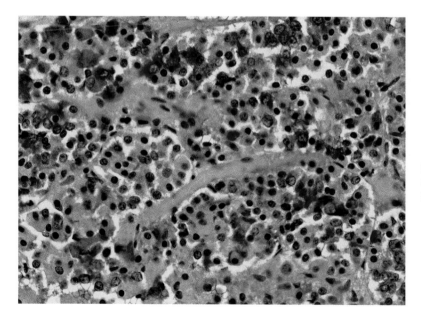

Figure 1-10

IMMUNOHISTOCHEMISTRY
OF PRL CELLS

Immunohistochemical staining for PRL in the anterior pituitary. These cells constitute 10 to 30 percent of anterior pituitary cells.

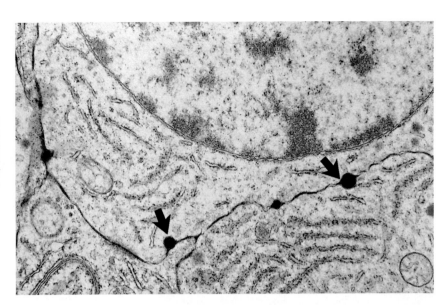

Figure 1-11

ULTRASTRUCTURE
OF PRL CELLS

Ultrastructural examination shows "misplaced" exocytosis in a prolactinoma (arrows). The secretory granules are secreted into the extracellular space away from the capillary (X14,000) (diaminobenzidine chromogen).

Corticotroph (ACTH) Cells

ACTH cells are basophilic cells representing 10 to 20 percent of anterior pituitary cells (fig. 1-12). They are present mainly in the mucoid wedge, the area that on horizontal cross section is the central portion of the gland that abuts the pars nervosa. Clusters of ACTH cells may be seen in the posterior pituitary, a phenomenon known as basophil invasion (fig. 1-13). The importance of recognizing this condition is to distinguish it from corticotrophic adenomas (11,13). ACTH cells stain for periodic acid–Schiff (PAS). In contrast, the GH and PRL cells are PAS negative. At the ultrastructural level, they contain 300- to 500-nm secretory granules and large perinuclear vacuoles known as enigmatic bodies; the latter are large phagolysosomes.

The pro-opiomelanocortin (POMC) gene is located on chromosome 2 and consists of three exons. ACTH is a 39 amino acid single-chain peptide derived from the 31-kd POMC glycoprotein. Perinuclear clusters of type 1, 6- to 9-nm keratin filaments, which react with antibodies directed against keratins of 54 to 60 kd, are commonly present in the cytoplasm.

ACTH stimulates the adrenal cortex to secrete glucocorticoids, mineralocorticoids, and sex steroids. The hypothalamus produces corticotropin-releasing hormone (CRH) which stimulates ACTH secretion. Glucocorticoids exert a direct negative feedback effect on both hypothalamic CRH and anterior pituitary ACTH secretion. When ACTH cells are suppressed by high levels of glucocorticoids from endogenous or exogenous sources, type 1 intermediate filaments accumulate in the cytoplasm and the secretory granules are pushed to the cell periphery adjacent to the cell membrane (fig. 1-14). These distinctively pathognomonic changes are known as *Crooke's hyalinization* or *Crooke's hyaline changes.*

Thyrotroph (TSH) Cells

TSH cells comprise less than 5 percent of anterior pituitary cells and are located principally in the anteromedial portion of the mucoid wedge (fig. 1-15). TSH cells are angular and contain cytoplasmic PAS-positive droplets. Ultrastructurally, TSH cells have small spherical secretory granules, 100 to 200 nm in diameter, usually located close to the cell membrane.

The TSH beta subunit gene is located on chromosome 1 and consists of three exons. The alpha subunit gene is found on chromosome 6 and is 9.4 kb long with four exons. The alpha subunit protein consists of 92 amino acids. The thyrotropin molecule is a 28-kd glycoprotein and the beta subunit which confers the specificity for TSH action ranges from 18 to 21 kd, depending on whether it contains one or two carbohydrate chains.

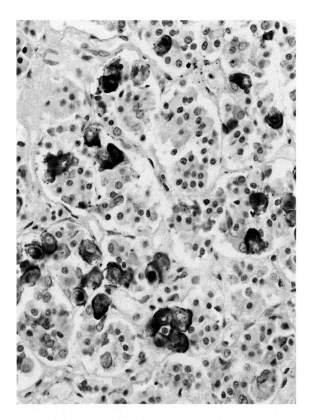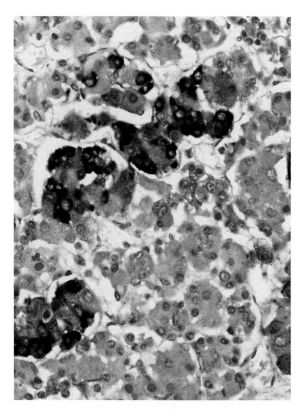

Figure 1-12

IMMUNOHISTOCHEMISTRY OF ACTH CELLS

Left: Immunohistochemical staining for ACTH.

Right: Another area of the anterior pituitary stained for pro-opiomelanocortin (POMC) messenger RNA by in situ hybridization shows a nodular cluster of POMC cells in the mucoid wedge. ACTH cells are present in 10 to 20 percent of anterior pituitary cells (alkaline phosphatase with NBT/BCIP).

The hypothalamic thyrotropin-releasing hormone (TRH) stimulates TSH secretion from the pituitary. Thyroid hormone feeds back on the hypothalamus and pituitary to regulate TSH secretion.

Gonadotroph (FSH/LH) Cells

Most gonadotropic cells produce both FSH and LH (fig. 1-16). FSH/LH cells are basophilic and are evenly distributed in the anterior pituitary. They comprise about 10 percent of anterior pituitary cells. Both FSH and LH share the same alpha subunit as TSH, while the beta subunit is unique for each molecule. The FSH beta gene is located on chromosome 11 and consists of three exons; the protein has 130 amino acids. The LH beta gene is located on chromosome 19 and consists of three exons; the LH beta protein consists of 145 amino acids.

Most gonadotroph cells contain both FSH and LH proteins which are located in small (200 nm) and larger (300 to 600 nm) secretory granules. FSH stimulates spermatogenesis and the growth of ovarian follicles while LH induces ovulation, luteinization of the ovarian follicles, and steroidogenesis. LH also stimulates Leydig cells to produce testosterone and the ovary to elaborate luteal phase hormones. Removal of the gonadal organs results in hypertrophy and hyperplasia of the pituitary gonadotropic cells with formation of "gonadectomy" cells (see fig. 1-7C).

Folliculostellate Cells

These are agranular cells located in the anterior pituitary (fig. 1-17) (5,15). They are irregular and somewhat star-shaped, hence the designation stellate. Folliculostellate cells have long cytoplasmic processes that extend between

11

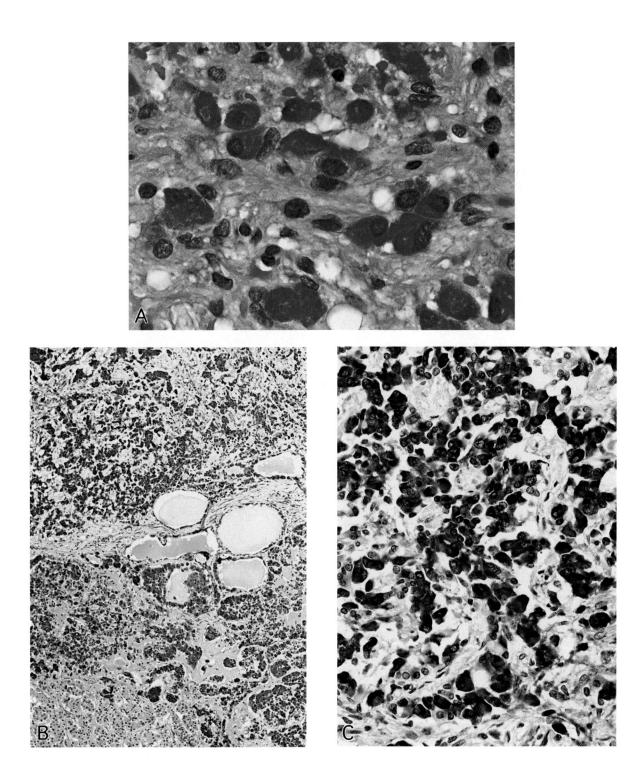

Figure 1-13

BASOPHIL INVASION

Basophil or corticotroph invasion into the pars nervosa. The "invading" cells have basophilic cytoplasm and are located among the processes of the pars nervosa (A). The relationship of the ACTH cells in the anterior pituitary (left) and the "invading" ACTH cells in the pars nervosa is shown in B. The two groups of cells are separated by the cystic spaces of the residual pars intermedia (B). Higher magnification of the ACTH-positive cells in the pars nervosa shows that some cells are in small clusters which could be misdiagnosed as an ACTH adenoma in a small biopsy (C).

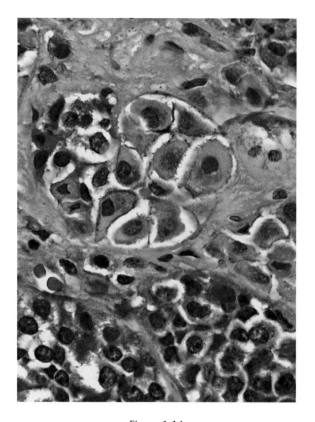

Figure 1-14

CROOKE'S CHANGES

Crooke's hyaline changes secondary to excess glucocorticoids leads to accumulation of type 1 intermediate filaments. The secretory granules are pushed to the periphery of the cells, and the hyaline-appearing keratin filaments are prominent in the cytoplasm.

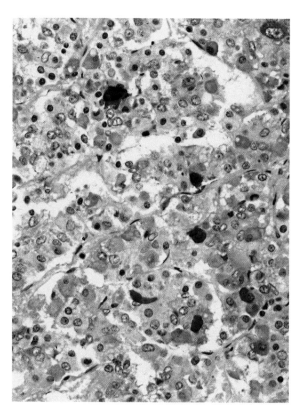

Figure 1-15

IMMUNOHISTOCHEMISTRY OF TSH CELLS

TSH cells in the anterior pituitary shown by immunostaining. These angular cells comprise less than 5 percent of anterior pituitary cells.

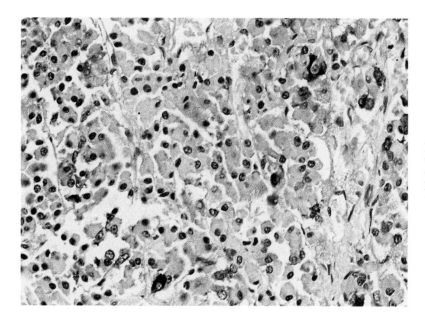

Figure 1-16

IMMUNOHISTOCHEMISTRY OF LH CELLS

Gonadotroph cells in the anterior pituitary immunostained for LH. These cells make up about 10 percent of anterior pituitary cells. FSH and LH are present in the same pituitary cells (diaminobenzidine chromogen).

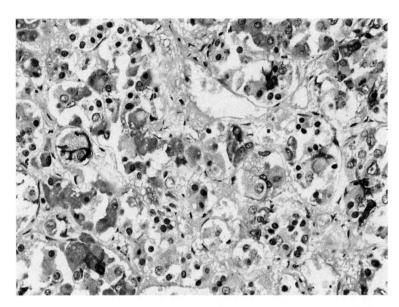

Figure 1-17

FOLLICULOSTELLATE CELLS

Folliculostellate cells revealed by immunopositivity for S100 protein. These cells have cytoplasmic processes that extend between the hormone-producing cells (diaminobenzidine chromogen).

hormone-producing cells. They are positive for S100 protein, glial fibrillary acidic protein (GFAP), and vimentin. Folliculostellate cells have several functions including phagocytosis, production of cytokines, and production of growth factors such as vascular endothelial growth factor and interleukin 6 in different species (8). These cells probably exert paracrine regulatory functions on the hormone-secreting anterior pituitary cells.

Neurohypophysis

The posterior pituitary is made up of pituicytes which are GFAP-positive glial cells, nerve fibers, and capillaries (fig. 1-18). The nerve fibers travel from the hypothalamic neurons which produce oxytocin, vasopressin, and neurophysin, along the axoplasm of unmyelinated nerve fibers, to the posterior lobe where they are stored by focal axonal dilatation in secretory granules (Herring bodies).

REACTIVE CHANGES

Pregnancy

During pregnancy the pituitary gland doubles in weight. This can be visualized by magnetic resonance imaging (MRI) (fig. 1-19). The increase in size is caused mainly by hyperplasia of the PRL cells (figs. 1-20, 1-21). There is an increase in the cells producing both PRL and GH with a concomitant decrease in the GH-producing cells (31,32). Because of the mark-

edly increased size of the gland, there is an increased risk of pituitary infarcts during pregnancy, especially during delivery, which may be associated with hypotension (*Sheehan's syndrome*). Although the pituitary gland decreases in weight after delivery, it remains larger in multiparous compared to nulliparous women.

Hormonal Syndromes

Hypofunction of endocrine target organs can lead to reactive changes in the pituitary gland, especially pituitary cell hyperplasias such as Addison's disease and Schmidt's syndrome (20,22). This is discussed later in the chapter. Most of the anterior pituitary cells producing trophic hormones directed at specific organs can be affected via a direct feedback effect due to decreased hormonal production.

Hyperfunction of specific endocrine target organs can also lead to reactive changes in the pituitary. Examples include hyperadrenocorticalism and hyperthyroidism.

Hyperadrenocorticalism. Excessive glucocorticoids from endogenous or exogenous sources lead to specific morphologic changes in the anterior pituitary; these are designated as Crooke's hyaline changes (21,23,24,28,29). In this process the cells have a glassy or hyalinized appearance on H&E-stained sections due to the accumulation of cytokeratin filaments in the cytoplasm. The secretory granules are pushed to the cell periphery, close to the cell membrane

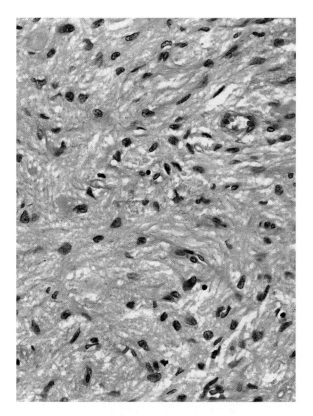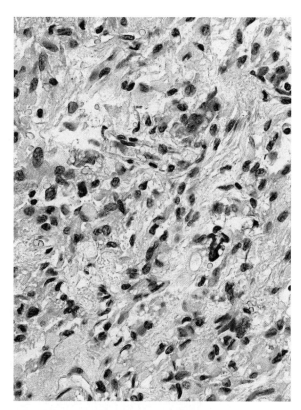

Figure 1-18

POSTERIOR PITUITARY

Left: Posterior pituitary made up of pituicytes, glial cells, and nerve fibers.
Right: The glial cells are positive for glial fibrillary acidic protein.

(see fig. 1-14). Specific conditions leading to Crooke's hyaline changes include: 1) adrenocortical hyperplasias, adenomas, and carcinomas; 2) ectopic production of ACTH or CRH by tumors such as small cell lung carcinomas, bronchial carcinoids, thymomas, pheochromocytomas, and others; 3) treatment with glucocorticoids for autoimmune diseases, organ transplantation, and other conditions; and 4) production of excessive ACTH by a pituitary adenoma. The latter leads to Crooke's change predominantly in the non-neoplastic ACTH cells, although such changes can also occur in adenomas. Crooke's changes are reversible once the stimulus is removed.

Hyperthyroidism. Patients with thyrotoxicosis may appear to have a decrease in the number of TSH cells, as detected by immunostaining (26,30). However, there usually are more TSH-positive cells with less immunoreactive hormone in this condition than previously realized, because the cells with small amounts of stored TSH do not stain with anti-TSH antibodies. The decreased immunostaining is probably related to the negative feedback effects of the increased triiodothyronine (T3) and thyroxine (T4) associated with hyperthyroidism.

Effects of Specific Drugs

Specific drugs used for various medical therapies may lead to reactive changes in the anterior pituitary (27). High dosages of estrogens are associated with PRL cell hyperplasia and hyperprolactinemia (29,34). In patients with PRL adenomas, estrogen may stimulate further growth of the tumor.

Somatostatin analogues such as octreotide are used in the treatment of many neuroendocrine tumors, including GH adenoma. In the normal pituitary, these drugs can inhibit GH

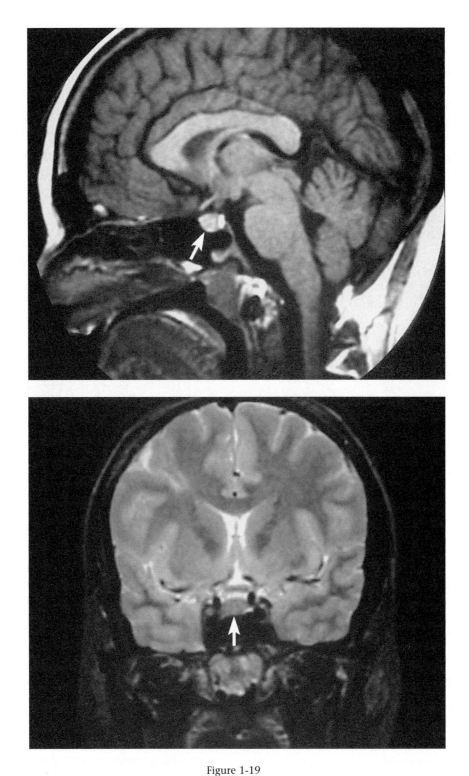

Figure 1-19

PITUITARY HYPERPLASIA

Top: Sagittal T1-weighted MRI in a 30-year-old pregnant female demonstrates a spherical, upwardly convex appearance of the pituitary gland.

Bottom: A similar appearance is seen on the coronal T2-weighted MRI. These findings are consistent with normal physiologic hyperplasia secondary to pregnancy.

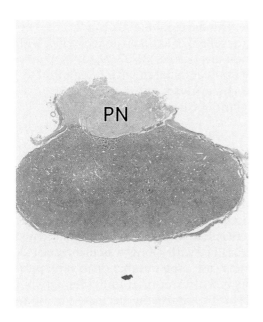
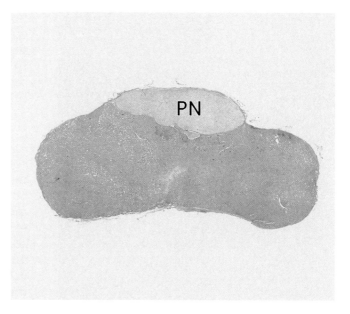

Figure 1-20

PITUITARY GLAND IN PREGNANCY

Comparison of gross section of the normal pituitary in a nulliparous woman (left) and the pituitary from a pregnant woman (right). During pregnancy, the pituitary increases two-fold in total weight and is more likely to undergo infarction. The pars nervosa present on top (PN) is not affected by the hyperplasia.

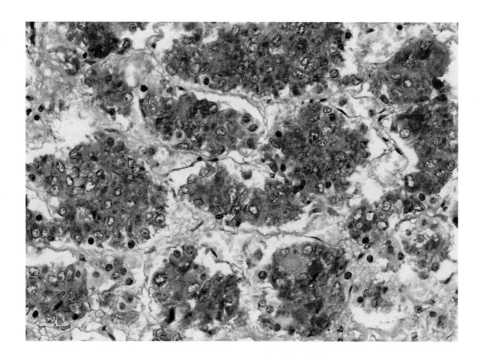

Figure 1-21

PRL CELLS IN PREGNANCY

PRL cell hyperplasia is prominent in this pituitary from a 5-month pregnant woman. Large clusters of PRL-positive cells are noted by immunostaining (diaminobenzidine chromogen).

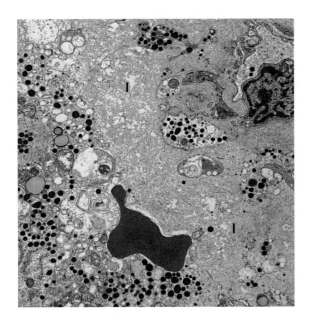

Figure 1-22

OCTREOTIDE EFFECT

GH adenoma from a patient treated with octreotide for 4 months shows increased collagen in the interstitium (I) of the anterior pituitary (X5,000).

secretion and may lead to a variable degree of anterior pituitary fibrosis (fig. 1-22) (19). Gonadotropin hormone–releasing hormone (GnRH) analogues used in the treatment of prostatic and other cancers can initially stimulate FSH and LH secretion, but with chronic treatment gonadotropin secretion is inhibited.

Dopamine agonists such as bromocriptine and parlodel are often used in the treatment of prolactinomas (33). They can inhibit PRL secretion in normal PRL cells as well as in tumor cells and lead to pituitary fibrosis (25,32).

HEREDITARY AND DEVELOPMENTAL DISORDERS

Agenesis of the Pituitary

Agenesis is a complete absence of the pituitary gland. Congenital absence of the pituitary gland is uncommon. Most neonates with pituitary aplasia survive only a few hours (41). There is usually an associated hypoplasia of the adrenal glands, thyroid gland, and gonads because of the effects of the lack of trophic hormone. This developmental disorder arises because of the failure of Rathke's pouch to fuse with the infundibular process (36,37,39,41,45,47,48). In many cases associated with congenital absence of the anterior pituitary, posterior pituitary gland tissue may be present.

Pituitary Hypoplasia

Pituitary hypoplasia is the defective or incomplete development of the pituitary gland. It may be developmental or result from atrophy.

Hypoplasia of the pituitary gland commonly occurs in association with anencephaly (42). Anencephaly is associated with a flattened sella turcica filled with spongy vascular tissue (43, 46). In most cases, the number of anterior pituitary cells is within normal limits for age, but the ACTH cells are usually decreased in number (43). Ultrastructurally, the ACTH cells have poorly developed organelles and the adrenal glands are hypoplastic (46). Consistent with the normal numbers of TSH and gonadotrophic cells, the weights of the thyroid and gonads are within normal limits in anencephalic neonates.

Ataxia-Telangiectasia Syndrome

Ataxia-telangiectasia syndrome, also known as *Louis-Bar syndrome,* is a complex autosomal recessive disorder associated with cerebellar ataxia, oculocutaneous telangiectasias, immunodeficiency, susceptibility to infection, and neoplasia. It is also associated with cytomegaly and nucleomegaly in multiple organ systems.

The ataxia-telangiectasia (AT) gene has been localized to the long arm of chromosome 11q (40,41). A mutated AT gene has been identified in this region and encodes a protein with close homology to protein kinase; this is regarded as the putative causative agent of the ataxia-telangiectasia syndrome. Recent studies of the pituitary glands of three patients with this syndrome showed variable numbers of pleomorphic bizarre cells with large nuclei that have GH and ACTH immunoreactivity (fig. 1-23) (40). These cytomegalic changes were also present in the posterior pituitary. DNA analysis showed that the bizarre cells were aneuploid, with many nuclei having a DNA content greater than 8N. However, pituitary tumors do not usually develop in these glands, so the bizarre cells should not be considered preneoplastic.

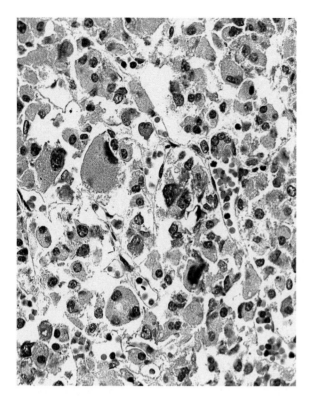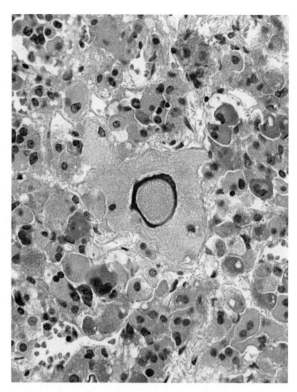

Figure 1-23

ATAXIA–TELANGIECTASIA

Anterior pituitary gland from a patient with ataxia-telangiectasia shows cells with enlarged nuclei (left) and other cells that are pleomorphic with marked cytomegaly (right). These cells usually stain for GH and ACTH. (Courtesy of Dr. B. Scheithauer, Rochester, MN.)

Empty Sella Syndrome

Empty sella syndrome is an intrasellar arachnocele resulting from an anomaly of the diaphragma sella. The empty sella syndrome may be primary or secondary depending on the etiology. In the primary type there is an incomplete or absent sellar diaphragm which leads to increased cerebrospinal fluid pressure in the sella; this results in compression of the sellar contents, with flattening of the pituitary gland and enlargement of the hypophyseal fossa. Cerebrospinal fluid is present and replaces the volume of the compressed pituitary by almost filling the sella turcica (fig. 1-24). In the primary empty sella syndrome, the pituitary gland is spread along the floor of the sella and the pituitary stalk reaches down to the compressed gland. The optic chiasm, which is anterior to the pituitary, forms a "V" shape as it descends with the hypothalamus into the sella. In spite

of the small gland and deformities, overt endocrine abnormalities are uncommon, as are visual symptoms. Immunohistochemical findings usually correlate with the lack of endocrine abnormalities, since all of the anterior pituitary cell types can be readily identified. Secondary empty sella syndrome can result from necrosis, infarct, or hypophysectomy leading to a small or absent pituitary within the hypophyseal fossa.

Isolated Hormone Deficiency

Deficiencies of individual anterior hormones are unusual. Gonadotropin deficiency may result from hypothalamic defects in patients with Kallmann's syndrome who have hypogonadism and anosmia. Isolated GH deficiency may have a genetic basis (49). A few cases of GH deficiency have been associated with deletion of the GH gene. Interestingly, morphological and immunohistochemical studies in patients with isolated

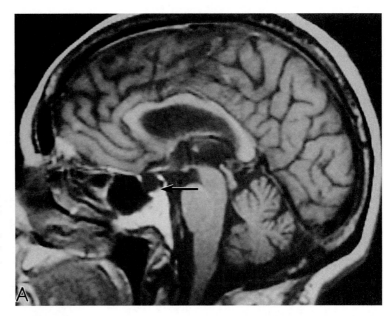

Figure 1-24

EMPTY SELLA SYNDROME

A: Sagittal T1-weighted MRI demonstrates a partially empty sella turcica. The sella is almost completely filled with cerebrospinal fluid, and the pituitary gland is flattened against the bony floor of the sella (arrow).

B: Axial T2-weighted image demonstrates the typical high signal intensity cerebrospinal fluid almost completely filling the sella turcica (arrow).

C: Low-power histologic section shows that the pituitary is compressed along the bottom of the enlarged sella. (Plate IC from Fascicle 21, 2nd Series.)

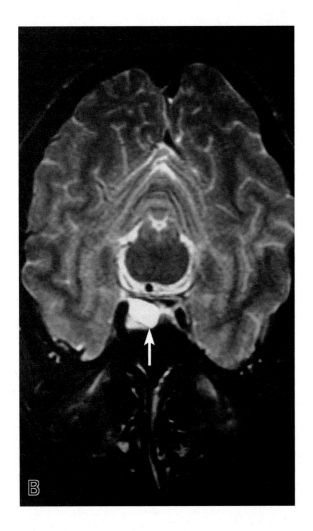

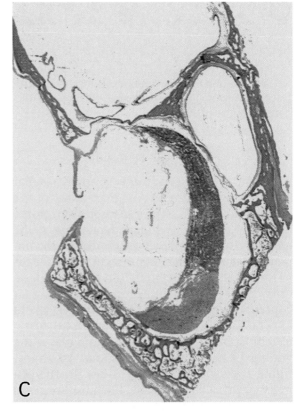

GH deficiency have shown abundant immunoreactive GH cells, suggesting another mechanism such as defective functional and biological activity of the secreted GH. Single cell-type "knock outs" or loss of a specific cell type can be found in patients with autoimmune hypophysitis.

Transcription Factor Deficiencies

Transcription factors are proteins present in the cell nucleus that help regulate normal gene function and also regulate growth and differentiation of specific genes. One of the pituitary transcription factors studied extensively is the Pit-1/GHF-1 (Pit-1) factor which is critical for the development of GH, PRL, and TSH cells. This transcription factor binds to the promoter regions of the GH-, PRL-, and TSH-beta genes to regulate normal gene activity and the development of these cell types. Mutations of the Pit-1 gene, including missense and nonsense mutations, have resulted in "transcription factor"–related diseases such as familial dwarfism and cretinism (35,38,44,48). With early diagnosis, these conditions can be treated with appropriate target-gland replacement therapy.

CIRCULATORY DISORDERS

Pituitary Apoplexy

This is an infarction of the pituitary gland usually secondary to hemorrhage. Pituitary apoplexy develops in pituitaries enlarged from pregnancy or adenomas.

Apoplexy was observed in 7 percent of 560 patients who had undergone surgery for pituitary tumors (62). In some autopsy series, infarctions involving 25 percent or more of the gland have been observed in up to 8 percent of patients (54,55, 57,59). Because the pituitary gland has tremendous reserve, patients may lose more than 50 percent of the anterior pituitary cells and still remain asymptomatic (53–55). Severe hypophyseal hormone deficiency becomes apparent when greater than 80 to 90 percent of the hormone-producing cells are destroyed (53). Changes in the serum levels of pituitary hormones can assist in the diagnosis (see Table 1-5). Pituitary apoplexy may be secondary to unusual circumstances such as heparin therapy for myocardial infarction (58). Clinically recognized pituitary apoplexy is usually seen in patients with pituitary macroadenomas.

Sheehan's Syndrome

Sheehan's syndrome is postpartum necrosis of the pituitary gland usually after hypotension secondary to blood loss during delivery. In some cases, vasospasm may initiate the ischemia, leading to the infarct in the anterior pituitary (60). The posterior pituitary is usually not affected since it has a rich arterial blood supply that is independent of the portal vasculature. As a result of infarction, there may be focal loss of anterior pituitary cells (fig. 1-25), or with more extensive infarction, more than 90 percent of the gland may be lost, leading to fibrosis of the gland after healing. In severe cases, the patient may have subclinical or overt hypofunction of the anterior pituitary.

Miscellaneous Conditions Causing Pituitary Infarction

A variety of conditions may lead to secondary pituitary infarction: head injury, massive cerebrovascular accidents, severe thrombocytopenia, and disseminated intravascular coagulation. In one form of coagulopathy caused by the Burmese Russell viper, fibrin deposits, hemorrhage, and necrosis of the anterior pituitary gland occur (61). If the patient survives, hypopituitarism often develops.

Exogenous Injury

Hypopituitarism may be caused by various physical injuries such as head trauma or surgical trauma (52). If these conditions disrupt the pituitary stalk, there is loss of specific neural and vascular connections to the hypothalamus. The loss of vascular connections can lead to infarcts of the anterior pituitary. Pituitary stalk section and head trauma are commonly associated with diabetes insipidus.

Injury from radiation to the hypothalamus or pituitary can lead to hypopituitarism (50, 51,56). In children who are irradiated because of leukemia or brain tumors, GH deficiency is a common finding (50). In adults who are treated with irradiation for pituitary tumors, the development of multiple endocrine deficiencies is common (51). The mechanism of injury may be related to direct injury to the pituitary or to the production of releasing and inhibitory hormones in the hypothalamic neurons. Damage to the

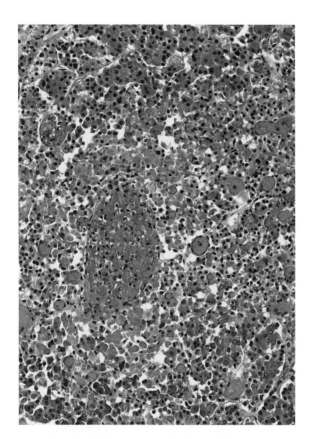 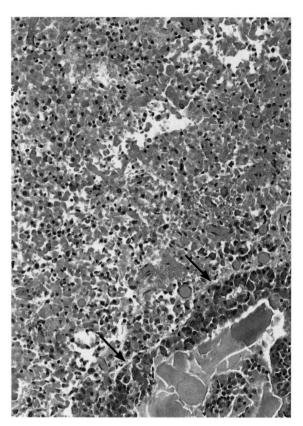

Figure 1-25

PITUITARY INFARCT

Left: There is a focal acute infarct with margination of neutrophils in the adjacent blood vessel in this pregnant patient (Sheehan's syndrome).

Right: The infarct was more extensive in the mucoid wedge, but some basophilic cells remain viable (arrows).

microvasculature or stroma may also contribute to these disorders. Studies suggest that cranial irradiation is more likely to cause hypothalamic than pituitary dysfunction (51).

METABOLIC DISORDERS

Amyloid Deposits

Amyloid is a pathologic, nonbranching, fibrillar protein with a beta-pleated sheet conformation that is deposited between cells of the pituitary gland. It can be deposited secondary to systemic disease or it may be associated with specific types of pituitary tumors (64–68,70,71). With systemic amyloidosis, the amyloid is usually found in the wall of blood vessels or in the interstitial connective tissue. Interstitial amyloid deposits may be associated with pituitary adenomas,

the most frequent of which are PRL tumors (fig. 1-26). Studies of pituitary amyloid have shown an amyloid P component. Local or organ-limited interstitial pituitary amyloid is usually considered a senile amyloid syndrome since it is an age-related disorder. Recent studies of senile interstitial amyloid deposits of the pituitary have noted glycosaminoglycans, basement membrane proteins, and apolipoprotein E, which are found in other amyloid syndromes such as AA-amyloidosis related to inflammatory conditions and Aß-amyloidosis related to Alzheimer's disease (66).

Iron Overload

Excessive accumulation of body iron leads to deposition in the parenchymal cells. Etiologic conditions leading to iron overload in the pituitary include idiopathic hemochromatosis,

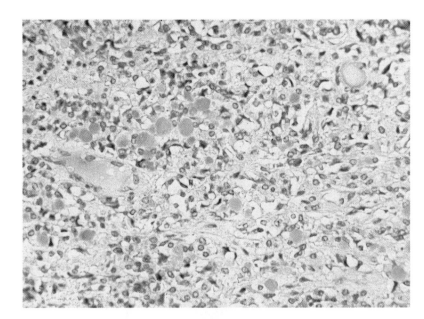

Figure 1-26

AMYLOID

Interstitial amyloid deposits in a prolactinoma. Nodular aggregates of amyloid are readily detected by Congo red stain. (Courtesy of Dr. B. Scheithauer, Rochester, MN.)

multiple blood transfusions, and chronic ingestion of iron supplements (63). These conditions can be associated with iron deposition in the anterior pituitary cells. Gonadotropic cells that produce FSH and LH usually contain more iron than other cell types (fig. 1-27). With severe iron deposition, the pituitary can develop extensive fibrosis which may lead to hypopituitarism. Prolonged excessive iron intake or absorption can cause pathological iron deposition in tissues and result in widespread organ damage.

Because the gonadotropin-producing cells are more commonly affected, iron deposition can lead to sexual dysfunction due to secondary hypogonadism, a result of damage to the FSH/LH cells of the anterior pituitary. The PRL cells are the second most common cell type affected by iron deposition (63). GH deficiency has also been associated with transfusion-induced iron overload syndromes in children.

Miscellaneous Metabolic Conditions

The pituitary gland may be affected by various familial metabolic conditions such as lysosomal storage diseases, Hurler's syndrome, or gargoylism, which are associated with abnormal storage of mucopolysaccharides in various tissues, including the anterior pituitary. Histologic examination shows membrane-bound vesicles with concentric osmophilic lamellae known as zebra bodies (69).

INFECTIOUS DISEASES

Acute Inflammation

In this condition, inflammatory cells acutely infiltrate the pituitary gland. Acute hypophysitis characterized by the presence of neutrophils and/or abscess formation may be associated with sepsis, purulent meningitis, otitis media, and thrombophlebitis of the cavernous sinus. Bacteria causing suppurative hypophysitis include *Pneumococcus*, group A *Streptococcus*, *Staphylococcus aureus*, *Enterococcus*, *Neisseria*, *Escherichia coli*, and others (72–74). The pituitary is infiltrated by sheets of polymorphonuclear leukocytes which may be walled off to form an abscess.

Granulomatous Inflammation

This inflammation of the pituitary gland is caused by multinucleated giant cells, lymphocytes, and plasma cells. Granulomatous inflammation involving the pituitary may be secondary to fungal infection or tuberculosis. Sarcoidosis can involve the anterior pituitary, although hypothalamic and posterior pituitary involvement is more common. Sarcoidosis can cause destruction of the hypothalamic neurons which produce regulatory peptides. Occasionally, the pituitary is involved with syphilis which can lead to extensive destruction of the gland (75). Granulomatous inflammation consists of a mixture of multinucleated giant cells, chronic

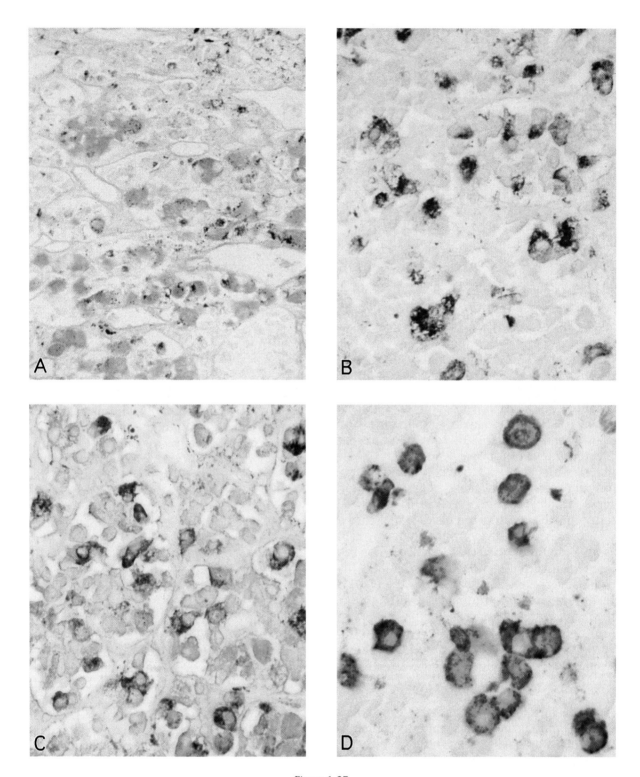

Figure 1-27

IRON DEPOSITION

Iron deposition in the anterior pituitary of a patient with idiopathic hemochromatosis. Prussian blue-PAS stain shows the iron within the cytoplasm (A). Combined Prussian blue staining and immunohistochemistry show a positive reaction for iron in LH (B) and alpha subunit (C) cells, while most ACTH cells are negative (D). (Courtesy of Dr. K. Kovacs, Toronto, Canada.)

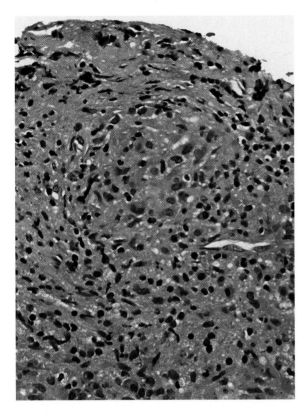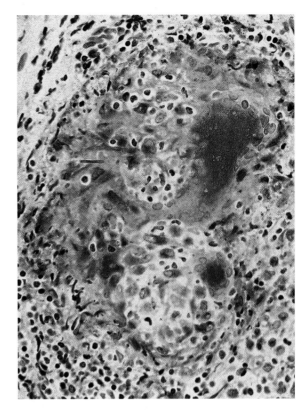

Figure 1-28

GRANULOMATOUS HYPOPHYSITIS

Left: Granulomatous inflammation of the anterior pituitary shows a mixed infiltrate of plasma cells, lymphocytes, and noncaseating granulomas.

Right: Staining for CD68 shows a positive reaction in the multinucleated cells. Stains for fungi and acid-fast organisms were negative (diaminobenzidine chromogen).

inflammatory cells including lymphocytes, and plasma cells in a background of fibrosis (fig. 1-28). Longstanding granulomatous inflammation with extensive scarring can lead to destruction of adenohypophyseal cells and hypopituitarism in some cases (fig. 1-28). Sarcoidosis can usually be distinguished from other granulomatous inflammatory conditions by the distinctive tight noncaseating granulomas (77). However, special stains for fungi and acid-fast organisms should be performed, since sarcoidosis is often a diagnosis of exclusion.

Giant Cell Granuloma

Giant cell granuloma is a rare idiopathic inflammatory disorder consisting of noncaseating granulomas, lymphocytes, and plasma cells (76). Similar findings may be seen in other endocrine tissues including the thyroid gland, adrenal cortex, and gonads. The differential diagnosis includes sarcoidosis since both conditions are associated with noncaseating granulomas. However, giant cell granuloma is confined to the pituitary and other endocrine tissues, while sarcoidosis commonly involves lymph nodes and other sites such as the lung. Giant cell granulomas may lead to progressive destruction of the adenohypophysis resulting in hypopituitarism.

Langerhans' Cell Histiocytosis

Definition. Langerhans' cell histiocytosis is a clonal proliferation of antigen-presenting dendritic cells.

General Remarks. Historically, Langerhans' cell histiocytosis was designated as *histiocytosis X* and divided into three groups: *Letterer-Siwe disease, Hand-Schüller-Christian disease,* and *eosinophilic granuloma* (78). The neoplastic cells are clonal antigen-presenting dendritic cells and express human leukocyte antigen (HLA)-DR and CD1a (79). This disorder can involve the hypothalamus, pituitary stalk, and posterior pituitary, leading to diabetes insipidus and hypothalamic dysfunction. The anterior lobe of the pituitary is usually not involved.

Microscopic Findings. The lesions consist of histiocytes with giant cells, lymphocytes, plasma cells, and eosinophils. Immunohistochemical staining is positive for S100 protein and usually positive for CD1a in the Langerhans histiocytes. Ultrastructural studies often show Birbeck granules in the cytoplasm of the Langerhans cells.

Differential Diagnosis. This condition may mimic granulomatous lesions such as sarcoidosis and giant cell granuloma (78). Like sarcoidosis, it involves the hypothalamus and posterior pituitary, so patients may develop diabetes insipidus. Destruction of hypothalamic neurons, leading to loss of regulation of hypothalamic-releasing and -inhibitory hormones, can occur as in sarcoidosis. The presence of eosinophils as well as histiocytes and lymphocytes, and immunoreactivity for S100 protein and CD1a allow one to make the diagnosis and distinguish Langerhans' histiocytosis from other granulomatous diseases.

AUTOIMMUNE DISEASES

The pituitary gland may be involved in systemic autoimmune diseases or autoimmune disorders that are restricted to the pituitary gland.

Lymphocytic Hypophysitis

Definition. Lymphocytic hypophysitis is an autoimmune disease in which lymphocytes and plasma cells infiltrate the pituitary gland.

General Remarks. Lymphocytic hypophysitis generally affects young women in late pregnancy or in the postpartum period (80,81, 85,87,88,90,91,94). Some patients have inflammatory conditions involving the thyroid gland, adrenal gland, and other endocrine tissues (82,84). Antipituitary antibodies have been identified in some cases of autoimmune hypophysitis, supporting an autoimmune etiology. However, immunofluorescence studies have failed to show immune complex deposits.

Clinical and Radiologic Findings. Although lymphocytic hypophysitis primarily affects young women in late pregnancy and in the postpartum period, cases have been reported in postmenopausal women and in men (90,94). In the study of Meichner et al. (91), all 18 patients were women but ranged from 22 to 74 years of age. Thirty-seven percent had preexisting endocrine disorders and 22 percent had associated autoimmune-related conditions. Most patients presented within 1 year postpartum or during pregnancy, although one 59- and one 74-year-old woman had the diagnosis established by biopsy. In a recent study by Thodou et al. (94), there were two males among the 16 cases studied; most of the women presented during pregnancy (71 percent). Nine patients (56 percent) presented with expanding pituitary sellar masses, 10 (63 percent) had anterior pituitary hypofunction, and 3 (19 percent) had diabetes insipidus. About 124 cases of lymphocytic hypophysitis have been reported since 1962 (85). Headache and visual field defects are the most frequent symptoms. Most patients show signs of isolated or multiple anterior pituitary hormone deficiencies. Secretion of ACTH is most frequently impaired, followed by TSH, gonadotropin, GH, and PRL. About one third of the cases involved hyperprolactinemia (85).

Radiologic studies by computed tomography (CT) and MRI with contrast enhancement usually show a mass lesion. These studies also show features of a pituitary mass lesion mimicking an adenoma (94). Thickening of the pituitary stalk may be present (85).

Macroscopic Findings. The pituitary gland is invariably enlarged in this condition, but it usually does not have the soft consistency of an adenoma.

Microscopic Findings. A mixed inflammatory infiltrate with predominant lymphocytes and some plasma cells is present (fig. 1-29). Lymphoid follicles with germinal centers are sometimes seen. Oncocytic metaplasia of the adenohypophyseal cells may be present, as well as occasional neutrophils, eosinophils, and macrophages. When the chronic inflammatory process results in focal or diffuse fibrosis, further destruction of anterior pituitary function can result.

Immunohistochemical Findings. Immunohistochemical staining shows a mixture of B- and T-lymphoid cells. The B cells are invariably polyclonal. The macrophages may stain for CD68.

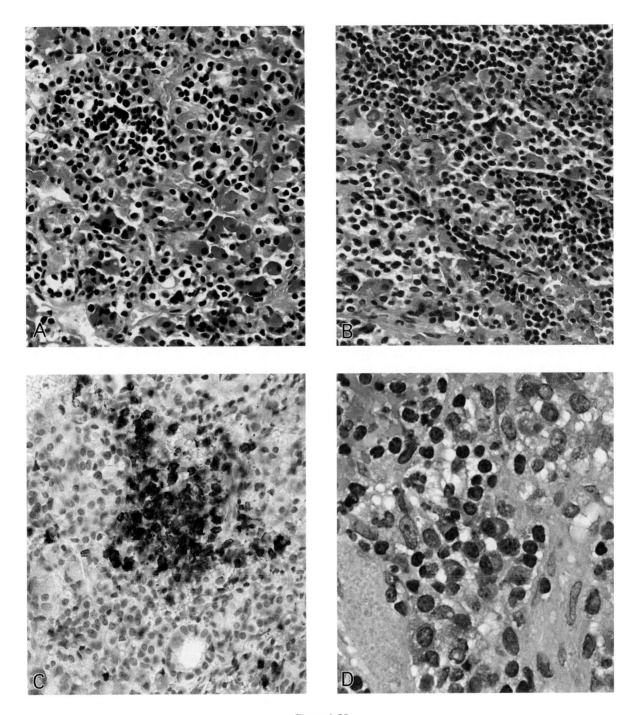

Figure 1-29

LYMPHOCYTIC HYPOPHYSITIS

A: A mixed inflammatory infiltrate of lymphocytes and plasma cells is present in this pituitary biopsy from a young woman with hyperprolactinemia.

B: The inflammatory infiltrate in another patient is denser and can lead to destruction of anterior pituitary cells.

C: Immunohistochemical staining often shows a mixed infiltrate of CD3-positive T cells and CD20-positive B cells. The B cells are polyclonal.

D: Lymphocytic hypophysitis associated with lymphocytes, plasma cells, and early fibrosis. These changes may also be seen in "secondary hypophysitis" which is usually associated with an adjacent neoplasm.

Differential Diagnosis. The findings of hyperprolactinemia and a pituitary mass usually raise the possibility of a prolactinoma. In small biopsies, the presence of a mixture of anterior pituitary cells and preservation of the reticulin pattern in early lesions helps to exclude an adenoma. Immunohistochemical staining for pituitary hormones shows a heterogeneous mixed pattern of staining which helps to exclude the diagnosis of an adenoma. Lymphomas of the adenohypophysis are extremely uncommon, and are diagnostically excluded by the cytologic features of the lymphocytes and analysis of B and T cells by immunohistochemistry. Other inflammatory conditions affecting the pituitary such as granulomatous disorders and sarcoidosis can usually be excluded by the presence of multinucleated giant cells, which should not be present in lymphocytic hypophysitis. A condition known as "secondary hypophysitis" in which the pituitary shows fibrosis, granulation tissue, and mixed B and T lymphocytes in equal amounts in the presence of a tumor in the sellar region, such as a craniopharyngioma or pituitary adenoma, has been reported and should be distinguished from lymphocytic hypophysitis (93). Detailed clinicopathologic studies and careful examination of all the biopsied tissues are needed to rule out this diagnosis. A recently described inflammatory disease, xanthomatous hypophysitis (83), may be confused with lymphocytic hypophysitis. However, the presence of predominantly foamy histiocytes in addition to lymphocytes and some plasma cells allows one to make the histologic distinction.

Treatment and Prognosis. Patients can develop diabetes insipidus with lymphocytic hypophysitis. Autoimmune diseases of the thyroid, adrenal, and parathyroid glands may occur concomitantly (85,94). Treatment with glucocorticoids has been reported to suppress the inflammatory response (94).

Observation and serial computerized imaging are reasonable if a pituitary mass is discovered in a clinical setting consistent with lymphocytic hypophysitis and if the symptoms of a mass (e.g., visual field defects) are absent. If the patient has visual field defects, decompression without hypophysectomy is the treatment of choice. However, if there is uncertainty about the diagnosis, multiple biopsies and extensive pituitary exploration should be performed. In patients with hormone deficiencies, appropriate replacement regimens should be initiated (85, 94). Recent studies have suggested that because of the compressive features of this condition and the transient endocrine features, if the clinical suspicion is high, conservative treatment may avoid the need for aggressive pituitary surgery.

Autoantibodies to Anterior Pituitary Cells

Autoantibodies to anterior pituitary cells have been detected in many disorders including the empty sella syndrome, specific hormone deficiencies, and hypopituitarism (82,92). Antibodies against specific pituitary cell lines have been detected in more than half of patients with primary empty sella syndrome (89).

Autoimmune Diabetes Insipidus

This idiopathic autoimmune disease involves the infundibulum and neurohypophysis. Diabetes insipidus may have various etiologies including an autoimmune basis. It may be familial with an autosomal-dominant inheritance or secondary to tumor, infections, trauma, and other lesions. In all these forms of diabetes insipidus, patients have polyuria and polydipsia from vasopressin deficiency. In autoimmune diabetes insipidus, the pituitary stalk is thickened or the neurohypophysis is enlarged, both of which can be recognized by MRI in many patients who have had the disorder for less than 2 years. Histologic examination may show an infiltration of T lymphocytes and plasma cells (86). As with autoimmune hypophysitis, patients may also have mild hyperprolactinemia, probably secondary to the disruption of the dopaminergic signal to the anterior pituitary PRL cells.

Autoimmune Polyglandular Syndromes

The autoimmune polyglandular disorders are autoimmune disorders associated with hypofunction of various endocrine tissues.

There are two types of autoimmune polyglandular syndrome. Type I includes adrenal insufficiency, mucocutaneous candidiasis, and hypoparathyroidism; the more common type II includes adrenal insufficiency, hyperthyroidism or hypothyroidism, insulin-dependent diabetes mellitus, primary hypogonadism, myasthenia gravis, hypophysitis, and celiac disease (82). Patients with the type II syndrome usually have two or more of these diseases. With hypofunction of the various organs, the pituitary can be secondarily affected, with hyperplasia of various cell types producing specific trophic hormones. These syndromes are discussed further in chapter 5.

PITUITARY CYSTS

Pituitary cysts are epithelial-lined structures that may be intrasellar or suprasellar in location. Several types of cysts occur in the region of the sella turcica. Many of these produce no specific clinical symptoms and are only discovered incidentally during autopsy or surgery for other conditions. Occasional cysts may reach a size large enough to cause local symptoms. Although in a few cases they may be associated with hypopituitarism and hyperprolactinemia from pressure effects on the pituitary stalk, in most cases the cysts do not produce any pituitary hormones and are not associated with endocrine symptoms or alterations in blood hormone levels.

Rathke's Cleft Cyst

Definition. Rathke's cleft cyst is an intrasellar or suprasellar cyst lined by ciliated cuboidal to columnar epithelium with goblet cells.

General Remarks. Rathke's cleft cysts are the most common cyst involving the pituitary (96,98, 99,101–103). They originate from the remnants of Rathke's pouch. Rathke's cleft remnants or small microscopic cysts can persist throughout life in the region of the intermediate lobe. Enlargement of the cysts can cause symptoms. On rare occasion, pituitary adenomas may be associated with Rathke's cyst and there may be a transition between the cells of the cyst and the adenoma, raising the possibility of a true transitional cell neoplasm from the hypophyseal duct.

Clinical and Radiologic Findings. Although Rathke's cleft cysts are often found incidentally at autopsy, larger lesions, especially cysts greater than 1 cm in diameter, may cause symptoms (such as visual disturbance) or changes in hypothalamic and/or pituitary function. In a recent study of 12 patients with Rathke's cleft cyst (98), 9 had visual symptoms and 8 had visual field defects. Three patients had panhypopituitarism, two of whom also had diabetes insipidus.

Rathke's cleft cysts vary considerably in radiologic appearance (fig. 1-30) (96,99,100).

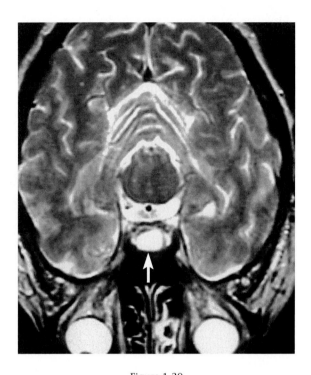

Figure 1-30

RATHKE'S CLEFT CYST

Axial T1-weighted MRI demonstrates a high signal intrasellar mass just to the left of midline (arrow). This did not enhance on postcontrast images (not shown).

The signal intensity varies with the architectural lining and the cyst content. Cysts lined by a simple epithelium which contain clear fluid may have a MRI density similar to cerebrospinal fluid, while cysts filled with mucus or more solid products have more heterogeneous signal characteristics (96,97,99,100).

Macroscopic Findings. The cysts are thin-walled structures with a great deal of variation in their content (fig. 1-31). The cyst wall may be difficult to find in small biopsy specimens and any adherent pituitary tissue should be carefully examined for a cyst lining.

Microscopic Findings. The cysts are lined by cuboidal to columnar epithelium with ciliated and goblet cells (fig. 1-32). Pituitary hormone cells may be present in or adjacent to the wall (fig. 1-33). The lining cells may undergo complete or partial squamous metaplasia. With complete squamous metaplasia, the ciliated epithelium and goblet cells may be absent. On occasion, xanthomatous change may obscure the epithelial nature of the lesion.

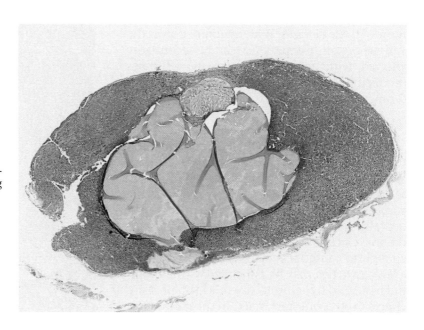

Figure 1-31

RATHKE'S CLEFT CYST

The Rathke's cleft cyst is a thick-walled epithelial-lined cyst containing eosinophilic proteinaceous fluid.

Cytologic Findings. Cytologic preparation of the cyst fluid may show the ciliated epithelium with goblet cells.

Immunohistochemical Findings. The epithelial lining cells are usually positive for keratin, epithelial membrane antigen, and carcinoembryonic antigen. Anterior pituitary cells may be present in the cyst wall and these most commonly stain for ACTH. Cells stain for S100 acidic protein and can be confused with the folliculostellate cells present in the normal adenohypophysis.

Ultrastructural Findings. Epithelial cells with cilia and goblet cells with desmosomal and apical junctional complexes are present on ultrastructural examination. In areas with squamous metaplasia, the goblet cells and ciliated epithelium are replaced by cells with tonofilament bundles and well-developed desmosomes (fig. 1-33).

Differential Diagnosis. In small biopsy specimens a craniopharyngioma, especially the papillary variant, may be confused with a Rathke's cleft cyst. The former consists of sheets of well-differentiated epithelial cells admixed with prominent areas of fibrovascular stoma. It may have focal areas with goblet or ciliated cells similar to the Rathke's cleft cyst. Unlike the adamatinomatous craniopharyngioma, papillary tumors are not usually calcified, so the absence of calcification on radiologic or histologic examination does not exclude this diagnosis.

Treatment and Prognosis. These benign cysts are usually cured by excision. Patients that have been treated by partial removal and drainage may have recurrences. In a recent study, 4 of 12 (33 percent) patients showed reexpansion of their cysts from 3 to 48 months after the initial surgery (99).

Epidermoid Cysts

Epidermoid cysts are slow-growing benign lesions lined by layers of flattened squamous epithelium. They occur throughout the neuraxis, but are mostly intracranial and lie within the cerebellopontine angle. Some may occur in the region of the pituitary, leading to confusion with a Rathke's cleft cyst or dermoid cyst. Some of these cysts resemble cystic craniopharyngiomas, although the other elements of craniopharyngioma are not present.

Dermoid Cysts

Dermoid cysts are lined by benign keratinizing squamous epithelium and often contain cutaneous adnexa. They may be seen occasionally in the sellar region (95). They are benign tumors lined by stratified squamous epithelium and contain other germ layers, including sweat glands, sebaceous glands, hair follicles, and connective and other tissues. The wall of the cyst may contain lymphocytes, macrophages, and occasional foreign body giant cells.

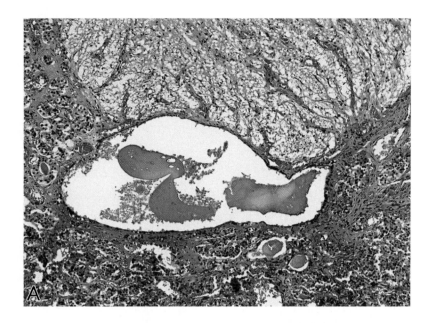

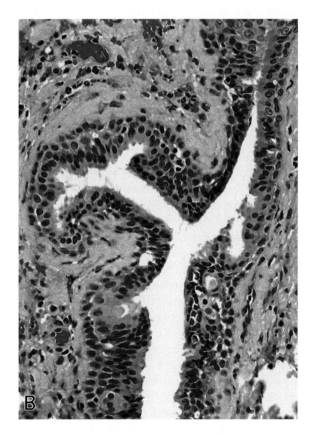

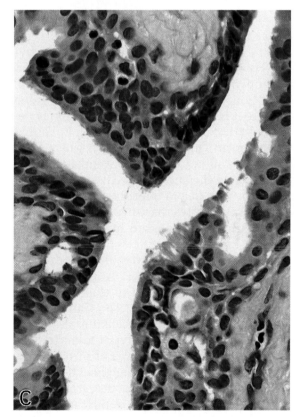

Figure 1-32

RATHKE'S CLEFT CYST

A: Microscopic simple Rathke's cleft cyst lined by cuboidal epithelium with proteinaceous material in the lumen.
B: A larger Rathke's cleft cyst with columnar epithelium admixed with goblet cells.
C: Higher magnification of the cyst wall shows the ciliated epithelium which is useful in establishing the diagnosis.

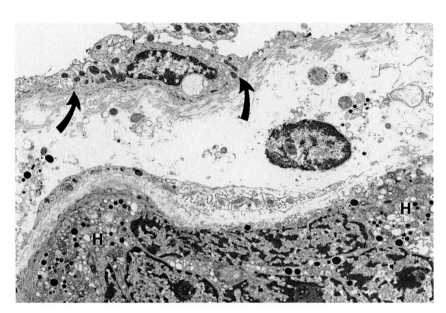

Figure 1-33

RATHKE'S CLEFT CYST: ULTRASTRUCTURE

Ultrastructure of the wall of a Rathke's cleft cyst showing lining cells (arrows). The hormone-producing anterior pituitary cells (H) are adjacent to the cyst wall (X4,000).

PITUITARY HYPERPLASIA

Pituitary hyperplasia is an absolute increase in the number of specific anterior pituitary cells. Although anterior pituitary hyperplasia may be preneoplastic, in most cases patients do not develop neoplasms, and the condition is often reversible if target-hormone treatment is initiated. The hyperplasia may be: 1) idiopathic (primary hyperplasia), 2) caused by end-organ failure and lack of negative feedback stimulation (secondary hyperplasia), or 3) caused by proliferation of specific anterior pituitary cell types due to direct hypothalamic hormone stimulation (tertiary hyperplasia). The hyperplasia may be related to hypothalamic dysfunction resulting in an excess of hypothalamic hormone production or to ectopic production of hypothalamic hormones from neoplasms such as endocrine tumors of the lungs, pancreas, and other sites (106,116). Gangliocytic hamartomas of the hypothalamus and other sites may also produce hypothalamic hormones, leading to hyperplasia of specific pituitary cell types (104,114). Gangliocytic hamartomas most commonly produce growth hormone–releasing hormone (GHRH) and gonadotropin hormone–releasing hormone (GnRH).

Histologically, hyperplasia can be readily recognized by reticulin staining (fig. 1-34) which may show a diffuse and/or nodular pattern of proliferation resulting from hypertrophy and hyperplasia of specific cell types. Immunohis-tochemical staining helps to identify the cell type undergoing hyperplasia.

ACTH Cell Hyperplasia

Secondary Hyperplasia. In longstanding Addison's disease, there is hyperplasia of ACTH cells (105,112,113). Histochemical stains show degranulated basophil cells while reticulin stains show preservation of the expanded acini. In a study of 18 patients with Addison's disease, the degree of diffuse and nodular hyperplasia of the ACTH cells was related to the duration of the disease (113). In occasional cases, ACTH-producing adenomas develop (115). An increased number of TSH cells has been noted in the pituitary of patients with Addison's disease, which may have an immunologic etiology when the adrenal and thyroid glands become atrophic (*Schmidt's syndrome*) (113).

Primary Hyperplasia. Primary ACTH cell hyperplasia may result from excessive secretion of corticotropin-releasing hormone (CRH) or may be idiopathic (fig. 1-35) (107,109,110). The hyperplasia is predominantly nodular, but may be diffuse if CRH is stimulated. Patients with excess CRH production from ectopic sources such as neoplasms or gangliocytic hamartomas may present with Cushing's syndrome; in many cases, such as with small cell lung carcinomas that commonly produce CRH and/or ACTH, a full-blown picture of Cushing's syndrome is not present because of the rapid course of the

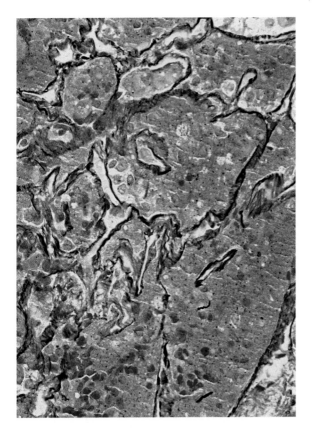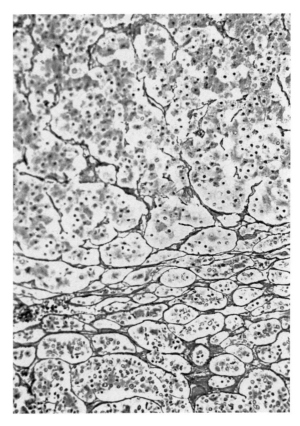

Figure 1-34

PITUITARY HYPERPLASIA

A comparison of the reticulin staining patterns in hyperplastic anterior pituitary (left), and (right) in adenoma (top of photo) with adjacent normal pituitary (bottom of photo). Hyperplasia is associated with an expansion but not a disruption of the reticulin pattern (left). The normal reticulin pattern is contrasted with the adjacent adenoma which shows disruption of this normal pattern (right).

disease. In pituitary hyperplasia due to ectopic hormone production, the adrenal glands become markedly enlarged and the combined weight may be up to 30 g.

ACTH cell hyperplasia may be difficult to diagnose in small biopsy specimens because of the variable pattern and distribution of ACTH cells in the normal pituitary. Because most ACTH cells are present in the mucoid wedge, if the biopsy is from this area, the pathologist should be very cautious when making a diagnosis of hyperplasia.

Biopsies from the pars nervosa may show basophil invasion with abundant ACTH-positive cells. ACTH cell hyperplasia and adenomas should not be diagnosed in a biopsy showing only basophil invasion.

GH Cell Hyperplasia

Secondary Hyperplasia. Secondary GH cell hyperplasia usually does not occur since there is no unique target organ failure associated with GH secretion.

Primary Hyperplasia. Primary GH cell hyperplasia is frequently associated with excess GHRH production from ectopic tumor–derived sources or gangliocytic hamartomas (116), or it may be idiopathic. It can be associated with gigantism or acromegaly (figs. 1-36, 1-37) (108, 117). The histologic features of childhood gigantism include a pattern of cells with GH and/ or PRL immunoreactivity, usually in a diffuse proliferation with some nodularity (fig. 1-38). The cells are very acidophilic. In cases of McCune-Albright syndrome associated with

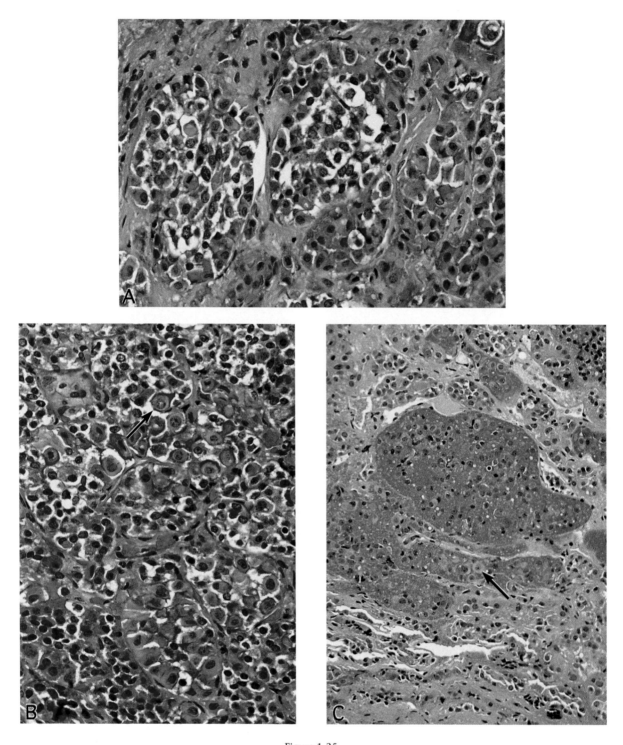

Figure 1-35

ACTH CELL HYPERPLASIA

A: ACTH cell hyperplasia secondary to a bronchial carcinoid secreting corticotropin-releasing hormone. A mixed pattern of hyperplasia is present with prominent nodularity and fibrosis in some areas.

B: Other areas of the biopsy show a diffuse pattern of hyperplasia and prominent Crooke's cell hyaline changes (arrow).

C: Another case of ACTH hyperplasia of unknown etiology (idiopathic) shows a prominent nodular pattern. Crooke's hyaline changes are also present (arrow).

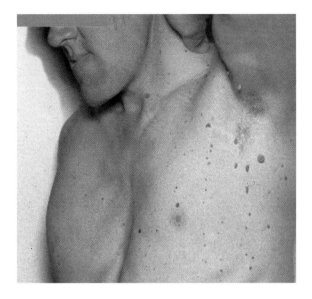

Figure 1-36

ACROMEGALY

This 30-year-old man presented with dental malocclusion. Mandibular extension, frontal bossing, and excessive skin tags are demonstrated.

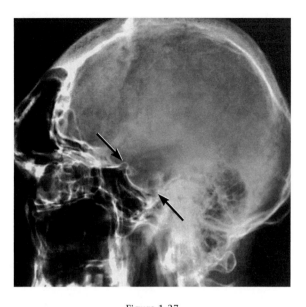

Figure 1-37

ACROMEGALY

Plain skull X ray demonstrating marked expansion of the frontal sinus and an enlarged sella turcica (arrows) in a patient with acromegaly.

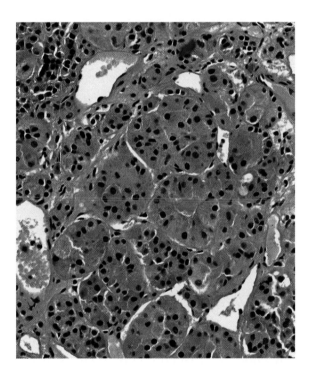

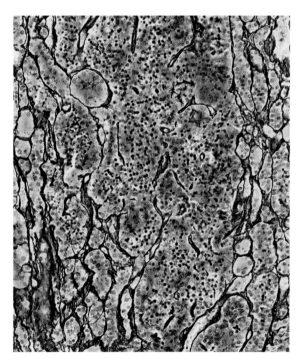

Figure 1-38

GH CELL HYPERPLASIA

Histologic section showing nodular and diffuse GH cell hyperplasia in an 8-year-old boy.
Left: The eosinophilic GH cells are increased in size and number.
Right: Reticulin stain shows the expanded acinar units.

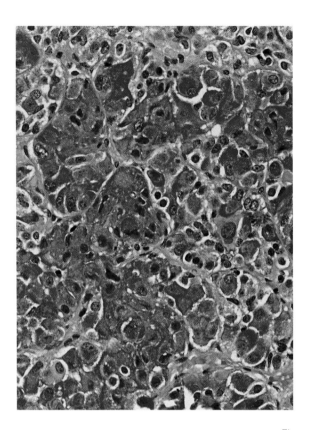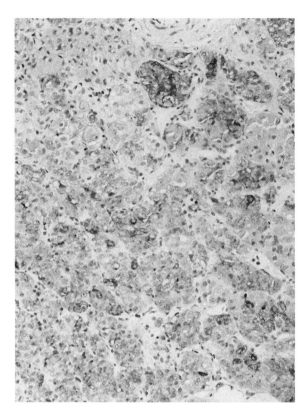

Figure 1-39

IDIOPATHIC TSH CELL HYPERPLASIA

Left: Prominent nodular aggregates of basophilic TSH cells are present.
Right: Immunostaining for TSH is usually weak because of the rapid secretion of newly produced hormone from the cells (diaminobenzidine chromogen).

GH hyperplasia, the anterior pituitary cells also produce GH and PRL.

When GH hyperplasia is associated with acromegaly, the cells are intensely immunoreactive for GH but may also stain for PRL. The pituitary acini in the lateral wings expand to give the gland a nodular appearance. Ultrastructural studies show densely granulated GH cells with larger secretory granules and a very prominent Golgi complex (107).

TSH Cell Hyperplasia

Secondary Hyperplasia. Secondary TSH cell hyperplasia is associated with primary hypothyroidism (111,115). In experimental animals, treatment with radioactive iodine, with drugs such as propylthiouracil, or surgical ablation of the thyroid gland can lead to TSH cell hyperplasia. In humans with secondary TSH cell hyperplasia, the pituitary gland shows a nodular enlargement and numerical increase of TSH cells (fig. 1-39); TSH adenomas may occasionally develop in these patients (112). Hyperplasia of PRL cells may be associated with hypothyroidism due to the depletion of hypothalamic dopamine stores. Enlargement of the pituitary gland, detected radiologically, may lead to the incorrect diagnosis of an adenoma.

Primary Hyperplasia. This is much rarer than secondary hyperplasia. The enlarged cells associated with thyroid deficiency contain an abundant dilated rough endoplasmic reticulum and prominent Golgi complexes with many vesicles and are known as "thyroidectomy" cells.

The secretory granules in primary and secondary TSH cell hyperplasia remain small, ranging from 150 to 250 nm in diameter (fig. 1-40) (107). With longstanding hypothyroidism,

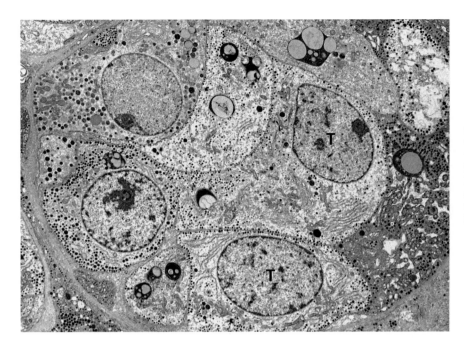

Figure 1-40

TSH CELL: ULTRASTRUCTURE

Ultrastructural appearance of prominent TSH cells (T) admixed with other cell types in the same acinar unit in the anterior pituitary. The hyperplastic TSH cells have small spare secretory granules and prominent dense lysosomes (X2,500).

there is weak immunoreactivity for TSH, associated with a decline in the numbers of cytoplasmic secretory granules.

Gonadotroph Hyperplasia

Secondary Hyperplasia. Most cases of gonadotroph hyperplasia are of the secondary type (107). In experimental animals, gonadotroph hyperplasia results from ablation of the testes or ovaries, leading to hypertrophy and hyperplasia of the gonadotropin hormone (GTH) cells. Ultrastructural studies show proliferation and dilatation of the rough endoplasmic reticulum, increasing prominence of the Golgi complex, and gradual reduction in the numbers of secretory granules (107). In patients with longstanding gonadectomy varying degrees of hyperplasia may be present.

PRL Cell Hyperplasia

Physiological hyperplasia of PRL cells during pregnancy and lactation has been discussed earlier.

Secondary Hyperplasia. PRL cell hyperplasia can also occur secondary to suprasellar space-occupying lesions such as craniopharyngioma, Rathke's cleft cyst, and meningioma, or secondary to large anterior pituitary tumors. All of these conditions can result in decreased delivery of dopamine to the anterior pituitary from the hypothalamus. Because dopamine has an inhibitory effect on the PRL cells, decreased delivery results in PRL cell hyperplasia.

Primary Hyperplasia. This form of hyperplasia is idiopathic and uncommon. The pattern of hyperplasia is diffuse.

Primary PRL cell hyperplasia is commonly diffuse, as can be seen by a diffuse immunohistochemical staining pattern for PRL cells with enlarged acini (107,108). Ultrastructural studies show sparsely granulated PRL cells with a well-developed rough endoplasmic reticulum and large Golgi complexes. Secretory granules are sparse, and there are few examples of reverse exocytosis or abnormal extrusion of secretory granules, a characteristic feature of PRL cells (107).

Differential Diagnosis of Pituitary Hyperplasia

The differential diagnosis of anterior pituitary hyperplasia includes a normal pituitary gland and pituitary adenomas (figs. 1-41, 1-42). The two conditions can be distinguished using the features outlined in Table 1-4. In patients with idiopathic anterior pituitary hyperplasia not associated with excessive hormone production, multiple techniques including imaging studies, H&E stains, reticulin stains, and immunohistochemical and ultrastructural analyses are usually needed to establish the diagnosis of hyperplasia.

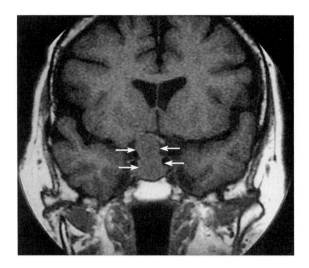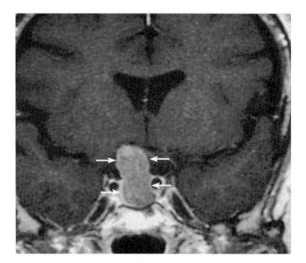

Figure 1-41

PITUITARY ADENOMA

Coronal T1-weighted MRIs before (left) and after (right) gadolinium contrast enhancement demonstrate a typical pituitary adenoma (arrows). Note the somewhat nonhomogeneous contrast enhancement in the right figure. This mass has the typical "figure 8" appearance seen with suprasellar extension.

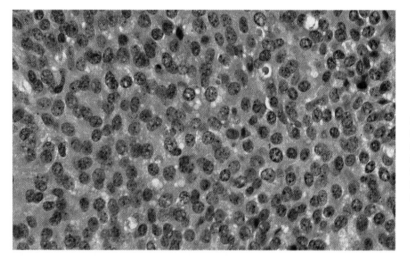

Figure 1-42

PITUITARY ADENOMA

Pituitary adenoma that is readily diagnosed on H&E-stained section. The cells are all uniform. There is loss of the acinar pattern. There are no acidophilic or basophilic cells admixed with the sheets of chromophobe cells. Immunostaining and ultrasound studies are used to characterize adenomas.

Table 1-4

DISTINCTION OF PITUITARY HYPERPLASIA FROM ADENOMA

	Hyperplasia	Adenoma
Reticulin stain	Preserved but expanded acini	Disruption of the acini
General microscopic appearance	Mixed diffuse and nodular pattern	Usually diffuse proliferation
Normal pituitary	Involved in hyperplastic processes	Compressed by expanding adenoma
Immunohistochemistry	Generally weak staining for hyperplastic hormone	Variable but generally strong staining for specific hormone
Electron microscopy	Evidence of hyperactivity, well-developed RER and Golgi, decreased numbers of secretory granules	Variable patterns of RER and Golgi, cells are usually well granulated

Table 1-5

NORMAL VALUES FOR PITUITARY HORMONES[a]

Hormone	SI[b]	Conventional
Argenine vasopressin (AVP), plasma, random fluid intake	2.3-7.4 pmol/L	18-23 mol/L
Corticotropin (ACTH), plasma	4-22 pmol/L	20-100 pg/mL
Gonadotropins, plasma		
women, basic		
FSH	5-20 IU/L	5-20 mIU/mL
LH	5-25 IU/L	5-25 mIU/mL
women, ovulatory peak		
FSH	12-30 IU/L	12-35 mIU/mL
LH	25-100 IU/L	25-100 mIU/mL
men		
FSH	5-20 IU/L	5-20 mIU/mL
LH	5-20 IU/L	5-20 mIU/mL
prepubertal boys and girls		
FSH	<5 IU/L	<5 mIU/mL
LH	<5 IU/L	<5 mIU/mL
Growth hormone, plasma		
After 100g glucose orally	<5 µg/L	<5 ng/mL
After insulin-induced hypoglycemia	>9 µg/L	>9 mg/mL
Human chorionic gonadotropin, beta-subunit, plasma, men and nonpregnant women	<3 IU/L	<3 mIU/mL
Oxytocin, plasma		
Random	1-4 pmol/L	1.25-5 ng/L
Ovulatory peak in women	408 pmol/L	5-10 ng/L
Prolactin, serum	2-15 µg/L	2-15 ng/mL

[a]Wilson JD, Foster DW, Kronenberg DW, Larsen PR., eds. Williams textbook of endocrinology. 9th ed. Philadelphia: WB Sanders, 1998: back cover.

[b]SI - system of international units.

REFERENCES

Embryology, Anatomy, and Physiology

1. Asa SL. Tumors of the pituitary gland. Atlas of Tumor Pathology, 3rd Series, Fascicle 22. Washington, DC: Armed Forces Institute of Pathology, 1998.

2. Baker BL, Jaffe RB. The genesis of cell types in the adenohypophysis of the human fetus as observed with immunocytochemistry. Am J Anat 1975;143:137–61.

3. Boyd JD. Observations on the human pharyngeal hypophysis. J Endocrinol 1956;14:66–77.

4. Gilbert MS. Some factors influencing the early development of mammalian hypophysis. Anat Rec 1935;62:337–59.

5. Girod C, Trouillas J, Dubois MP. Immunocytochemical localization of S-100 protein in stellate cells (folliculostellate cells) of the anterior lobe of the normal human pituitary. Cell Tissue Res 1985;241:505–11.

6. Goodyear CG, Guyda HJ, Giroud CJ. Development of the hypothalamic-pituitary axis in the human fetus. In: Tolis G, Labrie F, Martin JB, Natolin F, eds. Clinical neuroendocrinology: a pathophysiological approach. New York: Raven Press,1979:199–214.

7. Gorczyca W, Hardy J. Arterial supply of the human anterior pituitary gland. Neurosurgery 1987;20:369–78.

8. Ferrara N, Schweigerer L, Neufeld G, Mitchell R, Gospodarowicz D. Pituitary follicular cells produce basic fibroblast growth factor. Proc Natl Acad Sci USA 1987;84:5773–7.

9. Horvath E, Kovacs K. Fine structural cytology of the adenohypophysis in rat and man. J Electron Microsc Technique 1988;8:401–32.

10. Kovacs K, Asa SL. The adenohypophysis. In: Horvath E, Kovacs K, eds. Functional endocrine pathology. Boston: Blackwell Scientific, 1991:245–81.

11. Kovacs K, Horvath E. Tumors of the pituitary gland. Atlas of Tumor Pathology, 2nd Series, Fascicle 21. Washington, DC: Armed Forces Institute of Pathology, 1986.

12. Lloyd RV, Anagnostou D, Cano M, Barkan Al, Chandler WF. Analysis of mammosomatotropic cells in normal and neoplastic human pituitary tissues by the reverse hemolytic plaque assay and immunocytochemistry. J Clin Endocrinol Metabl 1988;66:1103–10.

13. Lloyd RV, D'Amato CJ, Thiny MT, Jin L, Hicks SP, Chandler WF. Corticotroph (basophil) invasion of the pars nervosa in the human pituitary: localization of pro-opiomelanocortin peptides, galanin and peptidylglycine-amidating monooxygenase-like immunoreactivities. Endocr Pathol 1993;4:86–94.

14. Lloyd RV, Chandler WF, Kovacs K, Ryan N. Ectopic pituitary adenomas with normal anterior pituitary glands. Am J Surg Pathol 1986;10:546–52.

15. Marin F, Kovacs K, Stefaneanu L, Horvath E, Cheng Z. S-100 protein immunopositivity in human nontumorous hypophyses and pituitary adenomas. Endocr Pathol 1992;3:28–38.

16. Osamura RY, Watanabe K. Histogenesis of the cells of the anterior and intermediate lobes of human pituitary glands: immunohistochemical studies. Int Rev Cytol 1985;95:103–29.

17. Thorner MO, Vance ML, Horvath E, Kovacs K. The anterior pituitary. In: Wilson JD, Foster DW, eds. Williams textbook of endocrinology, 8th ed. Philadelphia: WB Saunders, 1992:221–310.

18. Voss JW, Rosenfeld MG. Anterior pituitary development: short tales from dwarf mice. Cell 1992;70:527–30.

Reactive Changes Including Pregnancy, Hormonal Symptoms, and Drug Effects

19. Barkan AL, Lloyd RV, Chandler WF, et al. Preoperative treatment of acromegaly with long-acting somatostatin analog SMS 201-995: shrinkage of invasive pituitary macroadenomas and improved surgical remission rate. J Clin Endocrinol Metab 1988;67:1040–8.

20. Carpenter CC, Solomon N, Silverberg SG, et al. Schmidt's syndrome (thyroid and adrenal insufficiency). A review of the literature and a report of fifteen new cases including ten instances of coexistent diabetes mellitus. Medicine 1964;43:153–80.

21. Crooke AC. A change in the basophil cells of the pituitary gland common to conditions which exhibit the syndrome attributed to basophil adenoma. J Pathol Bacteriol 1935;41:339–49.

22. Crooke AC, Russell DS. The pituitary gland in Addison's disease. J Pathol Bacteriol 1935;40:255–83.

23. Halmi NS, McCormick WF. Effects of hyperadrenocorticism on pituitary thyrotropic cells in man. Arch Pathol 1972;94:471–4.

24. Halmi NS, McCormick WF, Decker DA Jr. The natural history of hyalinization of ACTH-MSH cells in man. Arch Pathol 1971;91:318–26.

25. Kovacs K, Stefaneanu L, Horvath E, et al. Effect of dopamine agonist medication on prolactin-producing pituitary adenomas: a morphological study including immunocytochemistry, electron microscopy, and in situ hybridization. Virchows Arch [A] 1991;418:439–46.

26. Murray S, Ezrin C. Effect of Graves' disease on the "thyrotroph" of the adenohypophysis. J Clin Endocrinol 1966;26:287–93.

27. Saeger W. Effect of drugs on pituitary ultrastructure. Microsc Res Tech 1992;20:162–76.

28. Saeger W: Surgical pathology of the pituitary in Cushing's disease. Pathol Res Pract 1991; 187:613–6.

29. Scheithauer BW, Kovacs KT, Randall RV, Ryan N. Effects of estrogen on the human pituitary: a clinicopathologic study. Mayo Clin Proc 1989;64:1077–84.

30. Scheithauer BW, Kovacs KT, Young WF Jr, Randall RV. The pituitary gland in hyperthyroidism. Mayo Clin Proc 1992;67:22–6.

31. Scheithauer BW, Sano T, Kovacs KT, Young WF Jr, Ryan N, Randall RV. The pituitary gland in pregnancy: a clinicopathologic and immunohistochemical study of 69 cases. Mayo Clin Proc 1990;65:461–74.

32. Stefaneanu L, Kovacs K, Lloyd RV, et al. Pituitary lactotrophs and somatotrophs in pregnancy: a correlative in situ hybridization and immunocytochemical study. Virchows Arch [Cell Pathol] 1992;62:291–6.

33. Tindall GT, Kovacs K, Horvath E, Thorner MO. Human prolactin-producing adenomas and bromocriptine: a histological, immunocytochemical, ultrastructural and morphometric study. J Clin Endocrinol Metab 1982;55:1178–83.

34. White MC, Anapliotou M, Rosenstock J, et al. Heterogeneity of prolactin responses to oestradiol benzoate in women with prolactinomas. Lancet 1981;1:1394–96.

Hereditary and Developmental Disorders

35. Aarskog D, Eiken HG, Bjerknes R, Myking OL. Pituitary dwarfism in the R271W Pit-1 gene mutation. Eur J Pediatr 1997;156:829–34.

36. Bergeron C, Kovacs K, Bilbao JM. Primary empty sella: a histologic and immunocytologic study. Arch Intern Med 1979;139:248–9.

37. Brewer D. Congenital absence of the pituitary gland and its consequences. J Pathol Bacteriol 1957;73:59–67.

38. Drolet DW, Scully KM, Simmons DM, et al. TEF, a transcription factor expressed specifically in the anterior pituitary during embryogenesis, defines a new class of leucine zipper proteins. Genes Dev 1991;5:1739–53

39. Kosaki K, Matsuo N, Tamai S, et al. Isolated aplasia of the anterior pituitary as a cause of congenital panhypopituitarism: case report. Horm Res 1991;35:226–8.

40. Kovacs K, Giannini C, Scheithauer BW, Stefaneanu L, Lloyd RV, Horvath E. Pituitary change in ataxia-telangiectasia syndrome: an immunocytochemical, in situ hybridization, and DNA cytometric study of three cases. Endocr Pathol 1997;8:195–203.

41. Moncrieff MW, Hill DS, Archer J, Arthur LJ. Congenital absence of pituitary gland and adrenal hypoplasia. Arch Dis Child 1972;47:136–7.

42. Mosier HD. Hypoplasia of the pituitary and adrenal cortex. Report of occurance in twin siblings and autopsy findings. J Pediatr 1956;48:633–9.

43. Osamura RY. Functional prenatal development of anencephalic and normal anterior pituitary glands. In human and experimental animals studied by peroxidase-labeled antibody method. Acta Pathol Jpn 1977;27:495–509.

44. Radovick S, Nations M, Du Y, et al. A mutation in the POU-homeodomain of Pit-1 responsible for combined pituitary hormone deficiency. Science 1992;257:1115–8.

45. Reid JD. Congenital absence of the pituitary gland. J Pediatr 1960;56:658–64.

46. Salazar H, MacAulay MA, Charles D, Pardo M. The human hypophysis in anencephaly. I. Ultrastructure of the pars distalis. Arch Pathol 1969;87:201–11.

47. Steiner MM, Boggs JD. Absence of pituitary gland, hypothyroidism, hypoadrenalism, and hypogonadism in a 17-year-old dwarf. J Clin Endocrinol Metab 1965;25:1591–8.

48. Tatsumi K, Miyai K, Notomi T, et al. Cretinism with combined hormone deficiency caused by a mutation in the Pit-1 gene. Nature Genet 1992;1:56–8.

49. Vnencak-Jones CL, Phillips JA III, Chen EY, Seeburg PH. Molecular basis of human growth hormone gene deletions. Proc Natl Acad Sci USA 1988;85:5615–9.

Circulatory Disorders

50. Clayton PE, Shalet SM. Dose dependency of time of onset of radiation-induced growth hormone deficiency. J Pediatr 1991;119:502–3.

51. Constine LS, Woolf PD, Cann D, et al. Hypothalamic pituitary dysfunction after radiation for brain tumors. N Engl J Med 1993;328:87–94.

52. Dugger GS, Van Wyk JJ, Newsome JF. The effect of pituitary-stalk section on thyroid function and gonadotropic-hormone excretion in women with mammary carcinoma. J Neurosurg 1962;19:589–93.

53. Horvath E, Kovacs K. Pathology of the pituitary gland. In: Ezrin C, Horvath E, Kaufman B, et al, eds. Pituitary diseases. Boca Raton, FL: CRC Press, 1980:1–83.

54. Kovacs K. Adenohypophysial necrosis in routine autopsies. Endokrinologie 1972;60:309–16.

55. Kovacs K. Necrosis of anterior pituitary in humans. Neuroendocrinology 1969;4:170–99.

56. Littley MD, Shalet SM, Beardwell CG, et al. Radiation-induced hypopituitarism is dose-dependent. Clin Endocrinol 1989;31:363–73.

57. McCormick WF, Halmi NS. The hypophysis in patients with coma depasse ("respirator brain"). Am J Clin Pathol 1970;54:374–83.

58. Oo MM, Krishna AY, Bonavita GJ, Rutecki GW. Heparin therapy for myocardial infarction: an unusual trigger for pituitary apoplexy. Am J Med Sci 1997;314:351–3.

59. Plaut A. Pituitary necrosis in routine necropsies. Am J Pathol 1952;28:883–99.

60. Sheehan HL. Postpartum necrosis of the anterior pituitary. J Pathol Bacteriol 1937;45:189–214.

61. Tun-Pe, Phillips RE, Warrell DA, et al. Acute and chronic pituitary failure resembling Sheehan's syndrome following bites by Russell's viper in Burma. Lancet 1987;2:763–7.

62. Wakai S, Fukushima T, Teramoto A, Sano K. Pituitary apoplexy: its incidence and clinical significance. J Neurosurg 1981;55:187–93.

Metabolic Disorders

63. Bergeron C, Kovacs K. Pituitary siderosis: a histologic, immunocytologic, and ultrastructural study. Am J Pathol 1978;93:295–309.

64. Bilbao JM, Kovacs K, Horvath E. Pituitary melanocorticotrophinoma with amyloid deposition. Can J Neurol Sci 1975;2:199–202.

65. Landolt AM, Kleihues P, Heitz PU. Amyloid deposits in pituitary adenomas: differentaition of two types. Arch Pathol Lab Med 1987;111:453–8.

66. Rocken C, Paris D, Steusloff K, Saeger W. Investigation of the presence of apolipoprotein E, glycosaminoglycans, basement membrane proteins, and protease inhibitors in senile interstitial amyloid of the pituitary. Endocr Pathol 1997;8:205–14.

67. Rocken C, Saeger W. Amyloid deposits of the pituitary in old age: correlation with histopathological alterations. Endocr Pathol 1994;5:183–90.

68. Rocken C, Uhlig H, Saeger W, Linke RP, Fehr S. Amyloid deposits in pituitaries and pituitary adenomas: immunohistochemistry and in situ hybridization. Endocr Pathol 1995;6:135–43.

69. Schochet SS Jr, McCormick WF, Halmi NS. Pituitary gland in patients with Hurler syndrome: light and electron microscopic study. Arch Pathol 1974;97:96–9.

70. Tan SY, Pepys MB. Amyloidosis. Histopathology 1994;25:403–14.

71. Tashima T, Kitamoto T, Tateishi J, Ogomori K, Nakagaki H. Incidence and characterization of age related amyloid deposits in the human anterior pituitary gland. Virchows Arch [A] 1988; 412:323–7.

Infectious Diseases

72. Domingue JN, Wilson CB. Pituitary abscesses. Report of seven cases and review of the literature. J Neurosurg 1977;46:601–8.

73. Doniach I. Histopathology of the pituitary. Clin Endocrinol Metab 1985;14:765–89.

74. Obenchain TG, Becker DP. Abscess formation in a Rathke's cleft cyst: case report. J Neurosurg 1972; 36:359–62.

75. Oelbaum MH. Hypopituitarism in male subjects due to syphilis. Q J Med 1952;21:249–66.

76. Rickards AG, Harvey PW. "Giant cell granuloma" and the other pituitary granulomata. Q J Med 1954;23:425–40.

77. Vesely DL, Maldonodo A, Levey GS. Partial hypopituitarism and possible hypothalamic involvement in sarcoidosis. Report of a case and review of the literature. Am J Med 1977;62:425–31.

Langerhans' Cell Histiocytosis

78. Favara BE. Langerhans' cell histiocytosis pathobiology and pathogensis. Semin Oncol 1991;18:3–7.

79. Willman CL, Busque L, Griffith BB, et al. Langerhans' cell histiocytosis (histiocytosis X)—a clonal proliferative disease. N Engl J Med 1994;331:154–60.

Autoimmune Diseases

80. Asa SL, Bilbao JM, Kovacs K, Josse RG, Kreines K. Lymphocytic hypophysitis of pregnancy resulting in hypopituitarism: a distinct clinicopathologic entity. Ann Intern Med 1981;95:166–71.

81. Beressi N, Cohen R, Beressi JP, et al. Pseudotumoral lymphocytic hypophysitis successfully treated by corticosteroid alone: first case report. Neurosurgery 1994;35:505–8.

82. Eisenbarth GS, Verge CF. Immunoendocrinopathy syndromes. In: Wilson JD, Foster DW, eds. Williams textbook of endocrinology, 9th ed. Philadelphia: WB Saunders, 1998:1651–62.

83. Folkerth RD, Price DL Jr, Schwartz M, Black PM, DeGirolami V. Xanthomatous hypophysitis. Am J Surg Pathol 1998;22:736–41.

84. Goudie RB, Pinkerton PH. Anterior hypophysitis and Hashimoto's disease in a young woman. J Path Bact 1962;83:584–5.

85. Hashimoto K, Takao T, Makino S. Lymphocytic adenohypophysitis and lymphocytic infundibuloneurohypophysitis. Endocr J 1997;44:1–10.

86. Imura H, Nakao K, Shimatsu A, et al. Lymphocytic infundibuloneurohypophysitis as a cause of central diabetes insipidus. N Engl J Med 1993;329:683–9.

87. Jensen MD, Handwerger BS, Scheithauer BW, Carpenter PC, Mirakian R, Banks PM. Lymphocytic hypophysitis with isolated corticotropin deficiency. Ann Intern Med 1986;105:200–3.

88. Karlsson FA, Kämpe O, Winqvist O, Burman P. Autoimmune disease of the adrenal cortex, pituitary, parathyroid glands and gastric mucosa. J Int Med 1993;234:379–86.

89. Komatsu M, Kondo T, Yamauchi K, et al. Antipituitary antibodies in patients with primary empty sella syndrome. J Clin Endocrinol Metab 1988;67:633–8.

90. Lee JH, Laws ER Jr, Guthrie BL, Dina TS, Nochomovitz LE. Lympocytic hypophysitis: occurrence in two men. Neurosurgery 1994;34:159–63.

91. Meichner RH, Riggio S, Manz HJ, Earll JM. Lymphocytic adenohypophysitis causing pituitary mass. Neurology 1987;37:158–61.

92. Pouplard A. Pituitary autoimmunity. Horm Res 1982;16:289–97.

93. Sautner D, Saeger W, Ludecke DK, Jansen V, Puchner MJ. Hypophysitis in surgical and autopsy specimens. Acta Neuropathologica 1995; 90:637–44.

94. Thodou E, Asa SL, Kontogeorgos G, Kovacs K, Horvath E, Ezzat S. Clinical case seminar. Lymphocytic hypophysitis: clinicopathological findings. J Clinical Endocrinol Metab 1995;80:2302–11.

Pituitary Cysts

95. Klonoff DC, Kahn DG, Rosenzweig W, Wilson CB. Hyperprolactinemia in a patient with a pituitary and an ovarian dermoid tumor: case report. Neurosurgery 1990;26:335–9.

96. Kucharczyk W, Peck WW, Kelly WM, Norman D, Newton TH. Rathke cleft cysts: CT, MR imaging, and pathologic features. Radiology 1987;165:491–5.

97. Lee BC, Deck MD. Sellar and juxtasellar lesions detection with MRI. Radiology 1985;157:143–7.

98. Matsushima T, Fukui M, Fujii K. Epithelial cells in symptomatic Rathke's cleft cysts. A light- and electron-microscopic study. Surg Neurol 1988;30:197–203.

99. Mukherjee JJ, Islam N, Kaltsas G, et al. Clinical, radiological and pathological features of patients with Rathke's cleft cysts and tumors that may recur. J Clin Endocrinol Metab 1997; 82:2357–62.

100. Ross DA, Norman D, Wilson CB. Radiologic characteristics and results of surgical management of Rathke's cysts in 43 patients. Neurosurgery 1992;30:173–8.

101. Steinberg GK, Koenig GH, Golden JB. Symptomatic Rathke's cleft cysts: report of two cases. J Neurosurg 1982;56:290–5.

102. Weber EL, Vogel FS, Odom GL. Cysts of the sella turcica. J Neurosurg 1970;33:48–53.

103. Yoshida J, Kobayashi T, Kageyama N, Kanzaki M. Symptomatic Rathke's cleft cyst: morphological study with light and electron microscopy and tissue culture. J Neurosurg 1977;47: 451–8.

Hyperplasia

104. Asa SL, Kovacs K, Tindall GT, Barrow DL, Horvath E, Vecsei P. Cushing's disease associated with an intrasellar gangliocytoma producing corticotrophin-releasing factor. Ann Intern Med 1984;101:789–93.

105. Crooke AC, Russell DS. The pituitary gland in Addison's disease. J Pathol Bacteriol 1935;40: 255–83.

106. Garcia-Luna PP, Leal-Cerro A, Montero C, et al. A rare cause of acromegaly: ectopic production of growth hormone-releasing factor by a bronchial carcinoid tumor. Surg Neurol 1987;27:563–8.

107. Horvath E, Kovacs K. Ultrastructural diagnosis of pituitary adenomas and hyperplasias. In Lloyd RV, ed. Surgical pathology of the pituitary gland. Philadelphia: WB Saunders, 1993:52–84.

108. Kovacs K, Ilse G, Ryan N, et al. Pituitary prolactin cell hyperplasia. Horm Res 1980;12:87–95.

109. Lloyd RV, Chandler WF, McKeever PE, Schteingart DE. The spectrum of ACTH-producing pituitary lesions. Am J Surg Pathol 1986; 10:618–26.

110. McKeever PE, Koppelman MC, Metcalf D, et al. Refractory Cushing's disease caused by multinodular, ACTH-cell hyperplasia. J Neuropathol Exp Neurol 1982;41:490–9.

111. Pioro EP, Scheithauer BW, Laws ER Jr, Randall RV, Kovacs KT, Horvath E. Combined thyrotroph and lactotroph cell hyperplasia simulating prolactin-secreting pituitary adenoma in longstanding primary hypothyroidism. Surg Neurol 1988;29:218–26.

112. Saeger W, Ludecke DK. Pituitary hyperplasia. Definition, light and electron microscopical structures and significance in surgical specimens. Virchows Arch [A] 1983;399:277–87.

113. Scheithauer BW, Kovacs K, Randall RV. The pituitary gland in untreated Addison's disease. A histologic and immunocytologic study of 18 adenohypophyses. Arch Pathol Lab Med 1983; 107:484–7.

114. Scheithauer BW, Kovacs K, Randall RV, Horvath E, Okazaki H, Laws ER Jr. Hypothalamic neuronal hamartoma and adenohypophyseal neuronal choristoma: their association with growth hormone adenoma of the pituitary gland. J Neuropathol Exp Neurol 1983;42:648–63.

115. Scheithauer BW, Kovacs K, Randall RV, Ryan N. Pituitary gland in hypothyroidism. Histologic and immunocytologic study. Arch Pathol Lab Med 1985;109:499–504.

116. Thorner MO, Perryman RL, Cronin MJ, et al. Somatotroph hyperplasia. Successful treatment of acromegaly by removal of a pancreatic islet tumor secreting a growth hormone-releasing factor. J Clin Invest 1982;70:965–77.

117. Zimmerman D, Young WF Jr, Ebersold MJ, et al. Congenital gigantism due to growth hormone releasing hormone (GRH) excess and pituitary hyperplasia with adenomatous transformation. J Clin Endocrinol Metab 1993;76:216–22.

2
PARATHYROID GLAND

NORMAL PARATHYROID GLAND

Embryology

The parathyroid glands are derived from branchial pouches III and IV, and can be recognized in the developing fetus around 5 to 6 weeks of development (41). They arise as diverticula of the pouch endoderm. Parathyroid III is derived from proliferations along the anterodorsal surface of pouch III and parathyroid IV is derived from the lateral portion of the dorsal extremity of pouch IV. Parathyroid III separates from the pharynx at the 18 mm stage of development when it is at the end of the lower pole of the thyroid gland. If parathyroid III does not separate from the thymus, which also forms from the third pouch, the gland is found within the thymic tongue in the lower neck, anterior mediastinum, or posterior mediastinum in adults. If parathyroid III separates from the thymus early, it may be localized cephalad to parathyroid IV and to the thyroid gland. Thus, there is some variation in the final location of parathyroid III depending on the level at which the separation occurs. Parathyroid III or remnants of this gland may be localized along the entire line of migration from the angle of the jaw to the pericardium (41).

Parathyroid IV, together with the ultimobranchial bodies, develops from the fourth branchial pouch. It acquires its adult position as an upper gland near the intersection of the recurrent laryngeal nerve and the medial thyroid artery. Because of its shorter migration path, parathyroid IV has a more constant location and is usually cephalad to parathyroid III.

Anatomy

The parathyroid glands are 4 to 6 mm in length, 2 to 4 mm in width, and 1 to 2 mm in thickness (fig. 2-1). They vary from yellow to tan depending on the percentage of stromal fat, oxyphil cells, and vascularity. They are ovoid or bean-shaped structures, but some glands may be elongated, bilobed, or multilobed. There is a dimorphic variation in gland weight, with the overall combined weight of 142 ± 5.2 mg in fe-

males and 120 ± 3.5 mg in males (15); the maximum total glandular weight should be 208 mg at the 95 percentile. Grimelius et al. (17) reported that the mean glandular weight was 32 mg with an upper limit of 59 mg in a large series of autopsy cases. Others (12) have noted that in hospitalized patients the mean weight of the glands was 46.2 mg compared to a lower weight (39.5 mg) in patients who died suddenly. The upper limit of gland weight was 73.1 mg for healthy white subjects and 91.6 mg for healthy black subjects (12), indicating the wide variation in parathyroid weight that may be encountered. In general, if a parathyroid gland weighs more than 40 mg it should be considered abnormal (8). The lower parathyroid glands are generally larger than the upper glands (12,17).

The parenchymal cell mass of the parathyroid gland is quite variable in cell number. It averages 74 percent of the adult gland weight, depending on the sex of the person, with an average parenchymal weight per gland of 21.6 mg and 18.2 mg for men and women, respectively (1,3,17,27). The mean total parenchymal weight for glands in women is greater (88.9 ± 3.9 mg) than men (82.0 ± 2.6 mg) (14). Total

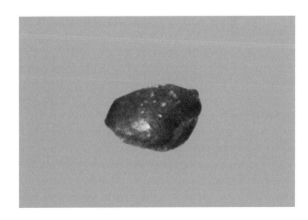

Figure 2-1

NORMAL PARATHYROID GLAND

Gross photograph of normal right superior parathyroid gland. The normal gland is 4 to 6 mm in length and weighs between 20 and 40 mg.

parenchymal weight is inversely related to serum calcium concentration in patients with secondary hyperparathyroidism and a direct relationship has been reported between gland weight, serum phosphorous concentration, and renal function when expressed relative to blood urea nitrogen in patients with secondary hyperparathyroidism (3,9).

The location of parathyroid III (inferior parathyroid gland) can be quite variable. The more common locations are inferior, posterior, or lateral to the lower pole of the thyroid gland and less commonly, high on the anterior aspect of the thyroid lobe (3). It may also be located in the lower thymus, anterior mediastinum below the thymus, and posterior mediastinum. In all of the aberrant locations and in the neck the glands are consistently bilaterally symmetrical.

In contrast to parathyroid III, parathyroid IV or the superior parathyroid gland is almost always present in the same anatomic location, approximately 1 cm above the intersection of the recurrent laryngeal nerve and the inferior thyroid artery. The superior parathyroid may on occasion be present in the thyroid capsule or within the thyroid parenchyma (3), and rarely, in the retropharyngeal and retroesophageal spaces. The variable location of the superior parathyroid should prompt the surgeon to perform a meticulous search for this gland in other locations if not readily localized in the region of the recurrent laryngeal nerve and inferior thyroid artery.

The superior thyroid artery is the main arterial supply of the superior parathyroid gland while the inferior thyroid artery supplies the inferior parathyroid gland. As with the aberrant location of the glands, the arterial supplies can be quite variable (9). Drainage of the superior parathyroid is via the superior or lateral thyroid vein and drainage of the inferior parathyroid occurs via the lateral or inferior thyroid vein. The lymphatic drainage of the parathyroid glands originates from a subcapsular plexus of the superior deep cervical, pretracheal, paratracheal, retropharyngeal, and inferior deep cervical nodes.

Supernumerary parathyroid glands, i.e., more than four glands located apart from the other glands and weighing more than 5 mg (18), are present in 2.0 to 6.5 percent of the population. The most frequent number of supernumerary glands is 5, although 6 to 12 glands have been noted in some patients (9). The supernumerary glands are most frequently located in the thymus, associated with the thyrothymic ligament, and are related to the migration of the inferior parathyroid glands (1), but they may be present in other locations as well. In a recent study of 32 children in the first years of life, 6 percent had supernumerary glands in the vagus nerve (6). Parathyroid tissues have been reported in very unusual locations such as the vaginal wall, in association with thyroid tissues and without evidence of teratomatous development (24).

The fibrous tissues of the parathyroid glands contain a vascular pole with an artery and a vein which branch into smaller vessels. The capsular arteries and veins are connected by arterioles, capillaries, and venules that are present in the fibrous septa between the parenchymal cells. The capillary network abuts on every parenchymal cell. As with other endocrine cells, the capillary endothelial lining cells have pores or fenestrations (34). The parathyroid gland is surrounded by two interconnecting plexuses of lymphatic capillaries which are located in the capsule. The loops of the lymphatic vessels dip into the gland from the inner plexus and the efferent lymphatic vessels arise from the outer plexus by special lymphatics or from those of the thyroid gland.

Nerve bundles are in close proximity to the parenchymal cells, indicating autonomic innervation (38). In other mammals that have been studied in some detail the nerves have been shown to originate from the medulla, the dorsal nucleus of the vagus nerve, and the vagus nerve itself (25).

Histology

The parenchymal elements of the parathyroid gland include chief cells, oncocytic cells, and transitional oncocytic cells which are arranged in a lobular pattern that is more prominent in adults (14). Each parenchymal cell is separated from the adjacent stroma by a prominent basement membrane. In infants and young children, chief cells are predominantly present (30). The chief cells of newborns and infants measure 6 to 8 μm in diameter, smaller than in adults. The membrane of the chief cell is poorly delineated in neonates and the cytoplasm is amphophilic with a lower content of intracellular fat compared to adults. About 30 to 40 percent of the chief cells of children contain large intracellular fat droplets (8,33). The chief cell nuclei in children often overlap, are centrally located, and have nucleoli.

In adults, the chief cells are 8 to 10 μm in diameter, and have round, centrally placed nuclei with course chromatin (fig. 2-2). Unlike children, those of adults have well-defined cytoplasmic as well as nuclear membranes. Mitotic figures are extremely uncommon in the normal adult parathyroid gland. The cytoplasm of the chief cells is amphophilic to slightly eosinophilic, with a vacuolated appearance due to intracytoplasmic glycogen and variable amounts of neutral lipid. In contrast to children, more than 80 percent of the chief cells in the normal adult gland contain large cytoplasmic fat droplets which can be readily visualized on frozen section with oil red O or azure A and Erie garnet B stains (35).

One variant of chief cells contains clear cytoplasm and must be distinguished from the Wasserhelle cells present in clear cell hyperplasia and rarely in clear cell adenoma. The Wasserhelle cells contain cytoplasmic vacuoles that are readily appreciated on ultrastructural studies, instead of the lipid and glycogen present in the clear cell variant of chief cells. Some parathyroid glands may contain chief cells that form acinar structures or larger glandular structures with eosinophilic periodic acid–Schiff (PAS)-positive material reminiscent of colloid material with thyroglobulin in the thyroid. The material may be congophilic and show the apple core birefringence characteristic of amyloid (17). It may be difficult to distinguish parathyroid tissue with abundant acinar formation and eosinophilic material in the central lumen from thyroid tissue without performing special stains (fig. 2-3). The presence of calcium oxalate crystals in the eosinophilic protein indicates thyroid tissue. If oxalate crystals are not present, stains for thyroglobulin and parathyroid hormone should readily resolve the question.

Oncocytic or oxyphilic cells are larger than chief cells, and range from 12 to 20 μm in diameter. They have granular eosinophilic cytoplasm with round to oval nuclei. These cells contain abundant mitochondria and high levels of oxidative enzymes. Oncocytic cells are not usually present in children, but appear around puberty and increase in number with age. In some cases of parathyroid hyperplasia, oncocytic cells become very prominent, forming clusters and nodules. It may be difficult to distinguish between oncocytic hyperplastic nodules and adenomas. Variants of oncocytic cells include the transitional oncocytic cells which are smaller and contain less eosinophilic cytoplasm than the mature oncocytic cells.

The interstitium of the parathyroid gland contains small amounts of collagen, capillaries, lymphatics, fibroblasts, pericytes, mast cells, and occasional lymphocytes. The amount of collagen increases with age: it is sparse in children, but in adults it gives the gland a lobulated appearance. Fat cells are sparse in the gland stroma in infants and children. They begin to appear just before puberty and increase in amount throughout life, reaching a maximum in the third to fifth decades. The amount of stromal fat is also determined by constitutional factors in adults.

The amount of stromal fat in the parathyroid gland of adults is probably less than the 50 percent reported in earlier studies (1,2,8, 10,13). Morphometric analyses have shown that most glands have less than 20 percent stromal fat while only about 9 percent of glands have more than 40 percent. In one study the average fat content of the parathyroid was 17 percent (10). Most studies show that fat is distributed unevenly in the gland, with the poles containing more fat than the central regions. Thus, if the location of a parathyroid biopsy is not known, an erroneous estimate of the fat: parenchyma cell ratio may result from a limited microscopic examination. Some investigations have utilized density measurements to estimate the parenchymal cell weight (9). An isometric gradient media such as Percoll or bovine serum albumin combined with the total weight of the gland is used to calculate the parenchymal cell weight of each parathyroid gland.

There are constitutional factors that cause variations in the amount of stromal fat. The nutritional state of the patient, genetic factors, chronic illness, and malignant diseases can affect the amount of parathyroid stromal fat; in addition, women have a higher percentage than men.

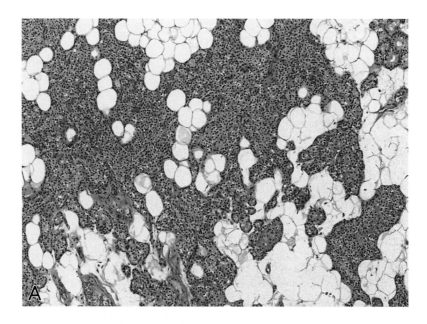

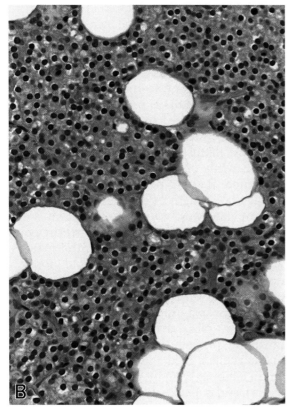

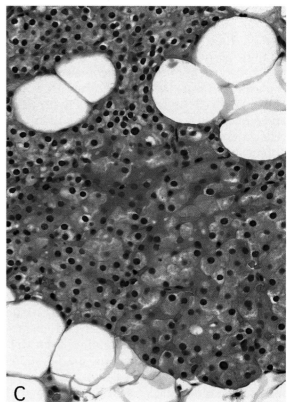

Figure 2-2

NORMAL PARATHYROID GLAND

Histologic views of normal parathyroid gland.
A: The low magnification shows the abundant stromal fat.
B: Higher magnification shows predominantly chief cells.
C: An oncocytic nodule with oncocytes and transitional oncocytes is present.

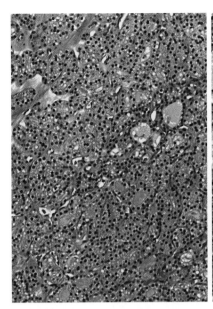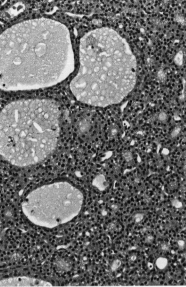

Figure 2-3

COMPARISON OF PARATHYROID AND THYROID GLANDS

Comparison of parathyroid (right) and thyroid cells from a hyperplastic nodule. It may be difficult to separate these two tissues without special stains, but the presence of calcium oxalate crystals helps to confirm thyroid tissue.

Histochemistry

Histochemical studies of parathyroid tissues often reveal moderate amounts of glycogen, which is readily demonstrated by PAS stain, with and without diastase digestion. Parathyroid chief cells often contain abundant intracytoplasmic neutral lipid droplets that can be rapidly demonstrated with the Azure B, Erie Garnet A procedure or with oil red O or Sudan IV stains (figs. 2-4, 2-5) (4,23,33,35,37). These latter stains require more time for completion. While the chief cells of normal parathyroid glands contain abundant lipid and moderate amounts of glycogen, the larger oncocytic cells have very little intracytoplasmic lipid or glycogen and abundant mitochondria.

Immunohistochemistry

Immunohistochemical studies can help to distinguish between parathyroid and thyroid or other endocrine tissues in difficult cases (Table 2-1). Low molecular weight keratins, keratins 8, 18, and 19, are commonly expressed in parathyroid tissues (28). Stains for high molecular weight keratins or with wide-spectrum keratin antibodies may be falsely negative, so it is important to use antibodies against low molecular weight keratins such as CAM5.2 or AE1 when staining parathyroid tissues (28,36).

Antibodies to parathyroid hormone have produced variable staining results in normal and

Table 2-1

IMMUNOHISTOCHEMICAL MARKERS FOR PARATHYROID CELLS

Parathyroid hormone	Neural cell adhesion molecules (NCAM) (CD56)
Chromogranin A	Proliferating cell nuclear antigen (PCNA)
Keratin-low molecular weight[a]	Parathyroid hormone–related peptide
Synaptophysin	Calcitonin
Ki67(MIB-1)	Calcitonin gene–related peptide

[a]For example, CAM5.2, AE1.

abnormal parathyroid tissues in the past. Various monoclonal and polyclonal antibodies are available today that produce satisfactory staining of parathyroid tissues (fig. 2-6) (11,43). Staining is consistently stronger in chief cells than oncocytic cells, indicating greater hormone storage in the former.

Broad-spectrum antibodies to neuroendocrine markers such as chromogranin A (also referred to as parathyroid secretory protein) and synaptophysin, are usually positive in parathyroid tissues (16,26,42), so these can also be used to separate parathyroid from thyroid follicular

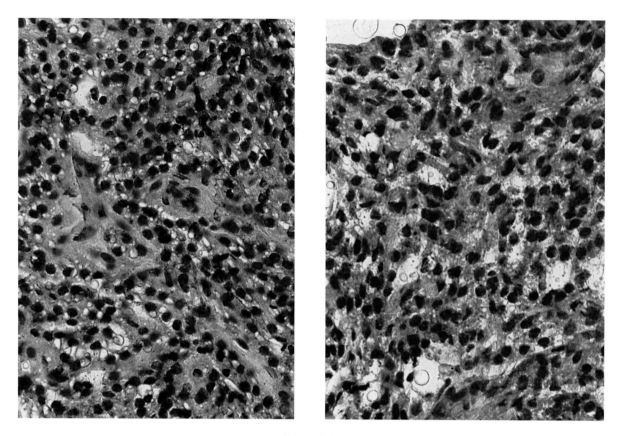

Figure 2-4

LIPID STAIN

Left: Rapid stain for intracellular lipid with azure A/Erie garnet B in normal parathyroid cells shows refractile cytoplasmic droplets.

Right: In contrast, a hyperplastic parathyroid gland has very little cytoplasmic lipid.

Figure 2-5

LIPID STAIN

Oil red O stain detects neutral lipid deposits in a normal parathyroid gland. (Plate IA from Fascicle 6, 3rd Series.)

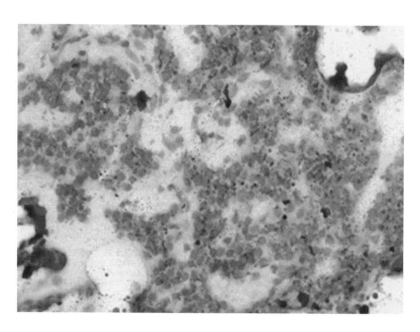

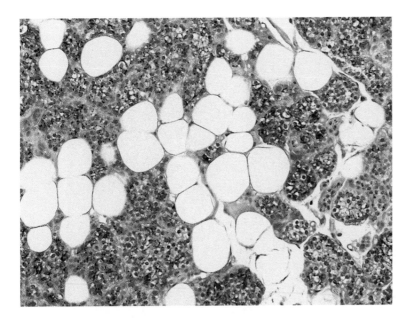

Figure 2-6

PARATHYROID HORMONE
(PTH) IMMUNOSTAIN

Immunohistochemical staining shows variable distribution of PTH immunoreactivity in normal parathyroid gland (diaminobenzidine chromogen).

tissues which are not members of the neuroendocrine system. Calcitonin staining is usually positive in thyroid C cells.

Recent studies have suggested that cytokeratin 14 is very useful and specific for oncocytic cells of the thyroid, and this may also apply to the parathyroid (36). Vimentin stains the stromal cells of the parathyroid gland, but not the parenchymal cells. Other intermediate filaments such as neurofilament have been reported by some investigators in parathyroid tissues (8). Antibodies to a parathyroid cell receptor involved in the sensing and gating of calcium have been developed (20,21). These antibodies react with chief cells to stain normal cells and cells in adenomas and hyperplasias with varying degrees of intensity; metastatic parathyroid carcinomas also stain.

In Situ Hybridization

In situ hybridization has been used to analyze parathyroid hormone gene expression. In one of the early studies, Stork et al. (39) studied the expression of preproparathyroid hormone messenger RNA in frozen and paraffin-embedded tissue sections. A strong hybridization signal for the gene product was present in some parathyroid cells including chief and transitional oncocytic cells while the oxyphil cells had a weaker signal (39). Similar findings were reported by Kendall et al. (22) with nonisotopic-labeled probes using digoxigenin as a reporter system.

Flow Cytometry

Flow cytometry has been used in the study of normal and abnormal parathyroid gland tissues (19). Earlier studies used fresh tissues in which the cell nuclei were stained with propidium iodide, but subsequent studies have used paraffin-embedded tissues for analysis, which is easier for most histopathologic retrospective studies (9). An early study of normal, hyperplastic, and adenomatous parathyroid tissue by Irvin and Bagwell (19) showed that flow cytometric analysis could distinguish between these conditions, although there was some overlap. A recent study of normal, hyperplastic, and adenomatous parathyroid tissue with DNA index and ploidy analyses showed that these parameters distinguished the normal from the abnormal glands (7).

Ultrastructure

The parathyroid glands have ultrastructural features that are similar to those of other endocrine glands (29,32). The chief cells are arranged in cords and nests, and are separated from the interstitium by basal lamina (fig. 2-7). The capillaries are lined by fenestrated endothelial cells (34,40). The functional activity of the parenchyma cells is associated with changes in the ultrastructural features. The chief cells have straight plasma membranes and are attached to other cells by desmosomes. With increased functional activity there is increased tortuosity

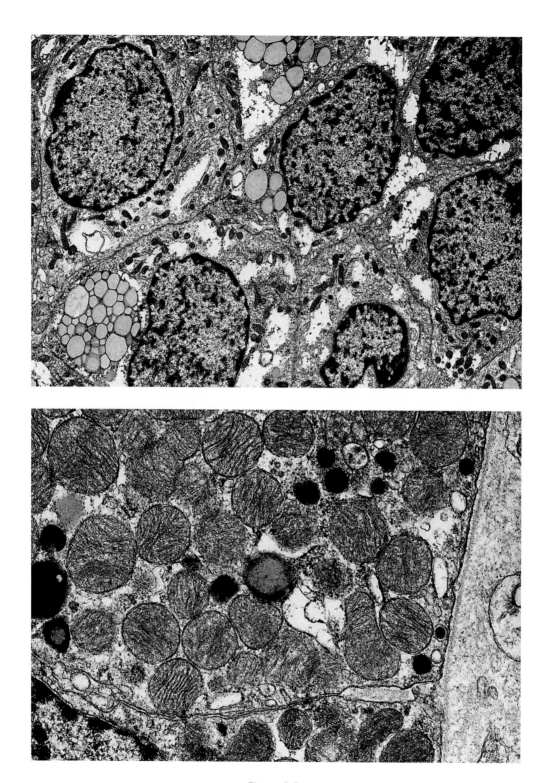

Figure 2-7

NORMAL PARATHYROID ULTRASTRUCTURE

Top: Normal parathyroid gland shows cells with round to oval nuclei, abundant intracellular cytoplasmic lipid, and occasional dense core secretory granules (X3,800).

Bottom: Oxyphil cells in the parathyroid gland have abundant cytoplasmic mitochondria (X13,000).

of the plasma membranes. Chief cells have moderate numbers of mitochondria, while oxyphil cells have abundant mitochondria that occupy most of the cytoplasm. Mitochondria in oxyphil cells are usually larger than those in chief cells.

The secretory granules in chief cells measure from 50 to 300 nm in diameter. They are round with dense core materials and have a limiting membrane with a slight lucent space. The mature secretory granules are generally more dense than the immature presecretory granules. A few secretory granules may be pleomorphic, ranging from oval to dumbbell in shape. Lysosomes are generally slightly larger than the secretory granules and are usually more pleomorphic.

Parathyroid chief cells contain abundant glycogen and lipid during the resting phase. Lipid droplets vary from 1 to 5 μm in diameter; the larger droplets are formed by aggregates of smaller droplets. During the active synthetic phase the chief cells contain less glycogen and lipid.

Oncocytic cells have smaller amounts of, and smaller sized, lipid droplets. In transitional oncocytic cells, the number of cytoplasmic mitochondria range between those in chief and in oncocytic cells. These transitional cells also have fewer secretory granules than the chief cells.

Chief cells in the active synthetic phase have a well-formed endoplasmic reticulum that forms multiple parallel stacks and prominent Golgi regions (33,34). In contrast, nesting phase chief cells have a less well-developed endoplasmic reticulum. Both oncocytic and transitional oncocytic cells have less well-developed endoplasmic reticulum and Golgi regions.

Molecular Biology and Physiology

Parathyroid hormone (PTH) is composed of 84 amino acids and has a molecular size of 9.5 kd (5,32). The PTH gene is located on chromosome 11p15 and is 4,200 base pairs in length (5). It has a 51 noncoding domain, a prepro sequence domain, and a domain containing the PTH sequence and the 31 noncoding region (5).

PTH is synthesized as a precursor molecule, preproparathyroid hormone, which is composed of 115 amino acids. It is subsequently processed in the endoplasmic reticulum where the first 25 N-terminal amino acids are clipped off to produce proparathyroid hormone. The 90 amino acid polypeptide is then processed in the Golgi complex by further cleavage of a hexapeptide at the N-terminal end of the molecule where it is converted to the active polypeptide. PTH is stored in secretory granules in association with members of the chromogranin/secretogranin family of polypeptides (6,7). The principal storage protein is chromogranin A which is present in the secretory granules of the parathyroid chief cells (42). Secretion of PTH is also associated with chromogranin A and the serum levels of chromogranin A are increased in parathyroid hyperplasia and adenomas.

PTH is degraded in the liver and kidney and breaks down to N- and C-terminal fragments. Immunoassays are used to measure these fragments. The biologically active site of the molecule is at the C terminus, so immunoassay measurement of this fragment more readily correlates with biologic activity than measurement of the N-terminal fragment.

The NH_2 terminal of the PTH molecule is essential for binding to its receptor, activation of adenyl cyclase, and biologic activity. Removal of a single NH_2-terminal amino acid leads to more than a 90 percent loss of biologic activity, with little loss of immunoreactivity (31).

Parathyroid hormone–related peptide (PTHrP) is a new class of peptide hormone with a marked amino-terminal homology to PTH, sharing eight of the first 13 amino acids. Both PTH and PTHrP bind to a common receptor (5).

The PTH and PTHrP genes probably arose from a common ancestral gene by chromosome duplication. The PTHrP gene is on the short arm of chromosome 12 and spaces more than 15 kb of genomic DNA (5). There are three isoforms of prepro PTHrP which give rise to three translation products of 139, 141, and 173 amino acids. Three major secretory forms of the proteins are present in different tissues. PTHrP is bioactively involved in calcium regulation. The PTH-like action, which is localized at the amino-terminal region, is the best characterized function. PTHrP also functions in epithelial growth and differentiation. PTHrP has a molecular weight of 16,000 to 17,000 daltons. It has been found in a variety of tumors associated with hypercalcemia as well as in normal cells such as keratinocytes, and in parathyroid glands, lactating mammary glands, smooth muscle, and placenta. Different alternatively spliced forms are also present in some of these sites (5).

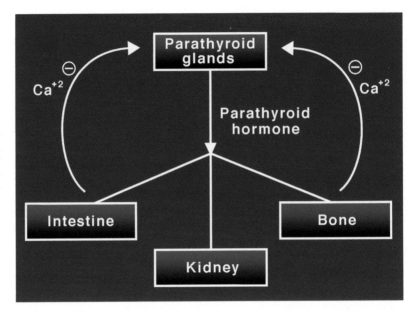

Figure 2-8

FEEDBACK REGULATION OF
PARATHYROID FUNCTION

PTH is secreted by the parathyroid glands. This hormone regulates serum calcium homeostasis at the level of the intestine, kidney, and bone. Serum calcium levels in the blood regulate PTH secretion by a feedback mechanism.

Table 2-2

CAUSES OF HYPERCALCEMIA

Vitamin D intoxication	Aluminum intoxication
Sarcoidosis	Milk-alkali syndrome
Thiazide diuretics	Malignancy[a]
Immobilization	Primary hyperpara-
Vitamin A intoxication	thyroidism[a]
Adrenal insufficiency	Secondary hyperpara-
William's syndrome	thyroidism

[a]These categories account for 90 percent of cases of hypercalcemia.

OVERVIEW OF HYPERCALCEMIA AND HYPOCALCEMIA

Hypercalcemia

The normal level of serum calcium is relatively constant and abnormal levels may be secondary to many etiologies (Table 2-2) (45,47,50). The work-up of patients with hypercalcemia includes performing appropriate tests for PTH and PTHrP in addition to serum calcium. The classic negative feedback mechanism regulates PTH secretion and calcium uptake (fig. 2-8) (45).

Most causes of hypercalcemia are related to primary hyperparathyroidism and malignant diseases, which account for about 90 percent of cases (Table 2-2). The clinical history and physical examination can be very useful in suggesting an etiology for the elevated serum calcium. Chronic symptomatic hypercalcemia is more likely related to primary parathyroid disease, while patients with hypercalcemia secondary to malignancies are often asymptomatic and have hypercalcemia for a much shorter duration in the course of their disease (Table 2-3).

Hyperparathyroidism

Hyperparathyroidism is a disruption in the PTH-serum calcium homeostasis resulting from a metabolic imbalance in which the serum PTH levels are increased (45). The serum calcium level can vary depending on the etiology of the metabolic disturbance (48). Patients with primary hyperparathyroidism usually have increased levels of serum calcium, although in a few conditions the level may be normal. Patients with secondary hyperparathyroidism, such as those with renal failure, usually are hypocalcemic and hyperphosphatemic, and have a compensatory increase in the serum PTH level. Patients with tertiary hyperparathyroidism usually develop an autonomously functioning parathyroid gland after a variable period of secondary hyperparathyroidism. Many forms of hyperparathyroidism have been reported; some of these are familial while others may be associated with specific drugs or disease entities (45,72).

Table 2-3

TUMORS ASSOCIATED WITH HYPERCALCEMIA

Solid Tumors
Breast carcinoma
Squamous cell carcinoma
Renal cell carcinoma
Urogenital tract carcinoma
Ovarian small cell carcinoma

Hematologic Malignancies
Multiple myeloma
Lymphomas

Hypercalcemia represents an imbalance in the flux of calcium in and out of the blood. The skeletal reserves of calcium are fairly large (about 1,000 g), so some calcium may be obtained from the bones in some pathologic conditions in which resorption may exceed formation, resulting in an increase net flow of calcium from bone to blood. Decreased renal calcium excretion and increased intestinal calcium absorption may contribute to increased serum calcium.

The clinical manifestations of hypercalcemia involve a wide variety of organs including the central nervous system with lethargy, confusion, and coma; the gastrointestinal tract with constipation, anorexia, nausea, and vomiting; the cardiovascular system with shortened S-T segment, bradycardia, and first degree heart block; and the renal system with impaired renal function (45). Other manifestations include soft tissue calcification, pruritus, and occasionally, widespread thromboses secondary to the activation of clotting factors by calcium.

Primary Hyperparathyroidism. The incidence of primary hyperparathyroidism has increased over the past 30 years due in part to the use of automated biochemical screening for serum calcium and other substances (62). The incidence of primary hyperparathyroidism between 1965 and 1974 was 7.8/100,000 people while it was 51.1 between 1974 and 1976. In patients under 40 years of age, the incidence was 10/100,000 and in males over 60 years old it was 92; the incidence was even higher in women older than 60 years of age at 188/100,000 (45,50).

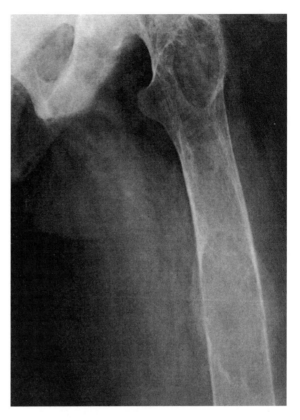

Figure 2-9

OSTEITIS FIBROSA CYSTICA GENERALISTA
This radiograph shows generalized osteopenia and multiple cysts. (Fig. 7 from Fascicle 15, 1st Series.)

The common presentation of patients with primary hyperparathyroidism today is with weakness and lethargy, while historically patients often presented with renal lithiasis or nephrocalcinosis. In large series of patients with primary hyperparathyroidism, hyperplasia accounts for 15 to 20 percent of cases; adenomas, 80 to 85 percent; and carcinomas, 2 to 3 percent (56,73). The neoplastic conditions (adenomas and carcinomas) will not be discussed, except in the differential diagnosis.

Bone Manifestations. The most common bone abnormality seen in patients with hyperparathyroidism is osteopenia (fig. 2-9) (45,50, 56,69). Historically, osteitis fibrosa cystica was a common finding at diagnosis, but is a relatively uncommon manifestation today, probably because of automated biochemical screening and earlier diagnosis.

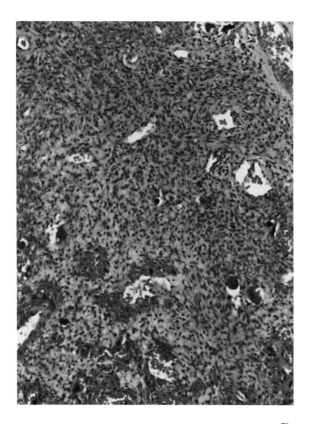 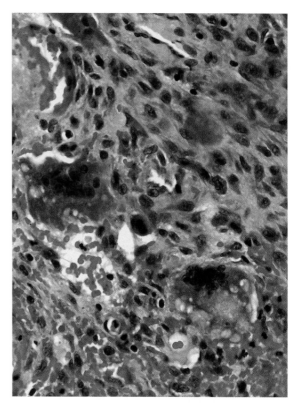

Figure 2-10

BROWN TUMOR OF HYPERPARATHYROIDISM

Left: Low-power view of a brown tumor in a patient with chronic hyperparathyroidism shows multinucleated osteoclasts with a fibrous stroma.

Right: Higher magnification shows the benign appearance of the giant cells. (Courtesy of Dr. K. K. Unni, Rochester, MN.)

In addition to diffuse osteopenia, patients with hyperparathyroidism may also have articular and periarticular problems including chondrocalcinosis, subchondral fractures, juxta-articular erosions, traumatic synovitis, calcific periarteritis, and gout. The bone disease may range from mild diffuse osteopenia to osteitis fibrosa cystica generalisata or von Recklinghausen's disease (51).

Histopathology. Early histologic changes include osteoclastic resorption of endosteal and subperiosteal bone surfaces and replacement of resorbed bone by fibrous connective tissue. A condition known as dissecting osteitis in which the bony trabeculae are cleared out by multinucleated osteoclasts and replaced by fibrous connective tissue occurs. Dissecting osteitis is almost pathognomonic for hyperparathyroidism. Two conditions are commonly associated with chronic longstanding hyperparathyroidism: brown tumors and giant cell reparative granulomas. Brown tumors develop when the bony trabeculae are resorbed and a fibrous response occurs secondarily to microfractures in the partially resorbed bone (fig. 2-10). This is usually associated with ruptured capillaries and bleeding, deposition of hemosiderin, and coalescence of macrophages to form giant cells. Foreign body and osteoclastic giant cells cluster into nodular areas in the sites with abundant deposition of hemosiderin. The histopathologic spectrum of brown tumors can be quite variable. Some areas may show reactive bone with dispersed giant cells, while other areas may contain numerous multinucleated stromal cells and degenerative changes. Giant cell reparative granulomas are similar to brown tumors, but are located in the jaw. In these lesions the giant

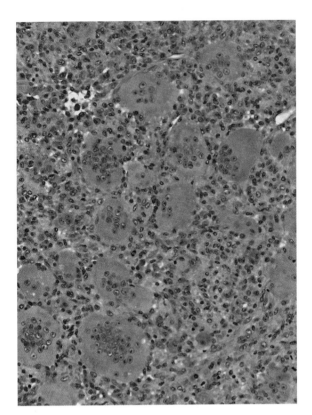 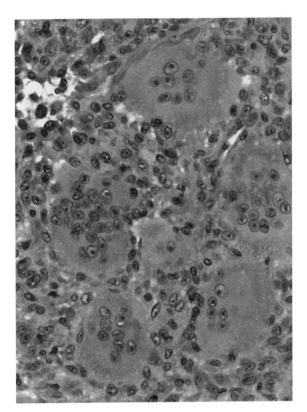

Figure 2-11

GIANT CELL TUMOR OF BONE

Left: In contrast to the brown tumor, the giant cell tumor of bone is made up of neoplastic giant cells with spindle cells in the stroma.

Right: Higher magnification shows the large nuclei and prominent nucleoli of the giant cells. (Courtesy of Dr. K. K. Unni, Rochester, MN.)

cells are more evenly spaced, the stromal cells are more reactive looking, and there is less osteoblastic activity. These lesions should be distinguished from true giant cell tumors of bone (fig. 2-11).

Electron microscopic studies of giant cell reparative granulomas and brown tumors have shown that the giant cells look like inactive osteoclasts. They contain dilated endoplasmic reticulum, few lysosomes, many mitochondria, and variable numbers of Golgi complexes. Short filopodia may be present (51). The giant cells often lack the striking ruffled borders that are commonly seen in active osteoclasts.

Secondary hyperparathyroidism is associated with osteomalacia. The histopathologic features include wider osteoid seams and dissecting osteitis along with increased osteoclastic activity.

Other Conditions Associated with Hyperparathyroidism. Renal stones are often as-sociated with hyperparathyroidism and may be the presenting symptom in some patients. Recurrent nephrolithiasis is seen in a small percentage of patients with primary hyperparathyroidism (45). Other manifestations of renal disease include increased urine creatinine and blood urea nitrogen, a decreased glomerular filtration rate, and tubular diseases including aminoaciduria and glycosuria.

There may be evidence of neuromuscular difficulties including weakness, fatigability, and psychiatric manifestations such as depression, psychomotor retardation, and personality changes. Severe hyperparathyroidism may rarely lead to coma and death if the condition is not ameliorated.

Gastrointestinal manifestations associated with hyperparathyroidism include peptic ulceration, acute and chronic pancreatitis with pancreatic calcification, vomiting, and constipation.

Deposits of calcium may occur in the conjunctiva resulting in band keratopathy and conjunctivitis (45).

Laboratory Diagnosis. Primary hyperparathyroidism results from excessive production of PTH in the absence of an appropriate physiological stimulus (45). The serum calcium concentration is elevated and the serum phosphorus concentration is decreased. Serum measurement of PTH levels can be problematic due to the heterogeneity of circulating hormone (61,67,68). PTH is cleaved at position 34 in the liver to produce an amino-terminal molecule that has a great deal of biologic activity and a short half-life. In contrast, the carboxyl-terminal fragment has less biologic potency but a longer half-life. In healthy individuals with normal renal function, the intact PTH molecule is made up mainly of PTH-like bioactivity; in patients in chronic renal failure, the amino-terminal fragment makes up to 60 percent of the biologic activity.

Immunoassays for PTH utilize various antisera (49,50). Assays with antibodies that recognize the amino portion of the molecule in contrast to the carboxyl-terminal can give discrepant results. The newer assays recognize intact PTH. Assays using the sandwich technique use one antibody to extract peptides at the amino-terminal with an N-terminal antibody. This is followed by a second antibody which recognizes the midportion of the molecule. The assay becomes highly specific by measuring an N-terminal fragment attached to an intact midportion of the molecule.

Measurement of ionized serum calcium levels provides the most useful information about the parathyroid gland and calcium homeostasis. The regulated component of serum calcium is the portion that is not bound to plasma proteins. Thus, total serum calcium should be normalized to the plasma protein concentration.

Measurement of serum phosphorus and detection of excess phosphorous diuresis can be useful in separating primary hyperparathyroidism from other causes of hypercalcemia. Measurement of renal tubular reabsorption of phosphate or renal phosphate clearance in a hypercalcemic patient will determine whether hyperparathyroidism exists. Urinary cyclic adenine monophosphate (AMP) levels can also help to determine the etiology of the hypercalcemia. In patients with primary hyperparathyroidism and humoral hypercalcemia associated with malignancy the urinary cyclic AMP levels are usually elevated (45).

Calcium and phosphorus constitute about 65 percent of the weight of bones. About 99 percent of the total body calcium is present in bone and most of this is localized in the crystal structure of the mineralized bone. The other 1 percent is rapidly exchangeable with the rest of the body calcium pool and is in equilibrium with intracellular calcium. Approximately 50 percent of circulating total calcium is bound to proteins (mainly albumin and globulins) and the ionized calcium concentration is about 1.2 mmol/L (5 mg/dL). This fraction is biologically active and is tightly controlled by hormone actions. More than 99 percent of intracellular calcium is found in the mitochondria or the inner plasma membrane, or associated with the endoplasmic reticulum. The release of these calcium sources is tightly regulated.

Most of the total body phosphorus is present in bone (85 percent in mineral phase). Circulating inorganic phosphorus is present at a 1 mmol/L (3 mg/dL) concentration, mostly in the ionized form. About 12 percent of serum phosphate is bound to protein.

PTH is best measured by two-site immunoassays which require both the amino-terminal and carboxyl-terminal sequences of PTH 1-84 on the same molecule. A slight diurnal variation is observed with blood PTH concentrations and there is also a slight pulsatile secretion; however, random measurements of serum PTH generally provide accurate information.

Parathyroid hormone–related peptide (PTHrP) is more difficult to measure clinically than PTH, since the blood levels are low even in patients with malignant hypercalcemia secondary to increased PTHrP (45,46,50). An immunoassay for the amino-terminal portion of PTHrP or the two-site immunoassay for the amino-terminal and midregion of the molecule can be used to separate normal subjects and individuals with nonmalignant hypercalcemia from those with hypercalcemia associated with malignancy. Normal subjects usually have circulating PTHrP concentrations of less than 5 pmol/L while patients with malignancy-associated hypercalcemia have mean values slightly over 20 pmol/L (70,71).

Vitamin D metabolites can be measured, but require sophisticated laboratory analysis including high pressure liquid chromatography or related procedures. The assay is most useful in detecting subnormal values of these metabolites. Measurement of the plasma concentration of 25(OH) vitamin D can be used to detect vitamin D deficiencies, however, the levels are not tightly regulated and usually reflect body stores of vitamin D (45). Laboratory measurement of this metabolite is recommended only when vitamin D deficiency is being considered. Measurement of the other metabolite, 1,25(OH)$_2$ vitamin D, may be useful if sarcoidosis or lymphomas are suspected (45).

Secondary and Tertiary Hyperparathyroidism. Patients with secondary hyperparathyroidism have an increase in the production of PTH due to hypocalcemia (Table 2-4) (45,54,55, 73). The initial stimulus of hypocalcemia, which is most commonly due to renal failure, stimulates parathyroid cell proliferation and an increase in gland size. In addition to renal failure other conditions, such as vitamin D deficiency and pseudohypoparathyroidism, may lead to secondary hyperparathyroidism (Table 2-4).

Tertiary hyperparathyroidism is rare. In this condition, a patient with chronic secondary hyperparathyroidism develops an autonomously functioning gland which may behave like an adenoma (45,73).

Neonatal Hyperparathyroidism. In this rare condition infants develop severe hypercalcemia within the first few weeks of life. The severe bone demineralization and periosteal resorption lead to pathologic fractures (44,63). Nephrolithiasis may also develop along with renal calcinosis. This condition is a surgical emergency since the infants will die in a few months if untreated by total parathyroidectomy (44). The histologic feature of the gland is that of diffuse chief cell hyperplasia.

The etiology of neonatal hyperparathyroidism is probably related to familial benign hypocalciuric hypercalcemia (see below) (44,45).

Familial Benign (Hypocalciuric) Hypercalcemia. This is a rare hereditary disorder in which patients develop hypercalcemia early in life. It is inherited in an autosomal dominant pattern (54,57,63).

Table 2-4

**ETIOLOGIES OF
SECONDARY HYPERPARATHYROIDISM**

Chronic renal failure	Severe hypomagnesemia
Dietary deficiency of vitamin D or calcium	Pseudohypoparathyroidism
Tissue resistance to vitamin D	

Patients have normal PTH levels, mild hypercalcemia, and hypermagnesemia, while the phosphorous levels are usually lower than normal. The urinary excretion of calcium relative to creatinine is also low.

The histopathologic appearance of the parathyroid gland shows diffuse hyperplasia with an increased parathyroid parenchymal area (76). Some investigators have reported that the glands may be within normal limits or only minimally enlarged (45,59).

Physiologic studies have shown that the glands are abnormal in their regulation of calcium homeostasis. This may be related to an abnormal set point for the level of calcium which is manifested at a supernormal level. Another possibility is that the kidneys have an increased sensitivity to the effects of PTH. Patients with two copies of the gene have severe hypercalcemia and parathyroid hyperplasia from birth (59,60).

Vitamin D Intoxication. Vitamin D intoxication may be associated with severe medical problems. The etiology is usually inadvertent ingestion of excess vitamin D. Patients have nausea, vomiting, weakness, and an altered state of consciousness. The plasma PTH level is suppressed (45). The hypercalcemia results from increased intestinal absorption of calcium and increased resorption of bone.

Lithium-Associated Hypercalcemia. A small percentage (about 10 percent) of patients on lithium therapy develop hypercalcemia associated with increased PTH levels (45,55,60,65). The hypercalcemia usually subsides after the medication is discontinued.

Granulomatous Diseases. Patients with sarcoidosis usually have high levels of 1,25(OH)$_2$ vitamin D which is probably the direct cause of the resultant hypercalcemia. There is an associated increased intestinal absorption of calcium and PTH levels are suppressed. Isolated macrophages from patients with sarcoidosis have been reported to synthesize $1,25(OH)_2$ vitamin D from $25(OH)$ vitamin D as do normal macrophages when stimulated by gamma interferon (45).

Hypercalcemia can also be associated with tuberculosis, fungal disease, and berylliosis. It has been reported in patients with Wegner's granulomatosis, pneumocystosis, and acquired immunodeficiency syndrome (AIDS). Hypercalcemia has also been associated with extensive foreign body granulomas (45).

Other Causes of Hypercalcemia. *William's syndrome* is a rare developmental disorder associated with supravalvular aortic stenosis, elfin facies, and mental retardation. Hypercalcemia may develop during the first few years of life due to increased intestinal absorption of calcium and elevated levels of $1,25(OH)_2$ vitamin D. The molecular basis of this disease has been localized to deletion or translocation of the distal portion of the elastin gene (64,77).

Patients with *hyperthyroidism* may have mild hypercalcemia and low PTH levels caused by direct stimulation of bone resorption by thyroid hormones. The hypercalcemia may be associated with adrenal insufficiency due to increased ionized calcium, hemoconcentration, and increased albumin levels. Thiazide diuretics do not cause hypercalcemia by themselves, but they exacerbate the hypercalcemia of primary hyperparathyroidism. The mechanism is probably related to increased distal tubular resorption of calcium (45).

Milk-alkali syndrome, which is characterized by hypercalcemia, metabolic acidosis, and renal failure, usually results from the massive ingestion of calcium and absorbable alkali. Immobilization can lead to hypercalcemia from bone resorption.

Hypercalcemia may also be seen in patients with malignancies of various types (see Table 2-3) (52,58,66,74,75).

Parathyroid Glands in Nonparathyroid Hormone–Related Hypercalcemia. A few studies have examined the parathyroid glands of patients who had surgical exploration for hypercalcemia and were found to have nonparathyroid causes of hypercalcemia (53). In one study of 12 patients, the gland size and weight were within normal limits. Histologi-

cally, the glands are composed of chief cells arranged in cords and nests, with some vacuolated cells present that are more prominent at the periphery of the gland. Intracellular fat is detected after staining with Sudan IV, indicating that these glands are similar to normal glands.

HEREDITARY AND DEVELOPMENTAL DISORDERS

Hypoparathyroidism

Hypoparathyroidism is the decreased or absent production of PTH caused by congenital or acquired conditions, leading to hypocalcemia. It is characterized by hypocalcemia and hyperphosphatemia (79,92,94). Hypoparathyroidism may be transient (such as occurs after surgical excision of a parathyroid adenoma or carcinoma), or permanent from other surgical procedures to the neck or from radiation therapy (85). Profound and symptomatic hypocalcemia may indicate hypoparathyroidism but may be seen after total parathyroidectomy and autotransplantation of parathyroid tissue (91).

Idiopathic hypoparathyroidism has various etiologies. In neonates it may be familial or secondary to hypoplasia or aplasia of the parathyroid glands associated with other malfunctions of the third and fourth branchial pouches (96). Idiopathic hypoparathyroidism in older children and adults may be familial and associated with autoimmune disorders. Some of these individuals have circulating antibodies to the parathyroid glands (80,83). Histologically, the parathyroid glands may vary from hypoplastic to absent, or may be infiltrated by lymphocytes.

DiGeorge's Syndrome

DiGeorge's syndrome is a selective T-cell deficiency that results from failure of development of the third, fourth, and sometimes fifth pharyngeal pouches. The third and fourth pharyngeal pouches give rise to the thymus, the parathyroid glands, and some cells in the thyroid gland and ultimobranchial bodies (87). Patients with DiGeorge's syndrome have a total absence of cell-mediated immune responses secondary to thymic hypoplasia. They also have hypocalcemia secondary to a lack of parathyroid glands, along with congenital defects of the heart and great vessels. The mouth, ears, and facies may be abnormal. Because of the low levels of circulating T lymphocytes there is poor defense against fungal and viral infections. Levels of immunoglobulins or B cells, as well as plasma cells, are normal. DiGeorge's syndrome appears to result from intrauterine fetal damage around the eighth week of gestation. Microdeletion of 22q11.21-q11.23 and a t(2;22) (q14;q11) balance translocation suggest that a gene at chromosome 22q11 may be the cause of this syndrome (84,93,99).

The "partial" DiGeorge's syndrome is a variant associated with a small but histologically normal thymus and some T-cell functions that improve with age. The parathyroid glands can be identified in patients with the partial syndrome. In most cases remnants of thymic tissue may be found. Almost all cases show deletion of chromosomal segment 22q11.21.

Kearns-Sayre Syndrome

This rare syndrome is also known as *oculocraniosomatic neuromuscular disease*. Ragged red fibers characterized by myopathic abnormalities lead to ophthalmoplegia and progressive weakness in association with endocrine abnormalities, including hypoparathyroidism.

In addition to hypoparathyroidism, other endocrine abnormalities include primary gonadal failure, diabetes mellitus, and hypopituitarism (98). Patients have abnormal mitochondrial inclusions on muscle biopsy. Antiparathyroid antibodies have not been reported, but antibodies to the pituitary gland and to striated muscle have been noted. The disease is thought to be autoimmune in part.

Autoimmune Polyglandular Syndrome

Autoimmune polyglandular syndrome is an insufficiency affecting two or more endocrine glands. There are two major types of autoimmune polyglandular syndrome (80,88,89, 92,95). Type I is associated with adrenal insufficiency, mucocutaneous candidiasis, and hypoparathyroidism. It is usually recognized in early childhood because of other associated conditions including Graves' disease, chronic active hepatitis, hypothyroidism, insulin-dependent diabetes mellitus, and hypophysitis.

Autoimmune polyglandular syndrome type II is the most common of the immuno-endocrinopathy syndromes and is associated with adrenal insufficiency, hyperthyroidism or primary hypothyroidism, insulin-dependent diabetes mellitus, primary hypogonadism, myasthenia gravis, and celiac disease. Circulating organ-specific antibodies are commonly present (89). Most patients are middle aged or older. Both types are associated with human leukocyte antigen (HLA)-B8 and HLA-DR3. Some elderly patients have an unusual hypoparathyroidism in which antibodies to the surface of parathyroid cells suppress parathyroid function. Hypoparathyroidism is more common with the type I than the type II syndrome (89).

Pseudohypoparathyroidism

Target organ unresponsiveness to PTH results in pseudohypoparathyroidism. This condition was described by Albright and coworkers in 1942 and is also known as *Albright's hereditary osteodystrophy* (78). It is associated with hypocalcemia, hyperphosphatemia, and a blunted response to PTH (78). The pathogenesis is resistance to PTH which may occur at different sites including an abnormal PTH receptor, abnormal adenylate cyclase component, circulating antagonists to PTH action, and others. Patients have distinct physical features that include short stature, round face, short thick neck, obesity, reduced intelligence, and subcutaneous deposits of calcium or bone.

Pseudopseudohypoparathyroidism

These patients have the phenotypic features of pseudohypoparathyroidism, but without demonstrable metabolic abnormalities. Some suggest that the term pseudopseudohypoparathyroidism should be used only to designate patients with clear-cut phenotypic features of pseudohypoparathyroidism, or first-degree relatives of patients with this condition who have a normal urinary cyclic AMP response to PTH, such as the mothers of patients with pseudohypoparathyroidism.

Parathyroiditis

Parathyroiditis is the extensive infiltration of lymphocytes into the parathyroid glands. This is a rare condition that may occur in patients with hypoparathyroidism and in those with primary chief cell hyperplasia.

It is thought to represent an autoimmune process (81,82,86,89,97).

Only a small series or single cases have been reported. Antibodies to parathyroid tissue were found in 28 of 74 patients (38 percent) with idiopathic hypoparathyroidism in one series (89).

The histologic appearance includes clusters of lymphoid cells, which may have lymphoid follicle function, between parathyroid cells. In addition, plasma cells and fibrosis may be present. Parenchymal destruction has been noted in some cases.

Although autoimmune parathyroiditis is usually associated with hypoparathyroidism, several of the reported cases have been associated with parathyroid gland hyperplasia. Both patients reported by Bondeson et al. (81) had parathyroid hyperplasia, but the glands were infiltrated by dense mixtures of lymphocytes and plasma cells. There were signs of parenchymal destruction in scattered areas. In a more recent study by Chelty and Forder (86), the parathyroid glands were enlarged, consistent with hyperplasia, but small cysts were present. Microscopic examination showed lymphocytes with follicles, and plasma cells; these cells effaced the parathyroid architecture (86).

Miscellaneous Conditions Causing Hypoparathyroidism

Postsurgical hypoparathyroidism may occur in a variable number of patients after neck surgery, especially on the thyroid and parathyroid glands (90). It may vary from transient hypocalcemia to more severe conditions. Injury to the parathyroid gland during thyroid surgery is the most likely etiology, especially when the hypocalcemia is permanent. Permanent hypoparathyroidism develops in about 1 percent of patients after initial surgery for primary hyperparathyroidism and the risk increases with surgery for recurrent disease (79).

Radioactive iodine (^{131}I) therapy can occasionally lead to hypoparathyroidism. It usually begins 5 to 18 months after therapy. Most cases are associated with therapy for Graves' disease rather than for thyroid carcinoma. Patients with intrathyroidal parathyroid glands are at greater risk, since the ^{131}I destroys tissues only to a depth of about 2 mm (85).

CYSTS AND HAMARTOMAS

Parathyroid Cyst

Definition. Parathyroid cyst is a thin walled structure lined by epithelial cells, usually containing thin watery fluid and PTH.

General Remarks. Parathyroid cysts are uncommon lesions that can be present in the neck or mediastinum (100–104,106–109,111); lesions occurring in the neck are more common than those in the mediastinum. The cysts may develop as remnants of the third or fourth branchial cleft along the embryologic migration path of the gland. It is also possible that the cysts develop from persistent Kursteiner canals which are found in association with developing parathyroid glands. Large parathyroid cysts may develop from the fusion of several microcysts (101,102).

Macroscopic Findings. Parathyroid cysts may vary in size from microcysts up to those of 10 cm or more (fig. 2-12). They are often loosely attached to the thyroid gland. The walls of the cysts are gray to white, translucent, very thin, and membranous. The fluid content is often thin, watery, and straw-colored, but may be blood tinged. The cyst fluid often contains PTH.

Microscopic Findings. The cyst wall is made of fibrous connective tissue with entrapped islands of parathyroid chief cells (figs. 2-13, 2-14). Some cysts may be lined by chief cells that secrete PTH directly into the cyst cavity.

Differential Diagnosis. The differential diagnosis includes a true cyst of the parathyroid gland, degenerative changes in an adenoma, or hyperplasia. The presence of hypercalcemia and elevated PTH is commonly associated with adenomas or hyperplasias, but not with many simple cysts. Extensive scarring in the cyst wall may obliterate evidence of preexisting adenomatous or hyperplastic cells.

Parathyroid Hamartoma

Definition. Parathyroid hamartoma is an enlarged parathyroid gland with unusual stromal changes which are usually either fatty, myxomatous, or fibrous.

General Remarks. Parathyroid hamartomas are considered to be benign neoplasms by most investigators (105,107,110). Because fatty infiltration is the most common finding they are often referred to as *lipoadenomas*.

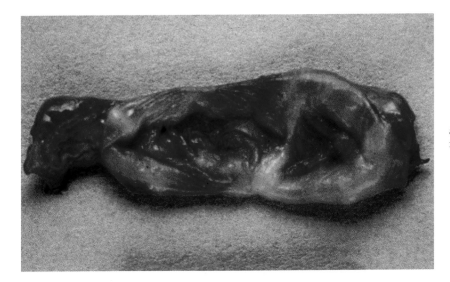

Figure 2-12

PARATHYROID CYST

Large parathyroid cyst in a patient with hyperparathyroidism and a benign cyst.

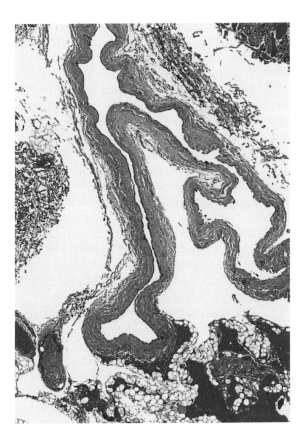

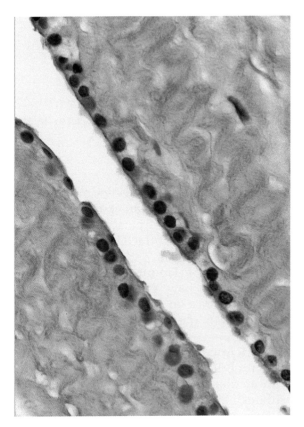

Figure 2-13

PARATHYROID CYST

Left: The cyst wall is lined by parathyroid cells and the fluid in the lumen is usually rich in PTH.
Right: Higher magnification shows that the lining cells are parathyroid chief cells.

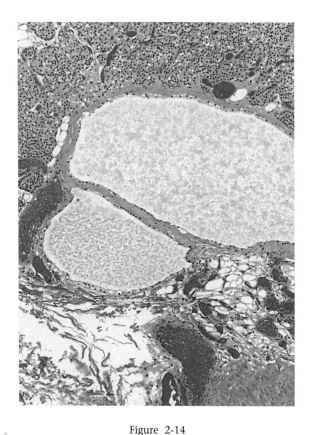

Figure 2-14

PARATHYROID MICROCYST

Microscopic cysts are present adjacent to the hyperplastic parathyroid gland.

Indeed, in a series with a review of the literature reported by LeGolvan et al. (105), there was only one enlarged parathyroid gland in the three patients in which other parathyroid glands were examined.

Macroscopic Findings. The lesions are encapsulated and have a soft, yellow-tan, lobulated appearance on cross section. They range in weight from normal parathyroid up to 400 g or more.

Microscopic Findings. The stromal component of the hamartoma is relatively unique, with an abundance of adipose tissue, with or without fibrosis and myxomatous changes. A prominent lymphoid cell infiltrate may be present in some areas. The parathyroid cells vary from chief cells, with or without oncocytic or water-clear cells, arranged in a thin, branching, cord-like manner.

Differential Diagnosis. Whether these lesions are true hamartomas (tumor-like proliferations of tissue indigenous to the organ but with a different structure) or true adenomas, remains somewhat controversial. Although most investigators favor a neoplastic process, clonality studies and other molecular analyses will be needed to resolve these issues. Since only one gland is enlarged in many patients, the suggestion is that they are really adenomas with metaplastic changes.

HYPERPLASIA

Primary Chief Cell Hyperplasia

Definition. This a proliferation of parathyroid parenchymal cells leading to an absolute increase in cell mass.

General Remarks. Parathyroid hyperplasia accounts for about 15 percent of cases of primary hyperparathyroidism. The most common cause of primary hyperparathyroidism is an adenoma (117,158), while carcinomas constitute less than 5 percent of cases. Since the early descriptions of chief cell hyperplasia as a cause of primary hyperparathyroidism, the difficulty in distinguishing between this condition and parathyroid adenomas simply on a histological basis has been recognized (133).

The prevalence of parathyroid hyperplasia is age-dependent, with an increasing prevalence in older individuals. A Swedish study reported hyperplasia in 7 percent of routinely examined cases at autopsy (113). The levels of serum calcium were above the normal range in glands that showed nodular hyperplasia. The patients in the study did not have clinical evidence of renal disease to invoke a possibility of secondary hyperparathyroid hyperplasia.

The main laboratory finding in patients with primary chief cell hyperplasia is an elevated serum level of PTH secondary to excessive synthesis and secretion. Serum chromogranin A levels are also elevated in many patients with primary hyperparathyroidism. The stimulus for the proliferation is not known, but earlier reports indicated that a serum mitogenic factor with a molecular weight between 50,000 and 55,000 daltons was identified in patients with multiple endocrine neoplasia type 1, implicating a hormonal cause of the hyperplasia (128,130).

Clinical and Radiologic Findings. Patients may be asymptomatic, especially with early hyperplasia. Symptoms are more common at calcium levels above 2.9 to 3.0 mmol/L (11.5 to 12.0 mg/dL), but some patients may still be asymptomatic at these levels. When the serum calcium exceeds 3.2 mmol/L (13 mg/dL), nephrolithiasis; calcification of skin, blood vessels, lungs, heart, and stomach; and renal insufficiency develop, especially if the blood phosphate level is normal or elevated secondary to renal failure. With severe hypercalcemia (above 3.7 mmol/L or 15 mg/dL) this becomes a medical emergency. When the serum calcium is 3.7 to 4.5 mmol/L (15 to 18 mg/dL) or higher, coma and cardiac arrest can readily develop.

More than 50 percent of patients with hyperparathyroidism are asymptomatic. Renal involvement due to calcium deposition in the renal parenchyma or recurrent nephrolithiasis was seen in 60 to 70 percent of patients prior to 1970. With today's earlier biochemical detection, renal complications are much less common. Renal stones are made up of calcium oxalate or calcium phosphate. Recurrent nephrolithiasis may be associated with urinary tract obstruction, infection, and loss of renal function. Bone disease, especially osteitis fibrosa cystica, is an uncommon complication of hyperparathyroidism today. However, progressive loss of bone mass leading to osteopenia can be seen with chronic disease. There is usually increased mineral turnover without a decrease in bone mass.

Neuromuscular manifestations include proximal muscle weakness, easy fatigability, and muscle atrophy. Correction of the hyperparathyroidism leads to complete regression of neuromuscular disease. Gastrointestinal complications include vague abdominal complaints and disorders of the stomach and pancreas. Pancreatitis may occur secondary to hyperparathyroidism. Other reported disorders include chondrocalcinosis, pseudogout, and neuropsychosomatic manifestations including depression.

Radiologic techniques can be used to monitor bone mineral density including computed tomography (CT); quantitative digital radiography can be used to evaluate spinal bone density. Single photon densitometry can be used to monitor cortical density in the extremities.

With hyperparathyroidism it is more common to selectively lose cortical rather than trabecular bone. Scintigraphic detection of hyperplastic glands can be extremely useful in planning surgery (fig. 2-15). This is especially true when the glands are in an abnormal location or are supernumerary. Technetium 99m sestamibi, an isonitrile radionuclide imaging agent, is used with subtraction ^{123}I thyroid scans for the imaging of abnormal parathyroid glands (137,170).

Molecular Biology Findings. Chief cell hyperplasia is associated with the multiple endocrine neoplasia (MEN) syndromes (138,139). About 20 percent of patients with primary chief cell hyperplasia have one of the MEN syndromes, most frequently MEN 1 (Table 2-5).

MEN 1, or Werner's syndrome, is associated with hyperplasia or adenomas of the parathyroid gland, pancreatic islets, and anterior pituitary gland. Patients may also have peptic ulcer disease secondary to a gastrin-producing tumor in the duodenum or pancreas (Zollinger-Ellison syndrome). There may be an increased incidence of bronchogenic, gastrointestinal and thymic carcinoids; adrenal cortical and thyroid follicular neoplasms; cutaneous leiomyomas; and cysts of moll (139). In most large series the parathyroid glands are most frequently affected (121). Initial studies with MEN 1 patients led to the identification of a region of chromosome 11 in which chromosome DNA was lost in some tumors in the normal parent. Linkage analyses with polymorphic DNA sequences from chromosome 11q confirmed the genetic localization (165). Loss of heterozygosity was subsequently shown in parathyroid tumors. More recent work has led to the cloning of the MEN 1 gene and has shown that it is associated with a tumor suppressor gene located on chromosome 11q which produces the protein product, menin (134). Abnormalities of this suppressor gene, including mutations, are associated with the hyperplasia and neoplasia of endocrine tissues involved in the MEN 1 syndrome.

MEN 2a, or Sipple's syndrome, is characterized by the development of bilateral C-cell hyperplasia and medullary thyroid carcinoma along with pheochromocytomas and parathyroid hyperplasia (132,139,142,168). MEN 2b, or Gorlin's syndrome, is characterized by the development of bilateral C-cell hyperplasia and medullary

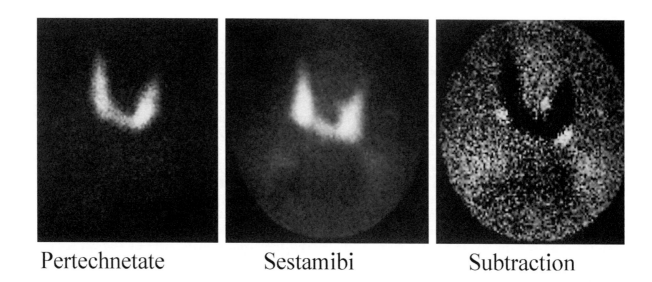

Pertechnetate   Sestamibi   Subtraction

Figure 2-15

PRIMARY PARATHYROID HYPERPLASIA

Scintigraphic detection of parathyroid hyperplasia. The pertechnetate (left) and sestamibi (middle) scans detect the enlarged parathyroid glands. After subtraction imaging three abnormal glands are seen (right). At surgery three hyperplastic glands, with the left inferior weighing 1.1 g, right superior weighing 2.4 g (displaced anteroinferiorly), and left superior weighing 0.16 g, were identified.

Table 2-5

MOLECULAR ABNORMALITIES ASSOCIATED WITH MULTIPLE ENDOCRINE NEOPLASIA SYNDROMES

Syndrome	Chromosome	Gene Involved	Mechanism
MEN 1	11q	Menin	Tumor suppressor
MEN 2a/2b	10q	RET proto-oncogene	Activating mutation of tyrosine kinase

thyroid carcinoma along with pheochromocytomas and oral and gastrointestinal ganglioneuromatosis. Abnormalities of the parathyroid gland have been noted in 10 to 35 percent of patients with MEN 2a, but are usually absent in MEN 2b patients.

The genetic defect in MEN 2a and 2b is a tyrosine kinase mutation of the RET proto-oncogene. The RET proto-oncogene mutation in MEN 2a usually affect exons 10 and 11 while in MEN 2b exon 918 of the RET tyrosine kinase receptor is commonly mutated (167).

The RET proto-oncogene encodes the tyrosine kinase receptors expressed in a variety of tissues, some of which are derived from the neural crest. RET tyrosine kinase is part of a multireceptor complex that includes glial-derived neu-rotrophic factor (GDNF) and its receptor GDNFR2. GDNF has been shown to be a ligand for the RET tyrosine kinase receptor.

In addition to MEN 1 and MEN 2, there are other mixed MEN syndromes associated with parathyroid hyperplasia or adenomas. Some of these include neurofibroma, medullary thyroid carcinoma, and parathyroid adenomas (144); pituitary adenomas and pheochromocytomas with or without parathyroid hyperplasia (122); and parathyroid hyperplasias with chemodectomas, bronchial carcinoid, pituitary adenomas, and gastrin cell hyperplasia.

Other familial-like lesions associated with parathyroid hyperplasia have been reported (114, 141,145,146,156). The genes for most of these less common associations have not been characterized.

Cyclin D1 (PRAD-1/BCL-1) Rearrangements and Other Molecular Abnormalities. Another molecular abnormality observed in parathyroid lesions is the PRAD-1 gene product, a cyclin D1 protein which has a critical regulatory role in the cell cycle (117,118). The promoter for PTH develops a reciprocal translocation on chromosome 11 which stimulates expression of the PRAD-1 gene product.

Other genetic defects in parathyroid disease include allelic loss of chromosome 1 in 40 percent of patients with parathyroid tumors and loss of both copies of the retinoblastoma (Rb) gene in some with parathyroid carcinomas. Recent studies of parathyroid adenomas with comparative genomic hybridization have also found abnormalities in chromosomes 16 and 19 (152).

Clonality of Parathyroid Hyperplasias. Clonality studies of parathyroid adenomas have shown that these lesions are monoclonal (116,118–120). One recent study of patients with primary and secondary parathyroid hyperplasias showed monoclonality in 38 percent (6 of 16) with primary parathyroid hyperplasia (119). These findings suggest that hyperplasia may be a precursor lesion for parathyroid adenoma in some patients.

Macroscopic Findings. The degree of enlargement of individual parathyroid glands in primary chief cell hyperplasia can be quite variable (fig. 2-16). In one study from Sweden, only two glands were enlarged in more than 65 percent of patients (112). In another study from the Massachusetts General Hospital, the total weight of all glands was less than 1 g in more than half the patients; no patient had any gland weighing over 10 g (173). Some investigators have reported different patterns of involvement of the glands in chief cell hyperplasia (123). In one study, three patterns were characterized: 1) a typical or classic pattern consisted of enlargement of all four glands; 2) a pseudoadenomatous pattern in which the degree of involvement varied from minimal to markedly enlarged; and 3) an occult pattern which consisted of minimal involvement of all four glands and a hyperplasia recognized primarily at the microscopic level (123). This subclassification is not frequently used today, but represents a thorough analysis of the gross variation that is encountered in primary chief cell hyperplasia.

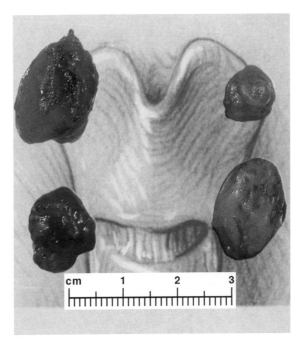

Figure 2-16

PRIMARY PARATHYROID HYPERPLASIA

Asymmetric hyperplasia shows marked enlargement of three glands with a smaller left superior gland.

These studies highlight some of the difficulties that are encountered in making a gross diagnosis of chief cell hyperplasia. In general, as the glands enlarge they became more irregular in configuration and have irregular projections. Cut sections of hyperplastic parathyroid glands are yellow-brown to tan-red, with a distinct homogenous appearance. In some glands nodularity may be a prominent feature and cystic changes may be evident (135,149).

Microscopic Findings. Histologic examination shows an increase in the proportion of parenchymal cells to stromal fat and a decrease in intracellular fat in most glands (figs. 2-17, 2-18) (159,160). The predominant cell type is a chief cell, although other cell types including oncocytic, transitional oncocytic, and clear cells may be present. The pattern of distribution of the residual stromal fat can be quite variable. A few fat cells may be admixed with hyperplastic chief cells or islets of chief cells may be present between abundant fat cells in some areas. These changes can be recognized at the time of frozen section (171).

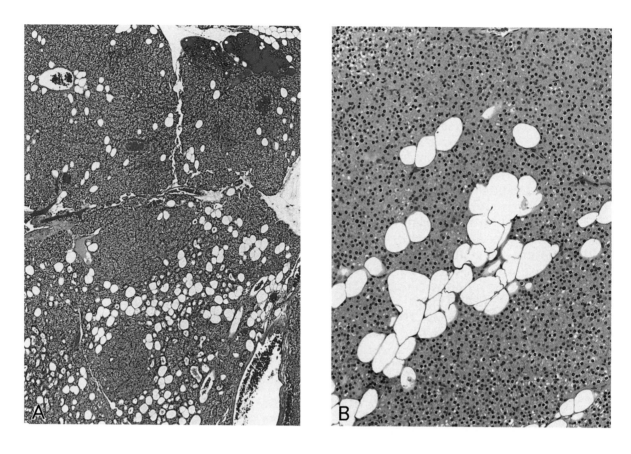

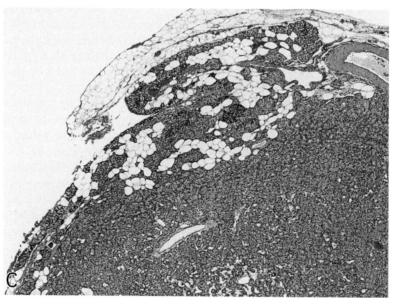

Figure 2-17

PRIMARY PARATHYROID HYPERPLASIA

A: Primary hyperplasia with an increase in the ratio of parenchymal cells to stromal fat and a decrease in intracellular fat.
B: Higher magnification shows a predominance of hyperplastic chief cells.
C: A more hypocellular area looks like a "rim of normal" parathyroid tissue.

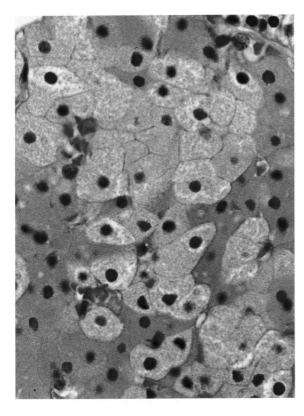

Figure 2-18

PARATHYROID HYPERPLASIA

An oncocytic nodule composed of oxyphil cells is present in this hyperplastic parathyroid gland from a patient with MEN 1a.

parenchyma, indicating a 500 percent increase in parathyroid tissue mass. Unfortunately, stains for intracellular fat were not done at the time of frozen section to determine its amount. However, all five patients had enlargement of all four glands.

The general appearance of hyperplastic glands includes follicles, cords, or solid sheets of parenchymal cells. Although a "rim of normal" parathyroid tissue is more characteristic of adenomas, these rims can also be observed in hyperplasia because of the irregular proliferative pattern in the glands.

The proliferative activity of the glands may be evident by occasional mitotic activity, noted on H&E-stained sections (163,166). In one study, up to 80 percent of parathyroid glands from patients with primary and secondary hyperplasia had a few mitotic cells per gland (166). Most had less than one mitotic figure per high-power field but five mitoses were found in one gland from a patient with MEN 2a. Nuclear pleomorphism is sometimes seen in hyperplastic glands and this finding is not associated with more aggressive features or malignancy. Chronic inflammatory cells may be present in glands with chief cell hyperplasia (138). In some cases, there is formation of lymphoid follicles with admixed plasma cells and lymphocytes. Although several investigators have speculated that this may represent an autoimmune condition, the etiology is unknown. In addition to lymphocytes, areas of fibrosis, myxoid degeneration, and old hemorrhage may be present. The possibility of a previous fine needle aspiration biopsy or previous surgery should be excluded when such histologic features are present.

In some hyperplastic glands microcysts or small macrocysts may be observed. This finding is more common in larger glands. One group of investigators reported on a rare familial variant of primary cystic chief cell hyperplasia (135).

Ultrastructural Findings. All of the principal cell types in hyperplastic parathyroid glands, including chief, oncocytic, and transitional oncocytic cells, have been studied ultrastructurally (115,123,126,128,148,151). The chief cells are larger than chief cells in normal glands (fig. 2-19). There are increased numbers of cytoplasmic organelles including mitochondria, rough endoplasmic

The general pattern of hyperplasia may be nodular or diffuse, with the former more common. Patients with MEN syndromes usually have a nodular pattern of hyperplasia. In some glands it is common to see hyperplastic nodules devoid of fat while the adipocytes are more common in the internodular and perinodular regions.

Lipohyperplasia is the term used by some investigators to describe hyperplastic parathyroid glands in patients with primary hyperplasia in which the predominant finding is that of fat cells (167). This lesion may be a hamartoma or a true adenoma. In a study of five patients (age 36 to 62 years), most of the glands ranged from 100 to 200 mg and the largest gland was 820 mg (167). The glands were up to five times the normal size and had approximately 50 percent fat and 50 percent

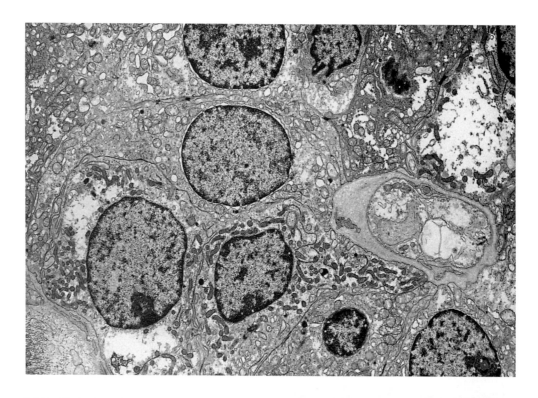

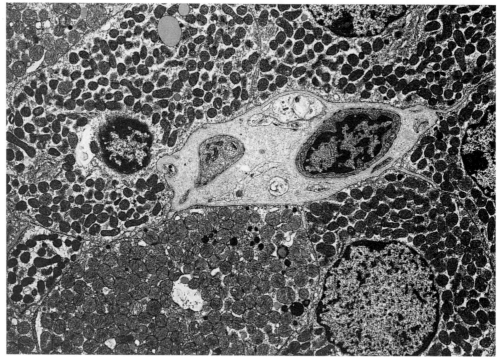

Figure 2-19

PARATHYROID HYPERPLASIA: ULTRASTRUCTURE

Top: Ultrastructure of hyperplastic parathyroid chief cells shows round nuclei and small nucleoli. The cytoplasm contains a few dense core secretory granules (X85,000).

Bottom: Clusters of oxyphil cells with abundant cytoplasmic mitochondria (X3,000).

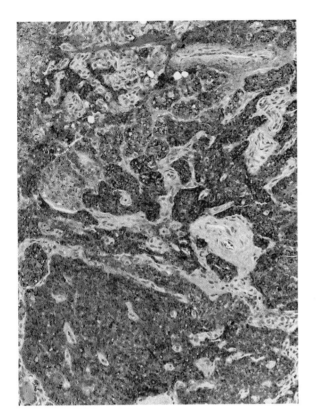 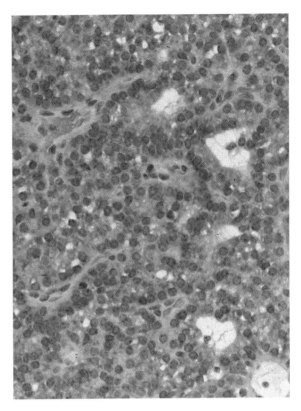

Figure 2-20

PARATHYROID HYPERPLASIA

Left: Immunostaining shows variable reactivity in the hyperplastic parathyroid cells as indicated by brown cytoplasmic staining.

Right: In situ hybridization for PTH messenger RNA shows a positive signal indicated by blue cytoplasmic staining (alkaline phosphatase-NBT/BCIP).

reticulum, and Golgi regions. Occasional secretory granules are present, but few cells have more than a few granules in spite of the abundant amounts of immunoreactive PTH and chromogranin that is seen in the cells. Moderate amounts of cytoplasmic glycogen are present.

Immunohistochemical Findings. Immunohistochemical studies often show diffuse staining for PTH and chromogranin A. However, very little chromogranin B is present in hyperplastic or normal parathyroid glands (147). Calcitonin may also be found in the parathyroid gland (164). In recent years, various investigators have used antibodies directed against cell cycle proteins to characterize parathyroid lesions. Retinoblastoma (Rb) protein is commonly expressed in parathyroid hyperplasias, as is cyclin D1. The proliferation rate assessed by Ki67 (MIB-1) immunostaining is low in both parathyroid hyperplasias and adenomas, but both lesions have a higher proliferation rate than normal glands. The cyclin-dependent kinase inhibitor p27^{Kip1} is also highly expressed in parathyroid hyperplasia. Recent studies suggest that parathyroid hyperplasias have a higher labeling index for p27 compared to parathyroid adenomas, so this finding may have some diagnostic utility (140). Staining for low molecular weight keratins (cytokeratins 8, 18, and 19) is positive in parathyroid glands. Flow cytometric analysis, immunostaining, and in situ hybridization analysis for PTH mRNA have been used in the study of parathyroid hyperplasia (fig. 2-20).

Differential Diagnosis. The principal lesions that should be distinguished from parathyroid hyperplasia at the time of frozen or permanent section analysis include normal

Figure 2-21

PARATHYROMATOSIS

Nests of normal and hyperplastic parathyroid tissue are present in the fibroadipose and skeletal muscle tissues. This condition can simulate parathyroid carcinoma or hyperplasia.

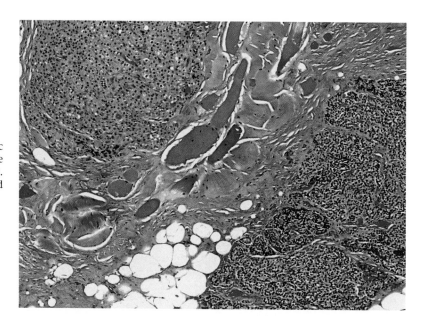

parathyroid glands, parathyroid adenomas, and parathyromatosis.

In adults, hyperplastic parathyroid glands usually have more parenchymal cells and less fat, and are larger than normal glands. However, in pediatric patients the normal glands usually contain very little stromal fat, so the total gland weight and size are more reliable indicators for separating normal from hyperplastic glands in these patients.

Examination of at least two parathyroid glands is necessary to separate adenomas from hyperplasias (124,125,133,137). As previously discussed, although a rim of normal tissue is more commonly seen in adenomas, one may see normal tissue in chief cell hyperplasia as well. Staining for intracellular lipid can be useful in distinguishing normal from hyperplastic glands, since hyperplastic glands have decreased amounts of intracellular lipid and generally have small lipid droplets. However, since both hyperplasia and adenomas have decreased intracellular lipid, fat stains are not helpful in distinguishing these two disorders.

The examination of a second gland is extremely useful. If one gland is enlarged while the second is normal in size and weight, the patient most likely has an adenoma. The presence of abundant intracellular fat in the chief cells is in keeping with this conclusion, since this suggests that the second smaller gland is suppressed.

Because asymmetric hyperplasia is a common finding, the surgical examination of at least three parathyroid glands and preferably all four, can help sort out difficult cases of hyperplasia (162). However, a common practice today is to examine only two glands in cases of suspected adenoma. Double adenomas, although uncommon, have been reported, so examination of more than two glands also helps in this distinction. In a study by Bondeson et al. (127), examination of at least two glands along with intraoperative lipid staining was useful in separating adenomas from hyperplasias, with equivocal findings reported in only 8 percent of cases.

Some investigators have used density gradient measurement to successfully evaluate the mass of parenchymal cells in parathyroid hyperplasia (169). The use of Ki67 (MIB-1) immunostaining does not help to distinguish hyperplasia from adenoma, but the p27^{Kip1} level has been reported to be useful in this differential diagnosis (140).

Parathyromatosis or small nests of parathyroid cells in the soft tissues of the neck and mediastinum may be difficult to distinguish from hyperplasia (fig. 2-21) (138–150,152), since these nests may enlarge with primary and secondary hyperplasia. In one study, 3 of 40 patients with primary chief cell hyperplasia had evidence of parathyromatosis (150). These nests may be responsible for recurrent or persistent hyperparathyroidism after subtotal parathyroidectomy for chief cell hyperplasia. Patients with supernumerary parathyroid glands may also have persistent or recurrent hyperparathyroidism if these extra glands are not removed during surgery.

Treatment and Prognosis. Subtotal parathyroidectomy is the treatment of choice for primary chief cell hyperplasia (131,136,150, 153,171). The general approach is to remove 3 1/2 glands, leaving a small portion of the fourth gland behind. Excision of the thymic tongue ensures that any extra parathyroid tissue is also removed. Another approach is to excise all four glands and immediately transplant a portion of one gland into the muscles of the forearm, which can be readily removed from this ectopic site in the future if necessary (154). Alternatively, cryopreservation of portions of the gland has been advocated by other investigators (157).

In one study with a long follow-up period, patients with hyperparathyroidism treated by subtotal parathyroidectomy had recurrent hypercalcemia in 16 percent of cases 1 to 16 years after surgery (161). The principal reason for recurrence was insufficient surgical excision of glands. Many patients with recurrence were cured by reoperation and removal of additional parathyroid gland tissue (161).

Recent studies have shown that a combination of technetium (Tc99m) sestamibi scintigraphy, intraoperative gamma probe detection, and rapid intraoperative PTH assay can be used to direct the operation in patients with hyperthyroidism (137). In one study, the rapid PTH assay led to successful surgery in all of 15 patients including those having a second operative procedure (137).

As discussed earlier, parathyromatosis (141, 155) and supernumerary parathyroid glands can be additional reasons for surgical failure in patients with primary hyperparathyroidism.

Primary Clear Cell Hyperplasia

Definition. This proliferation of vacuolated water clear (Wasserhelle) cells leads to an absolute increase in parathyroid parenchymal cell mass that involves multiple parathyroid glands.

General Remarks and Clinical Features. This is an extremely rare disorder which was first described by Albright and his colleagues in 1934 (172). More cases were reported between 1930 and 1975 than in subsequent years (172, 175–178). Historically, patients with primary clear cell hyperplasia presented with renal stones or had evidence of bone disease, as with the other forms of primary hyperparathyroidism before 1975. However, during the last two decades, most patients with primary clear cell hyperplasia have been asymptomatic at the time of diagnosis. The Massachusetts General Hospital had 19 cases between 1930 and 1975 (173,174). The Mayo Clinic reported 12 cases up to December 1951 which constituted 8.6 percent of their total cases (181).

To date, there have not been any reports linking clear cell hyperplasia to a distinct familial pattern or to an association with the MEN syndromes.

Macroscopic Findings. Diffuse and nodular enlargement of the parathyroid glands is a common feature of primary clear cell hyperplasia. The glands are usually irregular in shape, with foot-like processes extending to the adjacent adipose tissues of the neck. The glands may be slightly paler than in cases of chief cell hyperplasia, but the general color varies from tan to red-brown (fig. 2-22). Cystic degenerative hemorrhage and fibrosis may be present, especially in the larger glands. In one series from the Massachusetts General Hospital, the total gland weights ranged from 10 to 60 g in half the cases while the rest were less than 10 g (133). In the Mayo Clinic series, the average weight of parathyroid tissue was 19 g, with a range of 0.8 to 52.5 g; however, three patients had total gland weights of less than 5.0 g.

Microscopic Findings. The hyperplastic cells usually grow in a diffuse pattern, but a nodular growth pattern may also be seen (fig. 2-23). The cells are generally larger than chief cells, ranging in diameter from 10 to 40 µm. The nuclei are eccentric and may be multiple in some cells. Nuclei are generally placed at the pole of the cell adjacent to the stroma and vessel, giving the distinct "bunch of berries" appearance.

The architecture varies from a glandular to a trabecular or diffuse pattern. Cystic changes may be a prominent feature and the cysts often contain pale eosinophilic proteinaceous material that reacts with anti-PTH antibodies.

73

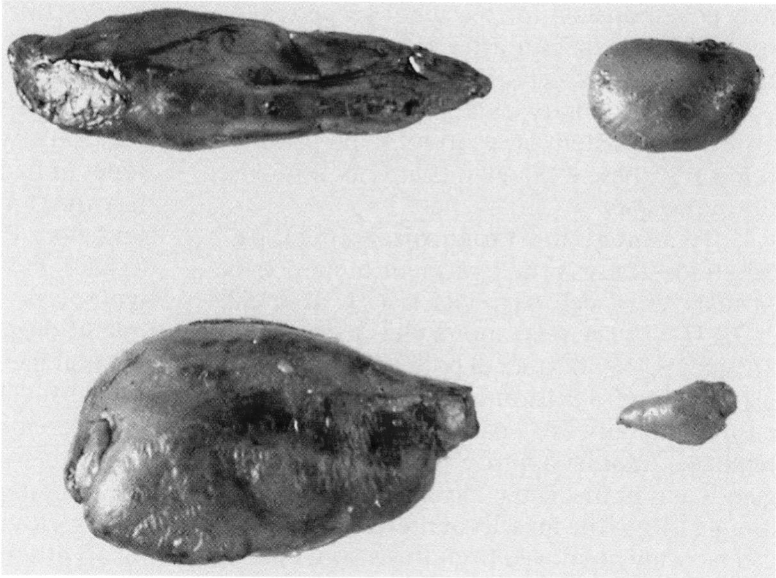

Figure 2-22

CLEAR CELL HYPERPLASIA

Asymmetric clear cell hyperplasia with variable enlargement of three parathyroid glands.

The individual cells have clear cytoplasm with many small vacuoles that range up to 0.8 µm in diameter. The large clear renal cell carcinoma–like pattern is rather distinctive. Histochemical stains are positive for glycogen, but usually very little stainable lipid is present.

Ultrastructural analysis shows abundant cytoplasmic small vacuoles which are probably derived from the Golgi vesicles (fig. 2-24) (179). Scattered dense core secretory granules with chromogranin A immunoreactivity and stored PTH with sparse rough endoplasmic reticulum and Golgi regions suggest that the cells are not very active metabolically (175). An analysis of PTH in tissues from clear cells and chief cell adenomas showed much lower levels of the hormone per milligram of fresh tissue than in normal tissue, supporting the ultrastructural observation that these cells are not very active metabolically.

Immunohistochemical studies show weak to absent immunoreactivity for PTH. Immunostaining for chromogranin A and low molecular weight keratin is usually positive. In situ hybridization for PTH shows staining of the mRNA in the cytoplasm.

Differential Diagnosis. The differential diagnosis of clear cell hyperplasia includes normal parathyroid glands and clear cell adenoma of the parathyroid. Clear cell adenomas have been reported in various series (178,179,181), so these

rare neoplasms must be separated from hyperplasia by biopsy of at least two glands. In cases of clear cell adenoma, the other parathyroid glands consist mainly of chief cells (178,181).

Treatment. As with other forms of hyperplasia, treatment is subtotal parathyroidectomy with removal of 3 1/2 glands and either reimplantation of parathyroid cells in the forearm or cryopreservation (180).

SECONDARY AND TERTIARY HYPERPARATHYROIDISM

Secondary Hyperparathyroidism

Definition. Secondary hyperparathyroidism is an increase in the parathyroid parenchymal mass in multiple parathyroid glands resulting from a known stimulus for PTH hypersecretion.

General Remarks. A variety of conditions can lead to secondary parathyroid hyperparathyroidism, but the most common cause is chronic renal failure (188–191,198,204,205, 208). Secondary hyperparathyroidism also occurs in patients with osteomalacia (due to vitamin D deficiency) and pseudohypoparathyroidism in which there is a deficient response to PTH at the level of the receptor. Hypocalcemia is the common denominator in all cases of secondary hyperparathyroidism. Secondary hyperparathyroidism results from an adaptive growth of

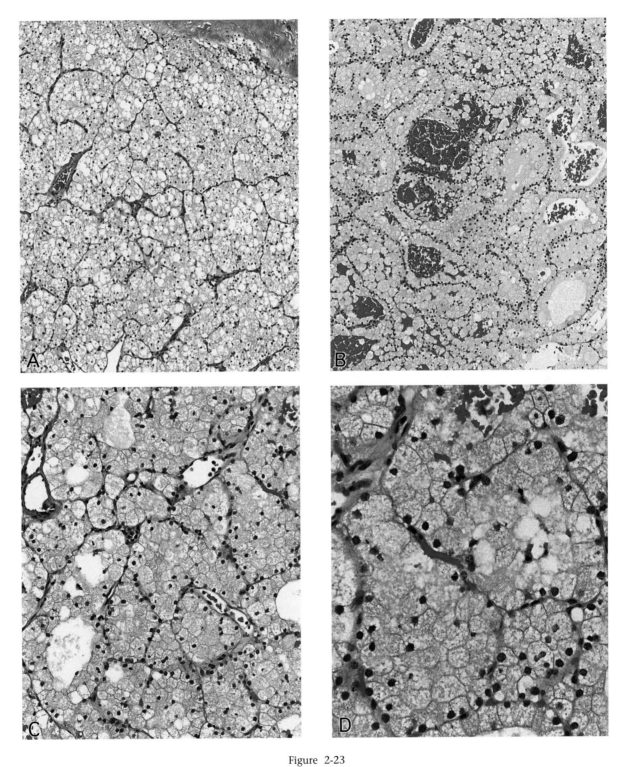

Figure 2-23

CLEAR CELL HYPERPLASIA

A: Clear cell hyperplasia showing cells with clear cytoplasm growing in a diffuse pattern.
B: Focal areas of congestion are present.
C: Higher magnification shows abundant clear cytoplasm.
D: The cells are larger than chief cells, and they may have central cystic spaces.

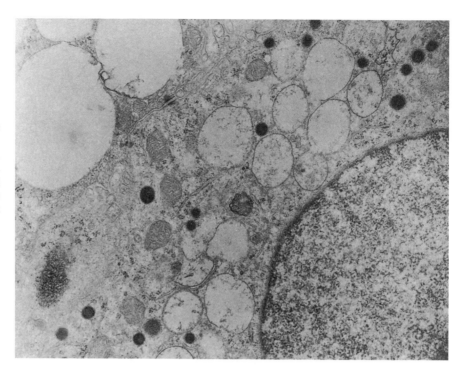

Figure 2-24

CLEAR CELL HYPERPLASIA: ULTRASTRUCTURE

Ultrastructural examination shows cells with membrane-limited vacuoles and scattered secretory granules (X22,720). (Fig. 76 from Fascicle 15, 1st Series.)

the glands because of decreased levels of ionized calcium and is presumably a reversible condition. In contrast, primary hyperparathyroidism is an autonomous growth of the parathyroid glands resulting from an unknown stimulus.

The mechanism of gland enlargement in secondary hyperparathyroidism is resistance to the normal level of PTH resulting in hypocalcemia; this leads to a hyperplastic stimulation of the gland resulting in an increased secretion of PTH (188,200).

In patients with renal failure, the initial stage of hypocalcemia is related to phosphate retention secondary to decreased phosphate excretion and reduced production of $1,25(OH)_2$ vitamin D due to the renal failure. This leads to reduced skeletal responsiveness to PTH while the lower levels of $1,25(OH)_2D$ prevent normal calcium absorption from the intestine.

Analysis of the causes of chronic renal failure in a recent series of 41 patients with secondary hyperparathyroidism showed that glomerulonephritis was the most common etiology (29 percent), followed by analgesic nephropathy (25 percent), reflux nephropathy (17 percent), and polycystic kidney disease (11 percent) (208). Surprisingly, diabetic nephropathy constituted only 3 percent of the cases.

Clinical Features. Patients with severe secondary hyperparathyroidism usually have hypercalcemia, hyperphosphatemia along with bone pain, ectopic calcification, and pruritus. Renal osteodystrophy is the term used to describe the bone disease in patients with secondary hyperparathyroidism and renal failure. At the same time, some patients may also have osteomalacia or vitamin D and calcium deficiencies, and osteitis fibrosa cystica may develop. Other skeletal disorders in patients with renal failure and secondary hyperparathyroidism who are on long-term dialysis include aluminum deposition associated with an osteomalacia-like picture and bone disease reflected by a low bone turnover state (188).

Ectopic calcification can involve the viscera, soft tissue, and periarticular surfaces (188), leading to arthritis with pain, swelling, and joint stiffness. Calcium may be deposited in the media of arteries and ischemic necrosis of the muscle, skin, and subcutaneous fat (calciphylaxis) can develop.

Macroscopic Findings. The weight and size of the glands vary with the stage of the disease (fig. 2-25). In the early stages, with mild secondary hyperparathyroidism, the glands are uniformly enlarged and have a yellow-tan appearance. Later, with more advanced disease, the glands are more variable in size and may be quite large (199). In a series of 200 patients with secondary hyperparathyroidism, the glands ranged from 120 to 6000 mg (199). The general appearance of the glands is similar to those seen in patients with primary chief cell hyperplasia, but the uniformity of glandular enlargement is more common early in secondary hyperplasia; however, asymmetric hyperplasia is often noted in both conditions.

Microscopic Findings. The hyperplastic glands contain increased numbers of parenchymal cells and decreased stromal fat cells (fig. 2-26) (182). The arrangement of the hyperplastic cells varies from diffuse sheets to trabecular, acinar, or cord-like growth patterns early in the disease. At later stages, a nodular pattern of proliferation is more common. In very large glands, it is not uncommon to see increased fibrosis, old hemorrhage, and cystic degeneration.

An admixture of different cell types is present in secondary hyperparathyroidism (fig. 2-26) (185). The most common is the chief cell which may appear vacuolated because of increased glycogen content. As in other forms of parathyroid hyperplasia, the intracellular lipid content is decreased. Oncocytic cells, usually growing in nodules, are a common finding. Transitional oncocytic cells are also present and are admixed with chief and oncocytic cells, growing in nodules or other patterns. Mitotic figures can be seen focally (201,203).

Ultrastructural Findings. Electron microscopic examination shows chief cells with some intercellular desmosomes and straight plasma membranes (194). There are scattered secretory granules with a granular endoplasmic reticulum and conspicuous Golgi regions (199); ultrastructural studies usually confirm the light microscopic impression that there are increased numbers of oncocytic and transitional oncocytic cells.

Immunohistochemistry and Flow Cytometry. Immunohistochemical studies often show PTH and chromogranin A in chief, oncocytic, and transitional oncocytic cells (191). The staining for PTH is reduced compared to normal glands.

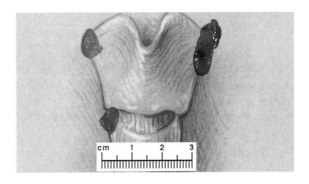

Figure 2-25

SECONDARY HYPERPLASIA

Variable enlargement of three parathyroid glands from a patient with renal failure.

Flow cytometric analysis shows an aneuploid population in some cases (186,193,195). Because aneuploid populations can be present in benign and malignant parathyroid glands, flow cytometric analysis does not allow a distinction between hyperplastic and neoplastic glands.

Differential Diagnosis. The differential diagnosis of secondary hyperparathyroidism includes an adenoma if only one gland is examined. Examination of at least two glands usually resolves this problem. However, asymmetric hyperplasia, which is more common with primary hyperplasia, may be present. The absence of a normal rim of a nodular pattern of growth in multiple glands is common in secondary hyperplasia.

Treatment and Prognosis. Removal of three entire parathyroid glands with a small portion of the fourth gland preserved in situ is a frequent surgical approach in secondary hyperparathyroidism (187). With continued chronic renal failure the remaining parathyroid gland continues to grow and may require future surgical intervention. Surgically induced parathyromatosis by implantation of parathyroid tissue into the neck leads to persistent or recurrent hyperparathyroidism (192).

Other surgical approaches for treating patients with secondary hyperparathyroidism include: 1) performing a total parathyroidectomy and implanting about 50 mg of parathyroid tissue into the forearm muscle to allow easy surgical access in case of recurrent hyperparathyroidism (196,207) and 2) performing a near total parathyroidectomy and cryopreserving

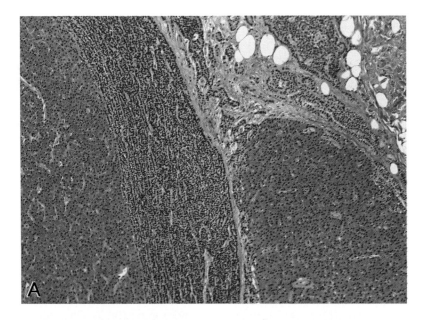

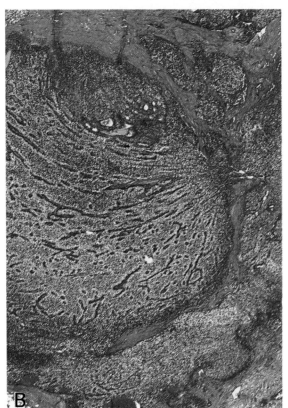

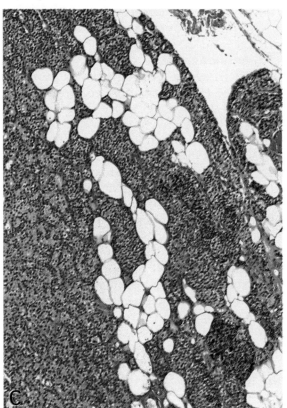

Figure 2-26

SECONDARY HYPERPLASIA

A: There is a nodular pattern of growth with chief cells and oxyphil cells.

B: A background of fibrosis is present.

C: A more sparsely cellular area suggests a "rim of normal" parathyroid tissue in this gland with secondary hyperplasia.

some parathyroid tissue for future reimplantation if the patient becomes hypoparathyroid. The surgical practice of performing parathyroid autotransplantation into the muscles of the forearm after total parathyroidectomy generally gives good results (196,206,207).

In some reports, a few patients have had graft failure or insufficient functioning of the graft, but this is usually only in a small percentage of cases. Another complication is recurrent hyperparathyroidism from the hyperplastic grafted tissue, but this is usually quite amenable to further surgical exploration. In one series, recurrent hyperparathyroidism was present in 6 of 42 (14 percent) patients with forearm autotransplants (196). Obvious mitotic activity and larger and more irregular nuclei with nodular hyperplasia were reported. In some cases, the autotransplanted tissue migrated to the skeletal muscles and connective tissues at sites distant from the original graft, indicating the potential for this grafted tissue to simulate malignant transformation.

Tertiary Hyperparathyroidism

Definition. Tertiary hyperparathyroidism is the development of autonomous parathyroid hyperfunction in a patient with a previously well-documented history of secondary hyperparathyroidism.

General Remarks. After renal transplantation, hypercalcemia secondary to hyperparathyroidism develops in about one third of patients (202). Transient hypercalcemia is the most common development and it usually resolves spontaneously. Persistent hypercalcemia may occur in up to 50 percent of patients with long-term grafts.

The mechanism of hypercalcemia in renal failure is thought to be related to partial resistance to the metabolic actions of PTH, leading to excessive production of the hormone and parathyroid gland hyperplasia. Hyperplasia develops because there is resistance to the normal level of PTH which results in hypocalcemia and this in turn leads to further stimulation of the parathyroid gland and to further increased PTH secretion. The "set point" of the ionizable serum calcium-PTH homeostasis changes and there is a higher concentration of immunoreactive PTH at any given level of calcium concentration (Table 2-6).

The nature of the changes in the parathyroid in tertiary hyperparathyroidism remains controversial. Some authors have referred to the changes as multiple adenomas (194), but they may represent adenomatous hyperplasia. The recent molecular characterization of clonality has shown that about 38 percent of cases of secondary hyperparathyroidism are monoclonal (184), providing strong evidence to suggest that an even higher percentage of glands would be clonal in tertiary hyperparathyroidism, thus representing true adenomas.

Macroscopic Findings. The most detailed analysis of parathyroid glands with tertiary hyperparathyroidism was done by Krause and Hedinger (197) who examined 128 glands from 41 patients. The gland weights varied form 0.1 to 7.0 g. Nodular hyperplasia was a common finding, but 44 percent of patients had diffuse hyperplasia. The average parathyroid weights for diffuse and nodular hyperplasia were 0.7 ± 0.4 g and 1.4 ± 0.7 g, respectively. A multinodular gland with a dominant nodule was a common finding (fig. 2-27).

Microscopic Findings. Analysis of the microscopic findings in the study of Krause and Hedinger (197) revealed three histologic patterns: diffuse hyperplasia, nodular hyperplasia, and adenoma development (figs. 2-28, 2-29). Diffuse hyperplasia showed predominantly chief cells with occasional oxyphil and water clear cells, giving a varied appearance to the hyperplastic glands. Fat cells were less than 5 percent of the total parathyroid mass. Areas of fibrosis, calcification, and hemosiderin deposition were not present with the nodular pattern. At least four nodules were present in one gland. Each nodule consisted of one type of cell, usually chief cells. Some oncocytic nodules were also present. Fibrosis and hemosiderin deposition were frequent findings. The two patients who had adenomatous changes in the hyperplastic glands had more fat cells (40 percent in one case in the three glands that were removed). The other patient had an adenomatous gland with a diffuse increase in clear cells while a second gland consisted of normal parathyroid tissue.

Ultrastructural Findings. Electron microscopy shows that the hyperplastic chief cells often have many interdigitating processes and desmosomes. There is evidence of high secretory

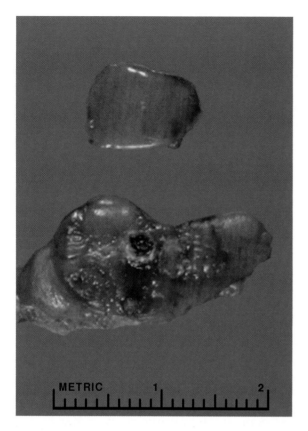 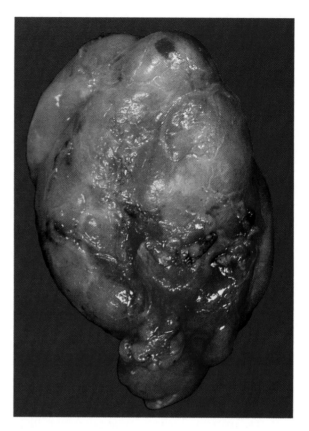

Figure 2-27

TERTIARY HYPERPLASIA

Left: Hyperplastic gland from a patient with tertiary hyperparathyroidism. The bisected gland shows nodular hyperplasia with foci of calcification and hemorrhage. (Plate XIV B from Fascicle 6, 3rd Series.)
Right: Markedly nodular growth pattern in tertiary hyperparathyroidism.

Table 2-6

NORMAL VALUES FOR PARATHYROID TESTS[a]

Test	SI[b]	Conventional
Calcium		
Ionized serum	1.0–1.4 mmol/L	4.0–5.6 mg/dL
Total serum	2.2–2.6 mmol/L	9.0–10.5 mg/dL
Magnesium, serum	0.8–1.3 mmol/L	1.8–3.0 mg/dL
Parathyroid hormone		
Intact parathyroid hormone assay		
Immunoradiometric assay (IRMA)	10–65 ng/L	10–65 pg/dL
Phosphorus		
Inorganic, serum	1.0–1.5 mmol/L	3.0–4.5 mg/dL

[a]Wilson JD, Foster DW, Kronengberg HM, Larsen PR, Williams textbook of endocrinology, 9th ed. Philadelphia: WB Saunders, 1998:back cover.

[b]SI - system of international units.

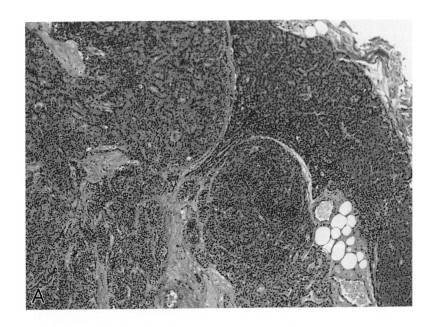

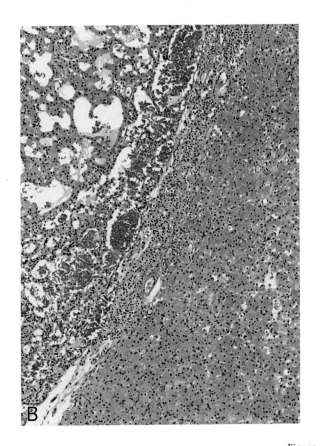

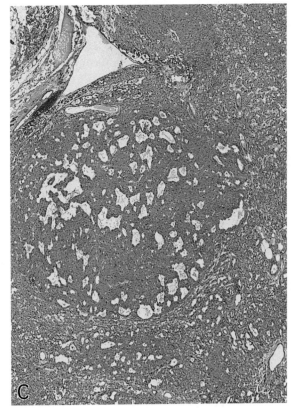

Figure 2-28

TERTIARY HYPERPLASIA

The gland shows a nodular growth pattern with chief and oxyphil cell hyperplasia (A). Two distinct nodular areas with microcystic chief cells (B) and oxyphil cells (C) are seen.

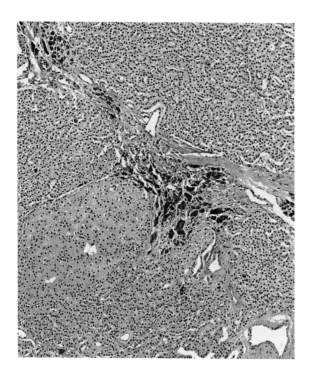

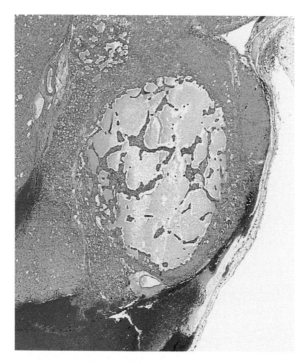

Figure 2-29

TERTIARY HYPERPLASIA

Left: Degenerative changes in a gland with tertiary hyperplasia include remote hemorrhage with hemosiderin-laden macrophages.

Right: Cystic degeneration in one of the nodules.

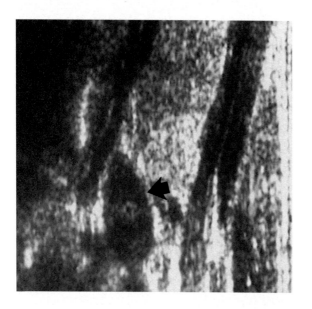

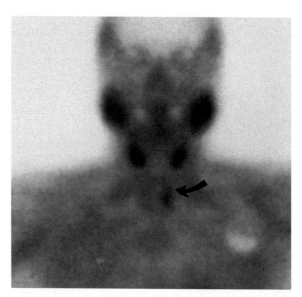

Figure 2-30

PARATHYROID ADENOMA

Left: Left inferior parathyroid adenoma shown by ultrasound as an oval hypoechoic mass posterior to the left lower pole of the thyroid (arrow).

Right: This corresponds to an area of persistent technetium 99m uptake by sestamibi imaging, confirming the adenoma (arrow).

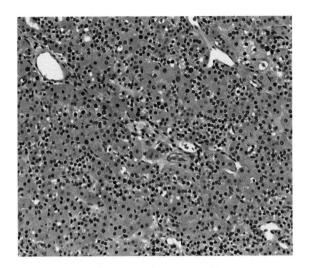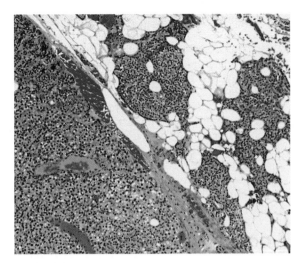

Figure 2-31

PARATHYROID ADENOMA

Left: An enlarged parathyroid gland composed of chief cells and transitional cells without stromal fat and with decreased intracellular lipid.

Right: A rim of normal parathyroid tissue is common in adenomas.

activity with an abundant rough endoplasmic reticulum, variable numbers of secretory granules, and prominent Golgi (183,197,199).

Differential Diagnosis. Comparison of the histopathologic findings in secondary and tertiary hyperparathyroidism reveals larger glands, more oncocytic cells, and more nodular glands in tertiary disease. However, clinicopathologic correlation, including a long history of secondary hyperparathyroidism, is needed to make a diagnosis of tertiary disease.

It may be difficult to distinguish tertiary hyperparathyroidism from an adenoma without the appropriate clinical history. However, nodularity is less common in adenomas, a feature that can be determined radiographically (fig. 2-30) or by gross examination of the gland. Adenomas usually have a rim of normal parathyroid tissue (fig. 2-31), while this is uncommon in tertiary hyperplasia.

Treatment and Prognosis. Subtotal parathyroidectomy with autoimplantation and/or cryopreservation is usually the treatment of choice. Recurrent hyperparathyroidism may be a complication of this approach.

REFERENCES

Normal Parathyroid Gland

1. Akerstrom G, Grimelius L, Johansson H, Lundqvist H, Pertoft H, Bergstrom R. The parenchymal cells in normal human parathyroid glands. Acta Pathol Microbiol Immunol Sc [A] 1981;89:367–75.
2. Akerstrom G, Grimelius L, Johansson H, Pertoft H, Lundqvist H. Estimation of the parathyroid parenchymal cell mass by density gradients. Am J Pathol 1980;99:685–94.
3. Akerstrom G, Malmaeus J, Bergstrom R. Surgical anatomy of human parathyroid glands. Surgery 1984;95:14–21.
4. Bondeson AG, Bondeson L, Ljungberg O, Tibblin S. Fat staining in parathyroid disease—diagnostic value and impact on surgical strategy: clinicopathologic analysis of 191 cases. Human Pathol 1985;16:1255–63.

5. Bringhurst FR, Demay MB, Kronenberg HM. Hormones and disorders of mineral metabolism. In: Wilson JD, Foster DW, Kronenberg HM, Larsen PR, eds. Williams textbook of endocrinology, 9th ed. Philadelphia: WB Saunders, 1998:1155–209.

6. Capen CC, Rosol TJ. Pathobiology of parathyroid hormone and parathyroid hormone-related protein: introduction and evolving concepts. Monogr Pathol 1993;35:1–33.

7. Chryssochoos JT, Weber CJ, Cohen C, et al. DNA index and ploidy distinguished normal human parathyroids from parathyroid adenomas and primary hyperplastic parathyroids. Surgery 1995;118:1041–9.

8. Dekker A, Dunsford HA, Geyer SJ. The normal parathyroid gland at autopsy: the significance of stromal fat in adult patients. J Pathol 1979; 128:127–32.

9. DeLellis RA. Tumors of the parathyroid gland. Atlas of Tumor Pathology, 3rd Series, Fascicle 6. Washington, DC: Armed Forces Institute of Pathology, 1993.

10. Dufour DR, Wilkerson SY. The normal parathyroid revisited: percentage of stromal fat. Human Pathol 1982;13:717–21.

11. Futrell JM, Roth SI, Su SP, Habener JF, Segre GV, Potts JT Jr. Immunocytochemical localization of parathyroid hormone in bovine parathyroid glands and human parathyroid adenomas. Am J Pathol 1979;94:615–22.

12. Ghandur-Mnaymneh L, Cassady J, Hajianpour MA, Paz J, Reiss E. The parathyroid gland in health and disease. Am J Pathol 1986;125:292–9.

13. Gilmour JR. Embryology of the parathyroid gland, the thymus and certain associated rudiments. J Pathol Bact 1937;45:507–22.

14. Gilmour JR. Normal histology of parathyroid glands. J Path Bact 1939;48:187–222.

15. Gilmour JR, Martin WJ. Weight of the parathyroid glands. J Path Bact 1937;44:431–62.

16. Gould VE, Lee I, Wiedenmann B, Moll R, Chejfec G, Franke WW. Synaptophysin: a novel marker for neurons, certain neuroendocrine cells, and their neoplasms. Human Pathol 1986;17:979–83.

17. Grimelius L, Akerstrom G, Johansson H, Bergstrom R. Anatomy and histopathology of human parathyroid glands. Pathol Ann 1981;16(pt 2):1–24.

18. Grimelius L, Akerstrom G, Johansson H, Juhlin C, Rastad J. The parathyroid glands. In: Kovacs K, Asa SL, eds. Functional endocrine pathology, vol 1, 2nd ed. Boston: Blackwell Science. 1998:381–414.

19. Irvin GL, Bagwell CB. Identification of histologically undetectable parathyroid hyperplasia by flow cytometry. Am J Surgery 1979;138:567–71.

20. Juhlin C, Akerstrom G, Klareokog L, et al. Monoclonal antiparathyroid antibodies revealing defective expression of a calcium receptor mechanism in hyperparathyroidism. World J Surg 1988;12:552–8.

21. Juhlin C, Holmdahl R, Johansson H, Rastad J, Akerstrom G, Klareskog L. Monoclonal antibodies with exclusive reactivity against parathyroid cells and tubule cells of the kidney. Proc Natl Acad Sci USA 1987;84:2990–4.

22. Kendall CH, Roberts PA, Pringle JH, Lauder I. The expression of parathyroid hormone messenger RNA in normal and abnormal parathyroid tissue. J Pathol 1991;165:111–8.

23. King DT, Hirose FM. Chief cell intracytoplasmic fat used to evaluate parathyroid disease by frozen section. Arch Pathol Lab Med 1979;103: 609–12.

24. Kurman RJ, Prabha AC. Thyroid and parathyroid glands in the vaginal wall: report of a case. Am J Clin Pathol 1973;59:503–7.

25. Lack EE, Delay S, Linnoila RI. Ectopic parathyroid tissue within the vagus nerve: incidence and possible clinical significance. Arch Pathol Lab Med 1988;112:304–6.

26. Lloyd RV, Wilson BS. Specific endocrine tissue marker defined by a monoclonal antibody. Science 1983;222:628–30.

27. Matsushita H, Hara M, Shishiba Y, Nakazawa H. An evaluation of the size of the parathyroid glands. Endocrinol Jpn 1984;31:127–31.

28. Miettinen M, Clark R, Lehto VP, Virtanen I, Damjanov I. Intermediate-filament proteins in parathyroid glands and parathyroid adenomas. Arch Pathol Lab Med 1985;109:986–9.

29. Nilsson O. Studies on the ultrastructure of the human parathyroid glands in various pathological conditions. Acta Pathol Microbiol Scand Suppl 1977;263:1–88.

30. Norris EH. The parathyroid glands and the lateral thyroid in man: their morphogenesis, histogenesis, topographic anatomy and prenatal growth. Contrib Embryol 1937;26:247–94.

31. Nygren P, Gylfe E, Larsson R, et al. Modulation of the Ca2+ sensing function of parathyroid cells in vitro and in hyperparathyroidism. Biochem Biophys Acta 1988;968:253–60.

32. Roth SI. The parathyroid gland. In: Silverberg SG, ed. Principles and practice of surgical pathology, vol 2, 2nd ed. New York: Churchill Livingstone, 1989:1923–55.

33. Roth SI, Abu-Jawdeh GM. Parathyroid glands. In: Sternberg SS, ed. Histology for pathologists, 2nd ed. Philadelphia: Lippincott-Raven, 1997: 1093–105.

34. Roth SI, Capen CC. Ultrastructural and functional correlations of the parathyroid gland. Int Rev Exp Pathol 1974;13:161–221.

35. Saffos RO, Rhatigan RM. Intracellular lipid in parathyroid glands. Hum Pathol 1979;10:483–5.

36. Santeusanio G, D'Alfonso V, Iafrate E, et al. Antibodies to cytokeratin 14 specifically identify oncocytes (Hurthle cells) in thyroid lesions and tumors. Appl Immunohistochem 1997;5:223–8.

37. Sasano H, Geelhoed GW, Silverberg SG. Intraoperative cytologic evaluation of lipid in the diagnosis of parathyroid adenoma. Am J Surg Pathol 1988;12:282–6.

38. Shoumura S, Iwasaki Y, Ishizaki N, et al. Origin of autonomic nerve fibers innervating the parathyroid gland in the rabbit. Acta Anat 1983;115:289–95.

39. Stork PJ, Herteaux C, Frazier R, Kronenburg H, Wolfe HJ. Expression and distribution of parathyroid hormone and parathyroid hormone messenger RNA in pathological conditions of the parathyroid [Abstract]. Lab Invest 1989;60:A92.

40. Theile J. Human parathyroid gland: a freeze fracture and thin section study. Curr Top Pathol 1977;65:31–80.

41. Weller GL Jr. Development of the thyroid, parathyroid and thymus glands in man. Contrib Embryol 1933;141:93–139.

42. Wilson BS, Lloyd RV. Detection of chromogranin in neuroendocrine cells with a monoclonal antibody. Am J Pathol 1984;115:458–68.

43. Winkler B, Gooding GA, Montgomery CK, Clark OH, Arnand C. Immunoperoxidase confirmation of parathyroid origin of ultrasound-guided fine needle aspirates of the parathyroid glands. Acta Cytol 1987;31:40–4.

Overview of Hypercalcemia and Hypocalcemia

44. Anast CS. Disorders of mineral and bone metabolism. In: Avery ME, Taeusch TW, eds. Schaffer's diseases of the newborn, 5th ed. Philadelphia: WB Saunders, 1984:464–79.

45. Bringhurst FR, Demay MB, Kronenberg HM. Hormones and disorders of mineral metabolism. In: Wilson JD, Foster DW, Kronenberg HM, Larsen PR, eds. Williams textbook of endocrinology, 9th ed. Philadelphia: WB Saunders, 1998:1155–209.

46. Capen CC, Rosol TJ. Pathobiology of parathyroid hormone and parathyroid hormone-related protein introduction and evolving concepts. Monogr Pathol 1993;35:1–33.

47. Castleman B, Roth SI. Tumors of the parathyroid glands. Atlas of Tumor Pathology, 2nd Series, Fascicle 14. Washington, DC: Armed Forces Institute of Pathology, 1978:1–94.

48. Cohn DV, MacGregor RR. The biosynthesis, intracellular processing and secretion of parathormone. Endocr Rev 1981;2:1–26.

49. Cohn DV, Morrissey JJ, Shofstall RE, Chu LL. Co-secretion of secretory protein-I and parathormone by dispersed bovine parathyroid cells. Endocrinology 1982;110:625–30.

50. DeLellis RA. Tumors of the parathyroid gland. Atlas of Tumor Pathology, 3rd Series, Fascicle 6. Washington, DC: Armed Forces Institute of Pathology, 1993.

51. Desai P, Steiner GC. Ultrastructure of brown tumor of hyperparathyroidism. Ultrastruct Pathol 1990;14:505–11.

52. Dickersin GR, Kline IW, Scully RE. Small cell carcinoma of the ovary with hypercalcemia: a report of 11 cases. Cancer 1982;49:188–97.

53. Dufour DR, Marx SJ, Spiegel AM. Parathyroid gland morphology in non-parathyroid hormone-mediated hypercalcemia. Am J Surg Pathol 1985;9:43–51.

54. Endres DB, Villanueva R, Sharp CF Jr, Singer FR. Measurement of parathyroid hormone. Endocrinol Metab Clin North Am 1989;18:611–29.

55. Greenspan FS. Basic and clinical endocrinology, 3rd ed. Norwalk, Conn: Appleton & Lange, 1991.

56. Heath DA. Primary hyperparathyroidism. Clinical presentation and factors influencing clinical management. Endocrinol Metab Clin North Am 1989;18:631–46.

57. Heath H III. Familial benign (hypocalciuric) hypercalcemia. A troublesome mimic of mild primary hyperparathyroidism. Endocrinol Metab Clin North Am 1989;18:723–40.

58. Insogna KL. Humoral hypercalcemia of malignancy. The role of parathyroid hormone-related protein. Endocrinol Metab Clin North Am 1989;18:779–94.

59. Law WM Jr, Carney JA, Heath H III. Parathyroid glands in familial benign hypercalcemia (familial hypocalciuric hypercalcemia). Am J Med 1984;76:1021–6.

60. Mallette LE. Regulation of blood calcium in humans. Endocrinol Metab Clin North Am 1989;18:601–10.

61. Marcus R. Laboratory diagnosis of primary hyperparathyroidism. Endocrinol Metab Clin North Am 1989;18:647–58.

62. Marx SJ. Genetic defects in primary hyperparathyroidism. N Engl J Med 1988;318:699–701.

63. Matsuo M, Okita K, Takemine H, Fujita T. Neonatal primary hyperparathyroidism in familial hypocalciuric hypercalcemia. Am J Dis Child 1982;136:728–31.

64. Mundy GR. Hypercalcemic factors other than parathyroid hormone related protein. Endocrinol Metab Clin North Am 1989;18:795–806.

65. Nussbaum SR, Zahradnik RJ, Lavigne JR, et al. Highly sensitive two-site immunoradiometric assay of parathyrin, and its clinical utility in evaluating patients with hypercalcemia. Clin Chem 1987;33:1364–7.

66. Omenn GS, Roth SI, Baker WH. Hyperparathyroidism associated with malignant tumors of nonparathyroid origin. Cancer 1969;24:1004–11.

67. Palmer M, Jakobsson S, Akerström G, Ljunghall S. Prevalence of hypercalcemia in a health survey: a 14-year follow-up study of serum calcium values. Eur J Clin Invest 1988;18:39–46.

68. Palmer M, Ljunghall S, Akerström G, et al. Patients with primary hyperparathyroidism operated on over a 24-year period: temporal trends of clinical and laboratory findings. J Chronic Dis 1987;40:121–30.

69. Parisien M, Silverberg SJ, Shane E, Dempster DW, Bilezikian JP. Bone disease in primary hyperparathyroidism. Endocrinol Metab Clin North Am 1990;19:19–34.

70. Rosenblatt M, Kronenberg HM, Potts JT Jr. Parathyroid hormone. Physiology, chemistry, biosynthesis, secretion, metabolism and mode of action. In: DeGroot LJ, ed. Endocrinology, vol. 2, 2nd ed. Philadelphia: WB Saunders, 1989:848–91.

71. Roskams T, Desmet V. Parathyroid hormone related peptides. A new class of multifunctional protein. Am J Pathol 1997;150:779–85.

72. Scholz DA, Purnell DC. Asymptomatic primary hyperparathyroidism. Ten year prospective study. Mayo Clin Proc 1981;56:473–8.

73. Segre GV, Potts JT Jr. Differential diagnosis of hypercalcemia: methods and clinical applications of parathyroid assays. In: DeGroot LJ, ed. Endocrinology, vol. 2, 2nd ed. Philadelphia: WB Saunders, 1989:984–1001.

74. Skrabanek P, McPartlin J, Powell D. Tumor hypercalcemia and "ectopic hyperparathyroidism." Medicine (Baltimore) 1980,59:262–82.

75. Stewart AF, Insogna KL, Broadus AE. Malignancy associated hypercalcemia. In: DeGroot LJ, ed. Endocrinology, vol. 2, 2nd ed. Philadelphia: WB Saunders, 1989:967–83.

76. Thorgeirsson U, Costa J, Marx SJ. The parathyroid glands in familial hypocalciuric hypercalcemia. Hum Pathol 1981;12:229–37.

77. Vasicek TJ, McDevitt BE, Freeman MW, et al. Nucleotide sequence of the human parathyroid hormone gene. Proc Natl Acad Sci 1983;80:2127–31.

Hereditary and Developmental Disorders

78. Albright F, Burnett CH, Smith PH, Parson W. Pseudo-hypoparathyroidism—an example of "Seabright-Bantam" syndrome, report of 3 cases. Endocrinology 1942;30:922–32.

79. Aurbach GD, Marx SJ, Spiegel AM. Parathyroid hormone, calcitonin and the calciferols. In: Wilson JO, Foster DW, eds. Williams textbook of endocrinology, 8th ed. Philadelphia: WB Saunders, 1992:1397–476.

80. Blizzard RM, Chee D, Davis W. The incidence of parathyroid and other antibodies in the sera of patients with idiopathic hypoparathyroidism. Clin Exp Immunol 1966;1:119–28.

81. Bondeson AG, Bondeson L, Ljungberg O. Chronic parathyroiditis associated with parathyroid hyperplasia and hyperparathyroidism. Am J Surg Pathol 1984;8:211–15.

82. Boyce BF, Doherty VR, Mortimer G. Hyperplastic parathyroiditis—a new autoimmune disease? J Clin Pathol 1982;35:812–4.

83. Brandi ML, Auerbach GD, Fattorossi A, Quarto R, Marx SJ, Fitzpatrick LA. Antibodies cytotoxic to bovine parathyroid cells in autoimmune hypoparathyroidism. Proc Nat'l Acad Sci USA 1986;83:8366–9.

84. Budarf ML, Collins J, Gong W. Cloning a balanced translocation associated with DiGeorge syndrome and identification of a disrupted candidate gene. Nat Genet 1995;10:269–78.

85. Burch WM, Posillico JT. Hypoparathyroidism after I-131 therapy with subsequent return of parathyroid function. J Clin Endocrinol Metab 1983;57:398–401.

86. Chetty R, Forder MD. Parathyroiditis associated with hyperparathyroidism and branchial cysts. Am J Clin Pathol 1991;96:348–50.

87. DiGeorge AM. A new concept of the cellular basis of immunity. J Pediatr 1965;67:907–11.

88. Eisenbarth GS, Jackson RA. Immunogenetics of polyglandular failure and related disease in HLA. In: Forid N, ed. Endocrine and metabolic disorders. New York: Academic Press, 1981:235–64.

89. Eisenbarth GS, Jackson RA. The immunoendocrinopathy syndromes. In: Wilson JD, Foster DW, eds. Williams textbook of endocrinology, 8th ed. Philadelphia: W.B. Saunders, 1992: 1555–66.

90. Gann DS, Paone JF. Delayed hypocalcemia after thyroidectomy for Graves' disease is prevented by parathyroid autotransplantation. Ann Surg 1979;190:508–13.

91. Grimelius L, Akerstrom G, Johansson H, Juhlin C, Rastad J. The parathyroid glands. In: Kovacs K, Asa S, eds. Functional endocrine pathology. Boston: Blackwell Scientific, 1998:381–414.

92. Irvine WJ, Barnes EW. Addisons' disease, ovarian failure and hypoparathyroidism. Clin Endocrinol 1979;4:379–434.

93. Kelly D, Goldberg R, Wilson D, et al. Confirmation that the velocardiofacial syndrome is associated with haplo-insufficiency of genes at chromosome 22q11. Am J Med Genet 1993;45:308–12.

94. Kopin IJ, Rosenberg IN. Idiopathic hypoparathyroidism: report of a case with autopsy findings. Ann Intern Med 1960;53:1238–49.

95. Neufeld M, Maclaren NK, Blizzard RM. Two types of autoimmune Addison's disease associated with different polyglandular autoimmune (PGA) syndromes. Medicine 1981;60:355–62.

96. Parfitt AM. Surgical, idiopathic and other varieties of parathyroid hormone-deficient hypoparathyroidism. In: DeGroot JL, Cahill GF Jr, Odell WD, et al, eds. Endocrinology, vol 2. London: Grune & Stratten, 1979:755–67.

97. Reiner L, Klayman MJ, Cohen RB. Lymphocytic infiltration of the parathyroid glands. Jew Mem Hosp Bull 1962;6-7:103–18.

98. Scully RE, ed. Case record of the Massachusetts General Hospital. Weekly clinicopathological exercises. A 30-year-old woman with an ocular motility disturbance, myopathy and hypocalcemia. Case 34. N Engl J Med 1987;317:493–501.

99. Wilson DI, Burn J, Scambler P, Goodship J. DiGeorge syndrome: part of CATCH 22. J Med Genet 1993;30:852–6.

Cysts and Hamartomas

100. Calandra DB, Shah KH, Prinz RA, et al. Parathyroid cysts: a report of 11 cases including two associated with hyperparathyroid crisis. Surgery 1983;94:887–92.

101. Castleman B, Roth SI. Tumors of the parathyroid glands. Atlas of Tumor Pathology, 2nd Series, Fascicle 14. Washington, D.C.: Armed Forces Institute of Pathology,1978:1–94.

102. DeLellis RA. Tumors of the parathyroid glands. Atlas of Tumor Pathology, 3rd Series, Fascicle 6. Washington, DC: Armed Forces Institute of Pathology, 1993.

103. Haid SP, Method HL, Beal JM. Parathyroid cysts. Report of two cases and a review of the literature. Arch Surg 1967;94:421–6.

104. Hoehn JG, Beahrs OH, Woolner LB. Unusual surgical lesions of the parathyroid gland. Am J Surg 1969;118:770–8.

105. LeGolvan DP, Moore BP, Nishiyama RH. Parathyroid hamartoma: report of two cases and a review of the literature. Am J Clin Pathol 1977;67:31–5.

106. Louis DN, Vickery AL Jr, Rosai J, Wang CA. Multiple branchial cleft-like cysts in Hashimoto's thyroiditis. Am J Surg Pathol 1989;13:45–9.

107. Ober WB, Kaiser GA. Hamartoma of the parathyroid. Cancer 1958;11:601–6.

108. Shields TW, Staley CJ. Functioning parathyroid cysts. Arch Surg 1961;82:937–42.

109. Wang C, Vickery Al Jr, Maloof F. Large parathyroid cysts mimicking thyroid nodules. Ann Surg 1972;175:448–53.

110. Weiland LH, Garrison RC, ReMine WH, Scholz DP. Lipoadenoma of the parathyroid gland. Am J Surg Pathol 1978;2:3–7.

111. Wick MR. Mediastinal cysts and intrathoracic thyroid tumors. Semin Diagn Pathol 1990;7:285–94.

Primary Chief Cell Hyperplasia

112. Akerstrom G, Bergstrom R, Grimelius L, et al. Relation between changes in clinical and histopathological features of primary hyperparathyroidism. World J Surg 1986;10:696–702.

113. Akerstrom G, Rudberg C, Grimelius L, et al. Histologic parathyroid abnormalities in an autopsy series. Hum Pathol 1986;17:520–7.

114. Allo M, Thompson NW. Familial hyperparathyroidism caused by solitary adenomas. Surgery 1982;92:486–90.

115. Altenahr E, Arps H, Montz R, Dorn G. Quantitative ultrastructural and radioimmunologic assessment of parathyroid gland activity in primary hyperparathyroidism. Lab Invest 1979;41:303–12.

116. Arnold A. Genetic basis of endocrine disease. 5. Molecular genetics of parathyroid gland neoplasia. J Clin Endocrinol Metab 1993;77:1108–12.

117. Arnold A. Parathyroid adenomas: clonality in benign neoplasia. In: Cossman J, ed. Molecular genetics in cancer diagnosis. New York: Elsevier, 1990:399–408.

118. Arnold A. Pathogenesis of endocrine tumors In: Wilson JD, Foster DW, Kronenberg HM, Larsen PR, eds. Williams textbook of endocrinology. Philadelphia: WB Saunders, 1998:145–52.

119. Arnold A, Brown MF, Ureña P, Gaz RD, Sarfati G, Drueke TB. Monoclonality of parathyroid tumors in chronic renal failure and not in primary parathyroid hyperplasia. J Clin Invest 1995;95:2047–53.

120. Arnold A, Horst SA, Gardella RJ, et al. Mutation of the signal peptide encoding region of the preproPTH gene in familial isolated hypoparathyroidism. J Clin Invest 1990;86:1087–7.

121. Benson L, Ljunghall S, Akerstrom G, Oberg K. Hyperparathyroidism presenting as the first lesion in multiple endocrine neoplasia type 1. Am J Med 1987;82:731–7.

122. Berg B, Biorklund A, Grimelius L, et al. A new pattern of multiple endocrine adenomatosis: chemodectoma, bronchial carcinoid, GH producing pituitary adenoma, and hyperplasia of the parathyroid glands, and antral and duodenal gastrin cells. Acta Med Scand 1976;200:321–6.

123. Black WC. Correlative light and electron microscopy in primary hyperparathyroidism. Arch Pathol 1969;88:225–41.

124. Black WC, Haff RC. The surgical pathology of parathyroid chief cell hyperplasia. Am J Clin Pathol 1970;53:565–79.

125. Black WC III, Utley JR. The differential diagnosis of parathyroid adenoma and chief cell hyperplasia. Am J Clin Pathol 1968;49:761–75.

126. Bombi JA, Nadal A, Muñoz J, et al. Ultrastructural pathology of parathyroid glands in hyperparathyroidism: a report of 69 cases. Ultrastruct Pathol 1993;17:567–82.

127. Bondeson AG, Bondeson L, Ljungberg O, Tibblin S. Fat staining in parathyroid disease—diagnostic value and impact on surgical strategy:clinicopathologic analysis of 191 cases. Hum Pathol 1985;16:1255–63.

128. Brandi ML. Multiple endocrine neoplasia type I: general features and new insights into etiology. J Endocrinol Invest 1991;14:61–72.

129. Brandi ML, Aurbach GD, Fattorossi A, Quarto R, Marx SJ, Fitzpatrick LA. Antibodies cytotoxic to bovine parathyroid cells in autoimmune hypoparathyroidism. Proc Natl Acad Sci USA 1986;83:8366–9.

130. Brandi ML, Aurbach GD, Fitzpatrick LA, et al. Parathyroid mitogenic activity in plasma from patients with familial multiple endocrine neoplasia type 1. N Engl J Med 1986;314:1287–93.

131. Bringhurst FR, Demay MB, Kronenberg HM. Hormones and disorders of mineral metabolism. In: Wilson JD, Foster DW, Kronenberg HM, Larsen PR, eds. Williams textbook of endocrinology, 9th ed. Philadelphia: WB Sanders, 1998:1155–209.

132. Carney JA, Go VL, Gordon H, Northcutt RC, Pearse AG, Sheps SG. Familial pheochromocytoma and islet cell tumor of the pancreas. Am J Med 1980;68:515–21.

133. Castleman B, Roth SI. Tumors of the parathyroid glands. Atlas of Tumor Pathology, 2nd Series, Fascicle 14. Washington D.C.: Armed Forces Institute of Pathology, 1978:1–94.

134. Chandrasekharappa SC, Guru SC, Manickam P, et al. Positional cloning of the gene for multiple endocrine neoplasia-type 1. Science 1997;276:404–7.

135. Clark OH. Hyperparathyroidism due to primary cystic parathyroid hyperplasia. Arch Surg 1978;113:748–50.

136. Cope O, Keynes WM, Roth SI, Castleman B. Primary chief-cell hyperplasia of the parathyroid glands: a new entity in the surgery of hyperparathyroidism. Ann Surg 1958;148:375–88.

137. Dackiw AP, Sussman JJ, Fritsche HA Jr, et al. Relative contributions of technetium Tc 99m sestamibi scintigraphy, intraoperative gamma probe detection, and the rapid PTH assay to the surgical management of hyperparathyroidism [Review]. Arch Surgery 2000;135:550–5.

138. DeLellis RA. Tumors of the parathyroid glands. Atlas of Tumor Pathology, 3rd Series, Fascicle 6. Washington DC; Armed Forces Institute of Pathology, 1993.

139. DeLellis RA, Dayal Y, Tischler AS, Lee AK, Wolfe HJ. Multiple endocrine neoplasia (MEN) syndromes: cellular origins and inter-relationships. Int Rev Exp Pathol 1986;28:163–215.

140. Erickson LA, Jin L, Wollan P, Thompson GB, van Heerden JA, Lloyd RV. Parathyroid hyperplasias, adenomas and carcinomas. Differential expression of p27^{kip1} protein. Am J Surg Pathol 1999;23:288–95.

141. Fitko R, Roth SI, Hines JR, Roxe DM, Cahill E. Parathyromatosis in hyperparathyroidism. Hum Pathol 1990;21:234–7.

142. Gagel RF, Tashjian AH Jr, Cummings T, et al. The clinical outcome of prospective screening for multiple endocrine neoplasia type 2a. An 18-year experience. N Engl J Med 1988;318:478–84.

143. Golden A, Canary JJ, Kerwin DM. Concurrence of hyperplasia and neoplasia of the parathyroid glands. Am J Med 1965;38:562–78.

144. Hansen OP, Hansen M, Hansen HH, Rose B. Multiple endocrine adenomatosis of mixed type. Acta Med Scand 1976;200:327–31.

145. Kramer WM. Association of parathyroid hyperplasia with neoplasia. Am J Clin Pathol 1970;53:275–83.

146. Larraza-Hernandez O, Albores-Saavedra J, Benavides G, Krause LB, Perez-Merizaldi JC, Ginzo A. Multiple endocrine neoplasia. Pituitary adenoma, multicentric papillary thyroid carcinoma, bilateral carotid body paraganglioma, parathyroid hyperplasia, gastric leiomyoma and systemic amyloidosis. Am J Clin Pathol 1982;78:527–32.

147. Lloyd RV, Iacangelo A, Eiden LE, Cano M, Jin L, Grimes M. Chromogranin A and B messenger ribonucleic acids in pituitary and other normal and neoplastic human endocrine tissues. Lab Invest 1989;60:548–56.

148. Mallette LE, Bilezikian JP, Ketcham AS, Aurbach GD. Parathyroid carcinoma in familial hyperparathyroidism. Am J Med 1974;57:642–8.

149. Mallette LE, Malini S, Rappaport MP, Kirkland JL. Familial cystic parathyroid adenomatosis. Ann Intern Med 1987;107:54–60.

150. Malmaeus J, Benson L, Johansson H, et al. Parathyroid surgery in the multiple endocrine neoplasia type 1 syndrome: choice of surgical procedure. World J Surg 1986;10:668–72.

151. Nilsson O. Studies on the ultrastructure of the human parathyroid glands in various pathologic conditions. Acta Pathol Microbiol Immunol Scand (A) 1977;263[Suppl]:1–88.

152. Palanisamy N, Imanishi Y, Rao PH, Tahara H, Chiganti RS, Arnold A. Novel chromosomal abnormalities identified by comparative genomic hybridization in parathyroid adenomas. J Clin Endocrine Metab 1998;83:1766–70.

153. Palmer JA, Brown WA, Kerr WH, Rosen IB, Watters NA. The surgical aspects of hyperparathyroidism. Arch Surg 1975;110:1004–7.

154. Rattner DW, Marrone GC, Kasdon E, Silen W. Recurrent hyperparathyroidism due to implantation of parathyroid tissue. Am J Surg 1985;149:745–8.

155. Reddick RL, Costa JC, Marx SJ. Parathyroid hyperplasia and parathyromatosis [Letter]. Lancet 1977;1:549.

156. Rode J, Dhillon AP, Cotton PB, Wolfe A, O'Riordan JL. Carcinoid tumour of the stomach and primary hyperparathyroidism—a new association. J Clin Pathol 1987;40:546–51

157. Roslyn JJ, Gordon HE, Mulder DG. Mediastinal parathyroid adenomas. A cause of persistent hyperparathyroidism. Am Surg 1983;49:523.

158. Roth SI. The parathyroid gland. In: Silverberg SG, ed. Principles and practice of surgical pathology, vol 2, 2nd ed. New York: Churchill Livingstone, 1990:1923–55.

159. Roth SI, Gallagher MJ. The rapid identification of "normal" parathyroid glands by the presence of intracellular fat. Am J Pathol 1976;84:521–8.

160. Roth SI, Munger BL. The cytology of adenomatous, atrophic and hyperplastic parathyroid glands of man. A light and electron-microscopic study. Virchows Arch [A] 1962;335:389–410.

161. Rudberg C, Akerstrom G, Palmer M, et al. Late results of operation for primary hyperparathyroidism in 441 patients. Surgery 1986;99:643–51.

162. Russell CF, Grant CS, Van Heerden JA. Hyperfunctioning supernumerary parathyroid glands. An occasional cause of hyperparathyroidism. Mayo Clin Proc 1982;57:121–4.

163. San Juan J, Montoeagudo C, Fraker D, Norton J, Merino M. Significance of mitotic activity and other morphologic parameters in parathyroid adenomas and their correlation with clinical behavior [Abstract]. Am J Clin Pathol 1989;92:523.

164. Schmid KW, Morgan JM, Baumert M, Fischer-Colbrie R, Bocker W, Jasani B. Calcitonin and calcitonin-gene-related peptide mRNA detection in a population of hyperplastic parathyroid cells also expressing chromogranin B. Lab Invest 1995;73:90–5.

165. Simpson NE, Kidd KK, Goodfellow PJ, et al. Assignment of multiple endocrine neoplasia type 2A to chromosome 10 by linkage. Nature 1987; 328:528–30.

166. Snover DC, Foucar K. Mitotic activity in benign parathyroid disease. Am J Clin Pathol 1981;75:345–7.

167. Straus FH, Kaplan EL, Nishiyama RH, Bigos ST. Five cases of parathyroid lipohyperplasia. Surgery 1983;94:901–5.

168. Takiguchi-Shirahama S, Kuyama K, Miyauchi AH, et al. Germ line mutations of the RET proto-oncogene in eight Japanese patients with multiple endocrine neoplasia type 2A (MEN2A). Hum Gen 1995;95:187–90.

169. Wang CA, Rieder SV. A density test for the intraoperative differentiation of parathyroid hyperplasia from neoplasia. Ann Surg 1978;187:63–7.

170. Wei JP, Burke GJ, Mansberger AR Jr. Prospective evaluation of the efficacy of technitium 99m sestamibi and iodine 123 radionuclide imagining of abnormal parathyroid glands. Surgery 1992;112:1111–6.

171. Westra WH, Pritchett DD, Udelsman R. Intraoperative confirmation of parathyroid tissue during parathyroid exploration: a retrospective evaluation of the frozen section. Am J Surg Pathol 1998;22:538–44.

Primary Clear Cell Hyperplasia

172. Albright F, Bloomberg E, Castleman B, Churchill ED. Hyperparathyroidism due to diffuse hyperplasia of all parathyroid glands rather than adenoma of one. Clinical studies on three such cases. Arch Intern Med 1934;54:315–29.

173. Castleman R, Roth SI. Tumors of the parathyroid glands. Atlas of Tumor Pathology. 2nd Series, Fascicle 14. Washington, DC: Armed Forces Institute of Pathology, 1978:1–94.

174. Dawkins RL, Tashjian AH Jr, Castleman B, Moore EW. Hyperparathyroidism due to clear cell hyperplasia. Serial determinations of serum ionized calcium, PTH and calcitonin. Am J Med 1973;54:119–26.

175. DeLellis RA. Tumors of the parathyroid gland. Atlas of Tumor Pathology, 3rd Series, Fascicle 6. Washington, DC: Armed Forces Institute of Pathology, 1993.

176. Dorado AE, Hensley G, Castleman B. Water clear cell hyperplasia of parathyroids: autopsy report of a case with supernumerary glands. Cancer 1976;38:1676–83.

177. Grenko RT, Anderson KM, Kauffman G, Abt AB. Water clear cell adenoma of the parathyroid. A case report with immunohistochemistry and electron microscopy. Arch Pathol Lab Med 1995;119:1072–4.

178. Kovacs K, Horvath E, Ozawa Y, Yamada S, Matushita H. Large clear cell adenoma of the parathyroid in a patient with MEN-1 syndrome. Ultrastructural study of the tumour exhibiting unusual RER formation. Acta Biol Hungarica 1994,45:275–84.

179. Roth SI. The ultrastructure of primary water clear cell hyperplasia of the parathyroid glands. Am J Pathol 1970;61:233–48.

180. Tisell LE, Hedman I, Hansson G. Clinical characterisics and surgical results in hyperparathyroidism caused by water-clear cell hyperplasia. World J Surg 1981;5:565–71.

181. Woolner LB, Keating FR Jr, Black BM. Tumors and hyperplasia of the parathyroid glands. A review of the pathological findings in 140 cases of primary hyperparathyroidism. Cancer 1952;5:1069–88.

Secondary and Tertiary Hyperparathyroidism

182. Akerström G, Malmaeus J, Grimelius L, Ljunghall S, Bergström R. Histological changes in parathyroid glands in subclinical and clinical renal disease. An autopsy investigation. Scand J Urol Nephrol 1984;18:75–84.
183. Altenähr E, Arps H, Montz R, Dorn G. Quantitative ultrastructural and radioimmunologic assessment of parathyroid gland activity in primary hyperparathyroidism. Lab Invest 1979;41:303–12.
184. Arnold A, Brown MF, Urena P, Gaz RD, Sarfati E, Drueke TB. Monoclonality of parathyroid tumors in chronic renal failure and in primary parathyroid hyperplasia. J Clin Invest 1995;95:2047–53.
185. Banerjee SS, Faragher B, Hasleton PS. Nuclear diameter in parathyroid disease. J Clin Pathol 1983;36:143–8.
186. Bowlby LS, DeBault LE, Abraham SR. Flow cytometric DNA analysis of parathyroid glands. Relationship between nuclear RNA and pathologic classification. Am J Pathol 1987;128:338–44.
187. Breslau NA. Update on secondary forms of hyperparathyroidism. Am J Med Sci 1987;294:120–31.
188. Bringhurst FR, Demay MB, Kronenberg HM. Hormones and disorders of mineral metabolism. In: Wilson JD, Foster DW, Kronenberg HM, Larsen PR, eds. Williams textbook of endocrinology, 9th ed. Philadelphia: WB Saunders, 1998:1155–209.
189. Castleman B, Mallory TB. Parathyroid hyperplasia in chronic renal insufficiency. Am J Pathol 1937;13:553–74.
190. Castleman B, Roth SI. Tumors of the parathyroid glands. Atlas of Tumor Pathology, 2nd Series, Fascicle 14. Washington, DC. Armed Forces Institute of Pathology, 1978:1–94.
191. DeLellis RA. Tumors of the parathyroid gland. Atlas of tumor Pathology, 3rd Series, Fascicle 6. Washington, DC: Armed Forces Institute of Pathology, 1993.
192. Fitko R, Roth SI, Hines JR, Roxe DM, Cahill E. Parathyromatosis in hyperparathyroidism. Hum Pathol 1990;21:234–7.
193. Harlow S, Roth SI, Bauer K, Marshall RB. Flow cytometric DNA analysis of normal and pathologic parathyroid glands. Mod Pathol 1991;4:310–5.

194. Hasleton PS, Ali HH. The parathyroid in chronic renal failure—a light and electron microscopical study. J Pathol 1980;132:307–23.
195. Irvin GL, Bagwell CB. Identification of histologically undetectable parathyroid hyperplasia by flow cytometry. Am J Surg 1979;138:567–71.
196. Klempa I, Frei U, Röttger P, Schneider M, Koch KM. Parathyroid autografts—morphology and function: six years' experience with parathyroid autotransplantation in uremic patients. World J Surg 1984;8:540–4.
197. Krause MW, Hedinger CE. Pathologic study of parathyroid glands in tertiary hyperparathyroidism. Hum Pathol 1985;16:772–84.
198. Pappenheimer AM, Wilens SL. Enlargement of the parathyroid glands in renal disease. Am J Path 1935;11:73–91.
199. Roth SI, Marshall RB. Pathology and ultrastructure of the human parathyroid glands in chronic renal failure. Arch Intern Med 1969;124:397–407.
200. Salusky IB, Coburn JW. The renal osteodystrophies. In: DeGroot LJ, ed. Endocrinology, vol 2, 2nd ed. Philadelphia: WB Saunders, 1989:1032–48.
201. San-Juan J, Monteagudo C, Fraker D, Norton J, Merino MJ. Significance of mitotic activity and other morphologic parameters in parathyroid adenomas and their correlation with clinical behavior [Abstract]. Am J Clin Pathol 1989;92:523.
202. Sitges-Serra A, Caralps-Riera A. Hyperparathyroidism associated with renal disease. Pathogenesis, natural history and surgical treatment. Surg Clin North Am 1987;67:359–77.
203. Snover DC, Foucar K. Mitotic activity in benign parathyroid disease. Am J Clin Pathol 1981;75:345–7.
204. St. Goar WT. Case records of the Massachusetts General Hospital (Case 29-1963). Castleman B, Kibbee BO, eds. N Engl J Med 1963;268:943–53.
205. Wallfelt CH, Larsson R, Gunnells E, Ljunghall S, Rastad J, Akerström G. Secretory disturbance in hyperplastic parathyroid nodules of uremic hyperparathyroidism—implication for parathyroid autotransplantation. World J Surg 1988;12:431–8.
206. Wells SA Jr, Ellis GJ, Gunnels JC, Schneider AB, Sherwood LM. Parathyroid autotransplantation in primary parathyroid hyperplasia. N Engl J Med 1976;295:57–62.
207. Wells SA Jr, Gunnells JC, Shelburne JD, Schneider AB, Sherwood LM. Transplantation of the parathyroid glands in man: clinical indications and results. Surgery 1975;78:34–44.
208. Young JL, Varga L, Warren BA. A study of parathyroid hyperplasia in chronic renal failure. Pathology 1994;26:99–109.

3
THYROID GLAND

NORMAL THYROID GLAND

Embryology

The thyroid anlage arises as bilateral vesicular tissue in the foramen cecum of the tongue. Specific proteins, termed transcription factors, are important for thyroid gland development (32) (discussed later). The anlage is visible by day 17 of fetal life as an endodermal structure in the fetal pharynx in close association with the embryonic heart (18,20,24,28). It subsequently descends as part of the thyroglossal duct to the neck. Although the thyroglossal duct usually becomes atrophic, remnants of thyroid tissue may persist along this path of descent. After the thyroglossal duct atrophies, the thyroid anlage begins to expand laterally. Around the seventh week of embryonic life, the median portion of the thyroid anlage meets the lateral thyroid. Between 9 and 12 weeks of development follicle formation continues, and colloid production ensues at 12 weeks. By 14 weeks, well-developed colloid-filled follicles are evident.

The C cells, which are derived from the neural crest (17,22), migrate to the ultimobranchial bodies and are subsequently incorporated into the thyroid gland. The ultimobranchial bodies are derived from branchial pouch complexes IV and V and develop during weeks 5 to 7 of fetal life. Before they regress, at about 9 weeks before term, parathyroid IV separates from the ultimobranchial component. The ultimobranchial bodies have a central and peripheral component consisting of a stratified epithelial cyst, and a more solid component of cells that transforms into a cystic structure.

Anatomy

The macroscopic appearance of the normal adult thyroid gland is that of a bilobate organ in the midportion of the neck, immediately in front of the larynx and trachea (fig. 3-1). The two lobes are joined by the isthmus. Each lobe has a pointed superior pole and a blunt inferior pole. The isthmus lies across the trachea anteriorly below the level of the cricoid cartilage. The right lobe may be longer than the

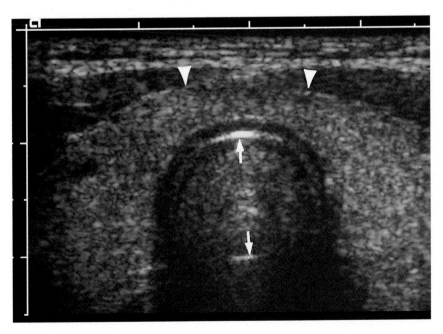

Figure 3-1

NORMAL ADULT THYROID GLAND

Ultrasound of the normal thyroid gland at the level of the isthmus (arrowheads) shows the homogeneous nature of the parenchyma. The gland surrounds the anterior aspect of the air-filled trachea (arrows) on this transverse view.

left and the isthmus may be quite wide in some individuals. About 40 percent of individuals have a pyramidal lobe which is a vestige of the thyroglossal duct.

The normal weight of the adult gland ranges from 15 to 25 g and varies with iodine intake, age, sex, functional status of the gland, size of the individual, and hormonal status. The gland is generally larger and heavier in women than in men and changes during pregnancy and the menstrual cycle, increasing up to 50 percent during the early secretory phase of the cycle (7,12,13).

The thyroid gland has a thin fibrous capsule and septa that divide the gland incompletely into lobules. Incidental nodules may be present in about 10 percent of adult thyroid glands (2). The different types of nodules present in the thyroid are discussed later in this chapter. The parathyroid glands are usually adjacent to the posterior surface of the thyroid gland while the recurrent laryngeal nerves run in the cleft between the trachea and esophagus medially. Enlargement of the thyroid gland can interfere with the normal functions of the recurrent laryngeal nerves and lead to alterations in phonation.

The left superior thyroid arteries, which are branches of the external carotid artery, supply blood to the thyroid gland along with the right and left inferior thyroid arteries, which are derived from the subclavian arteries. Venous outflow includes the internal jugular, the brachycephalic, and sometimes the anterior jugular veins. The lymphatic drainage of the thyroid coalesces in the subcapsular region, and the larger lymphatics leave the gland along with the veins.

The nerve supply to the thyroid originates from the superior and middle cervical sympathetic ganglia. Adrenergic nerve fibers that end near the follicles may also influence thyroid secretion (27).

Histology

The thyroid gland is divided into lobules composed of 20 to 40 follicles supplied by a branch of the thyroid artery. Each follicle can range from 50 to 500 μm, with an average size of 200 μm (figs. 3-2, 3-3). The shape of individual follicles is quite variable. Sanderson polster change is a condition in which a collection of small follicles bulges into the lumen of larger follicles. This can be seen in normal thyroid glands, but is accentuated in hyperplasia.

Follicles contain colloid in their lumina which consists of concentrated periodic acid–Schiff (PAS)-positive thyroglobulin. The tinctorial quality of the colloid may vary with the activity of the follicles, i.e., active follicles usually have weakly eosinophilic and flocculent colloid while inactive follicles tend to have more eosinophilic colloid. Calcium oxalate crystals are often found in normal colloid and consist of anisotropic crystalline material which may become abundant in less active glands or follicles (23).

Normal thyroid tissue may occasionally be encountered outside the thyroid gland. In one study of 56 young adults between 20 to 40 years of age, normal thyroid was found outside the gland in 40 (10). In addition, thyroid tissue was present in the skeletal muscle of the neck in six patients.

Patients with hyperplastic or inflammatory thyroid disease may have involvement of these ectopic foci as well (10). Benign thyroid nodules that are anatomically separate from the thyroid gland are referred to as parasitic nodules (discussed on page 105).

Follicular Cells

Follicular cells have a polar orientation, with the apex directed toward the lumen of the follicle and the base toward the basement membrane. Since the total number of acini does not change with age, any age-related changes probably reflect changes in individual or groups of acini.

Ultrastructural studies of follicular cells show microvilli at the apical portions of the cells (8,15) which enable cilia to project from the central portion of each cell (figs. 3-4, 3-5). The cells have a basement membrane 300 to 400 A° thick at the basal surface. Follicular cells have well-developed desmosomes with terminal bars between the cells. The nuclei of follicular cells are round with diffuse chromatin. Cytoplasmic organelles include small mitochondria, prominent lysosomes, and moderate amounts of rough endoplasmic reticulum.

Immunohistochemical findings in follicular cells include expression of thyroglobulin and low molecular weight keratin; vimentin may be co-expressed (3,6,16,26,27). In situ hybridization studies have shown mRNA for thyroglobulin

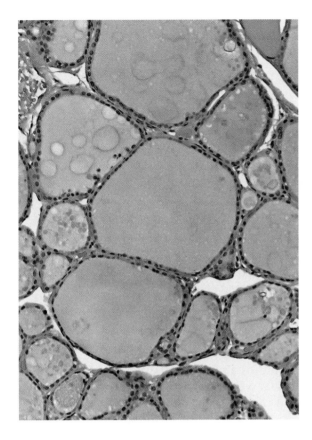

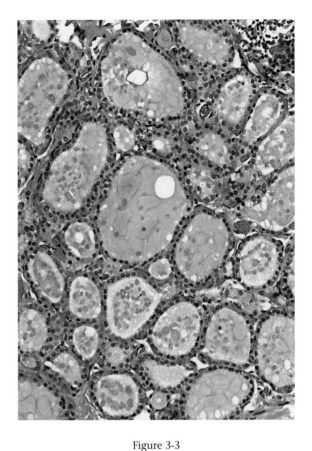

Figure 3-2

NORMAL ADULT THYROID GLAND

Histologic appearance of normal thyroid gland with round to oval follicles.

Figure 3-3

NORMAL ADULT THYROID GLAND

Thyroid gland from a 70-year-old patient. The colloid appears more flocculent and basophilic. These changes are within normal limits but are more common in older individuals.

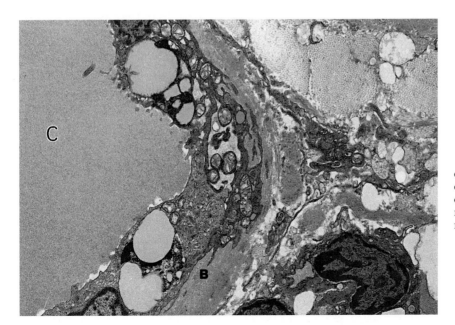

Figure 3-4

NORMAL ADULT THYROID GLAND

Ultrastructural appearance of thyroid follicle. The follicle cells surround the luminal colloid (C). Several follicle cells rest against the basement membrane (B) (X6,457).

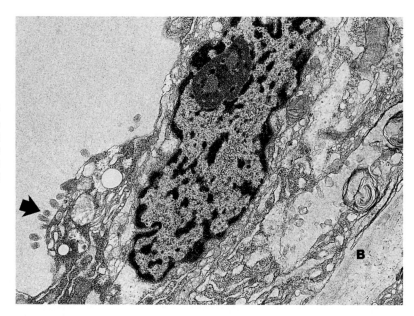

Figure 3-5

NORMAL ADULT THYROID GLAND

Ultrastructural features show follicle cells with low cuboidal epithelium. The basement membrane (B) is located towards the basal portion of the follicle. Luminal cilia (arrow) extend into the colloid (X8,000).

within normal and neoplastic follicular cells (1,21). Squamous metaplasia may be seen in the thyroid with inflammation, neoplastic conditions, and benign nodules (18). Squamous metaplasia may result from stem cell differentiation of inflamed or reparative follicular epithelium towards squamous type (18) and is discussed with Hashimoto's thyroiditis.

C Cells

Calcitonin-producing C cells are often difficult to identify on hematoxylin and eosin (H&E)-stained sections. These cells are usually intrafollicular rather than parafollicular. They have pale to clear cytoplasm and oval nuclei. They can be readily identified with argyrophilic stains such as the Grimelius reaction or with lead hematoxylin stains. C cells are located predominantly in the middle and upper third of the lateral lobes; the upper and lower poles are essentially devoid of C cells. They are more numerous in neonates, decrease in the adult thyroid gland, and increase after 60 years of age. C cells constitute about 0.1 percent of the mass of the normal adult gland.

Immunohistochemical stains can readily identify C cells. They are positive for broad-spectrum neuroendocrine markers such as chromogranin A and synaptophysin as well as for specific peptides including calcitonin, calcitonin gene–related peptide, somatostatin, gastrin-releasing peptide, or bombesin (5,25,30). Immunostaining may be positive for low molecular weight keratin, neuron-specific enolase, and carcinoembryonic antigen.

Ultrastructural examination supports the observation that the C cells are intrafollicular and are separated from the thyroid interstitium by the follicular basal lamina. They contain two types of secretory granules: type I measure 280 nm and are moderately electron dense while type II are smaller (130 nm) and more electron dense. Ultrastructural immunohistochemical studies show calcitonin in both type I and type II granules (4).

In situ hybridization studies have localized calcitonin and calcitonin gene–related product mRNA in C cells (9,31).

Solid Cell Nests

Solid cell nests (SCN) are a third cell type commonly seen in the normal thyroid gland. They are usually found in the posterolateral or posteromedial portion of the lateral lobes of the gland and probably represent ultimobranchial body rests (11,29). They are often small, measuring 0.1 mm or less in diameter. They consist of polygonal to oval cells with oval nuclei and finely granular chromatin; nuclear grooves may be present. Other cells may have round nuclei and clear cytoplasm (fig. 3-6). SCN are found in 3 percent of routinely examined thyroid

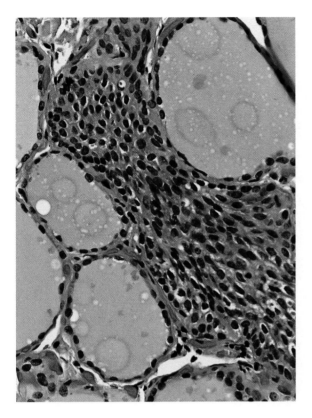 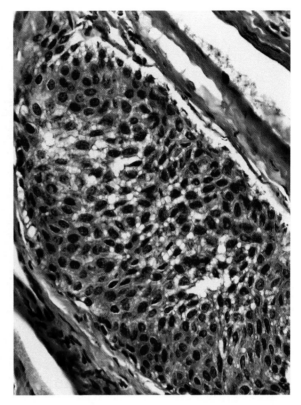

Figure 3-6

SOLID CELL NEST

Left: Solid cell nest in the normal thyroid gland. These ultimobranchial body nests are made up of polygonal to oval cells with oval nuclei.

Right: Higher magnification shows the granular chromatin of the nuclei.

glands and in one study in 61 percent of glands that were examined (11).

Ultrastructural studies show cells with desmosomes, intermediate filaments, and intraluminal cytoplasmic projections. Immunohistochemical studies show positive staining for low molecular weight keratin, and some expression of calcitonin, although this is not a consistent finding (14,19). Cells may also stain for polyclonal carcinoembryonic antigen.

In addition to the stromal elements, other types of cells and tissues that may be found in the thyroid include mature fat, cartilage, ectopic thymus, and intrathyroidal, parathyroidal, and skeletal muscle.

Physiology

The thyroid gland produces three hormones which have a wide range of effects on physiologic homeostasis. The follicular cells produce thyroxine (T4) and triiodothyronine (T3) (fig. 3-7), while the C cells produce calcitonin. The principal function of the thyroid gland is to produce thyroid hormones to meet the demands of the peripheral tissues. The feedback mechanism of the pituitary gland and hypothalamus helps to regulate thyroid function (fig. 3-8). The hypothalamus produces thyrotropin-releasing hormone which regulates thyroid-stimulating hormone (TSH) production and secretion by the anterior pituitary (44,56,63,65).

Exogenous iodine is required for the synthesis of about 100 μg of T4 daily by the thyroid gland (48). Iodine balance is maintained by dietary sources, but many conditions can modify the iodine intake, such as medications, dietary supplements, and food additives. A series of reactions govern the synthesis and production

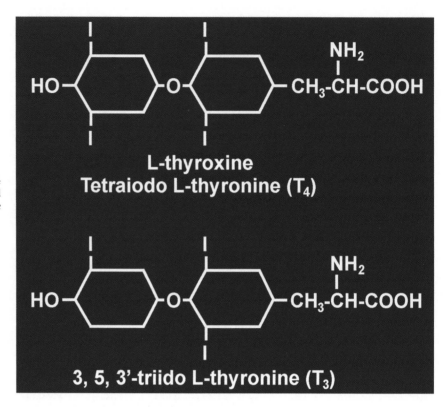

Figure 3-7

THYROXINE AND TRIIODOTHYRONINE

The chemical structures of T4 and T3 produced in the thyroid gland. T4 has one more iodine molecule than T3.

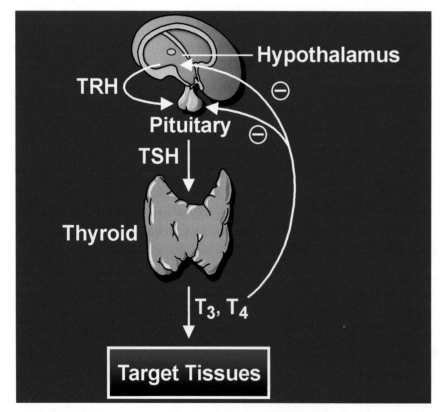

Figure 3-8

THYROID HOMEOSTASIS

The negative feedback mechanism between the hypothalamus, pituitary, thyroid, and end organs regulate thyroid homeostasis. The hypothalamus produces thyrotropin-releasing hormone (TRH) which stimulates the release of thyroid-stimulating hormone (TSH) from the pituitary. TSH in turn stimulates the synthesis of thyroxine (T4) and triiodothyronine (T3), and the T3 and T4 feedback on the pituitary and hypothalamus to help regulate the hypothalamic-pituitary-thyroid axis.

of thyroid hormone from dietary sources (see fig. 3-2). The first step involves trapping and concentrating iron from dietary sources and from the recycling of degraded thyroid hormone by the body. Iodine intake varies with geographic location. A minimum of 60 mg of iodine/day is required for thyroid hormone synthesis and it is estimated that at least 100 mg/day is required to eliminate all signs of iodine deficiency from the population (48).

In the body iodine is confined largely to the extracellular fluid, and most of it is cleared by the kidneys and thyroid gland. The thyroid gland contains the largest part of body iodine (about 8 mg), most of which is in the form of free iodine and amino acids.

Once iodine is in the thyroid gland, it is oxidized to the organic form. This reaction involves the enzyme thyroid peroxidase (TPO) located in the apical cell membrane of the follicle. Hydrogen peroxide (H_2O_2) and TPO iodinate tyrosyl residues within thyroglobulin (Tg) to yield hormonally inactive iodotyrosines. Iodotyrosines are coupled in Tg to iodothyronines, the hormonally active T3 and T4. Release of T3 and T4 during hydrolysis of Tg involves reuptake of colloid at the apical thyroid cell membrane. This is followed by proteolysis of Tg, which releases free iodinated amino acids and iodothyronines into the circulation. Intrathyroidal deiodination of the iodotyrosines released during Tg hydrolysis results in free iodine which is reutilized by the gland for further thyroid hormone synthesis. Various proteins are required for thyroid hormone synthesis, including Tg, TPO, and TSH receptors to regulate TSH signaling for optimum hormone synthesis. Transcription factors, which are nuclear proteins, are also required for thyroid hormone synthesis and include a thyroid transcription factor, PAX8. These factors regulate the activity of the Tg and TPO genes in the thyroid gland (57).

During thyroid hormone synthesis, iodine is oxidized and incorporated with monoiodotyrosine (MIT) and diiodotyrosine (DIT) (52,65a). Oxidation occurs in the large Tg molecule. Synthesis of T4 in the Tg molecule requires a coupling reaction in which two DIT molecules fuse. For T3 and T4 to be synthesized efficiently, Tg has to be present. The Tg gene is very large (more than 260 kb) and is located on chromosome 8 (40).

The thyroid gland has the largest store of hormones among endocrine glands, and it has a low rate of hormonal turnover (1 percent/day). Tg is present in the plasma of normal individuals and may range up to 50 ng/mL. The source of this Tg is from molecules that have leaked from the thyroid lymphatics. In patients with thyroid cancer, the plasma Tg concentration may be very elevated.

During the process of thyroid hormone release, colloid from the follicular lumen is endocytosed by the processes of macropinocytosis and micropinocytosis. The former process occurs by pseudopods at the apical membranes while the latter occurs by smaller coated vesicles at the apical surface. Both forms of pinocytosis are regulated by TSH. T4 is resorbed within the thyroid cells and then transferred into the plasma, and this process is also regulated by TSH (47).

Autoradiographic studies of the thyroid gland have provided insight into its anatomy and physiology. Variations in different areas of the gland and in different follicles are noted by this procedure.

The breakdown of Tg and the release of T4 and T3 are inhibited by various chemicals including iodine. Iodine is known to inhibit the stimulation of thyroid adenylate cyclase by TSH and by the thyroid-stimulating immunoglobulins that are present in Graves' disease. Calcitonin, which is produced by the C cells, has a general physiologic effect of lowering serum calcium by acting on bone, kidney, and gastrointestinal tract (34). Although calcitonin inhibits bone resorption and increases calcium and phosphate excretion, it probably has a minor role in calcium homeostasis in humans (34).

Drugs Inhibitory to Thyroid Hormone Synthesis

A wide spectrum of drugs can inhibit thyroid hormone synthesis. Because of the negative feedback mechanism, decreased levels of thyroid hormone lead to elevated TSH secretion and enlargement of the thyroid gland from TSH stimulation. Antithyroid agents generally belong to two groups: agents inhibiting thyroid iodine transport and agents inhibiting the organic binding and coupling reactions. Chemicals in the first group include thiocyanate and perchlorate which had been used clinically in the past. Chemicals in the second group include thioamides such as propylthiouracil, methimazole, and phenylbutazone.

Lithium has antithyroid activity. It inhibits organic binding reactions as well as thyroid hormone release, but its mechanism of action is not well understood (35,59). Certain natural foods also contain antithyroid chemicals. Members of the genus Brassica, including cabbage, rutabaga, turnips, and kohlrabi, contain thiocyanates (41). The vegetable cassava contains a cyanogenic glycoside, linamarin, which is metabolized to thiocyanate, so ingestion of cassava can lead to the development of goiters in areas of the world with endemic iodine deficiency.

Peripheral Effects of Thyroid Hormone

Thyroid hormone in plasma is bound to several proteins, mainly thyroxine-binding globulin (TBG) and transthyretin (TTR) or T4-binding prealbumin. T4 and T3 may also bind to albumin which has a low binding affinity for thyroid hormone. About 10 percent of the plasma thyroid hormone is associated with albumin.

T4 is converted to T3 by deiodination in the 5' position, which accounts for about 30 to 40 percent of secreted converted T4. It is T3 that regulates gene expression in thyroid hormone target tissues (62). The conversion of T4 to T3 may be impaired by various conditions including trauma and certain diseases like the euthyroid sick syndrome. This latter condition may be caused by fasting, malnutrition, and hepatic and renal dysfunction, as well as certain drugs such as propylthiouracil, glucocorticoids, propranolol, and amiodarone (38,61,62).

Abnormal Amounts of Iodine

Abnormalities can result from increased or decreased amounts of dietary iodine.

Iodine Excess. Increased amounts of iodine can lead to decreased yields of organic iodine or a relative blockage of organic iodine binding (Wolff-Chaikoff effect) (64). An increase in the iodine-trapping mechanism or impairment of organic iodine formation can lead to goiter or hypothyroidism in patients without Graves' disease or in those patients who have not received radioiodine therapy. Treatment with iodine leads to decreased vascularity and hyperplasia of the thyroid gland as is seen with Graves' disease before surgical resection (51).

Iodine Deficiency. Decreased amounts of iodine in the diet lead to a rapid decrease in serum thyroid hormone (48) and a compensatory increase in TSH. Although T4 levels are low, T3 synthesis is maintained during the development of a goiter (33). With iodine deficiency, other compensatory changes occur including an increase in the conversion of monoiodotyrosine to diiodotyrosine. TSH stimulates thyroid follicular cell replication leading to the development of a goiter (36,37).

Amiodarone Toxicity

Amiodarone is a drug used to treat patients with cardiac arrhythmias. Because it contains a large amount of iodine, it can lead to hyperthyroidism (43,46,51,53,58,61) as well as producing toxic side effects in many other organs including the lungs and liver.

The clinical manifestations of amiodarone toxicity in the thyroid gland range from myxedema to hyperthyroidism. It has been postulated that amiodarone interferes with thyroid hormone production and/or degradation. Morphologic changes in patients with hyperthyroidism include follicular disruption, vacuolization of follicular epithelial cells, and infiltration of macrophages and lymphocytes into areas of degenerating follicles (figs. 3-9, 3-10). Ultrastructural studies have shown lysosomes in the disrupted vacuolated cells with prominent lamellar configurations (figs. 3-11, 3-12) (58). It is thought that the release of colloid from the destroyed follicles may lead to increased thyroid hormone levels and hyperthyroidism.

Diphenylhydantoin (Phenytoin)

This drug is used to treat epileptic disorders. It competes with thyroxine for thyroxine-binding globulin-binding sites (55) and decreases T4 production (51). Diphenylhydantoin can induce thyroiditis possibly by inducing an autoimmune reaction with the thyroid gland as the target organ (48,49).

Reactive Changes

Pregnancy. The functioning of the thyroid gland undergoes marked changes during and after pregnancy (42,45). Total serum T4 and T3 levels increase to circulating concentrations twice as high as in nonpregnant women (39,45). The increased thyroid hormone levels

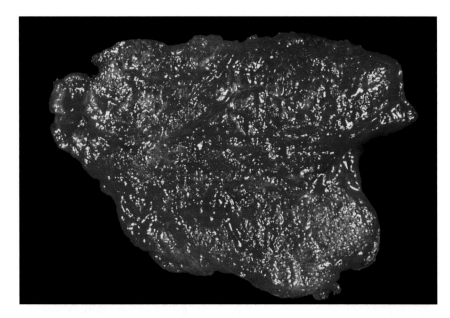

Figure 3-9

AMIODARONE TOXICITY

This patient was treated with amiodarone for cardiac arrhythmia and developed amiodarone toxicity which led to the removal of the thyroid gland. The gross appearance of the thyroid on cut section is beefy red and similar to normal thyroid.

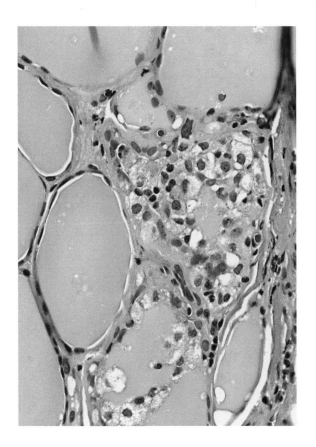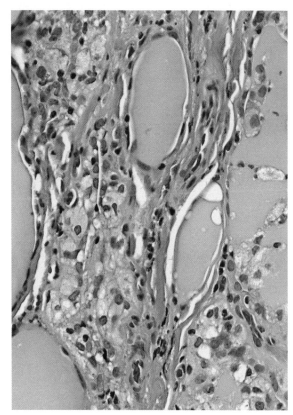

Figure 3-10

AMIODARONE TOXICITY

Left: Histologic change includes follicular disruption.

Right: There is also vacuolization of follicular epithelial cells with infiltrates of macrophages, and scattered lymphocytes.

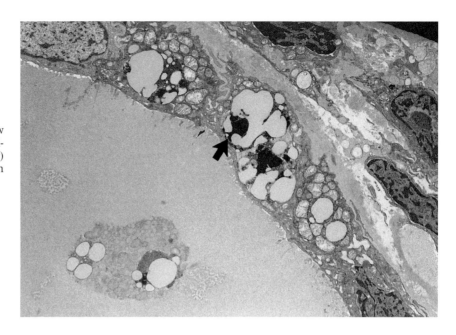

Figure 3-11

AMIODARONE TOXICITY

Ultrastructural studies show prominent cytoplasmic vacuolization with lysosomes (arrow) and a lamellar configuration (X3,000).

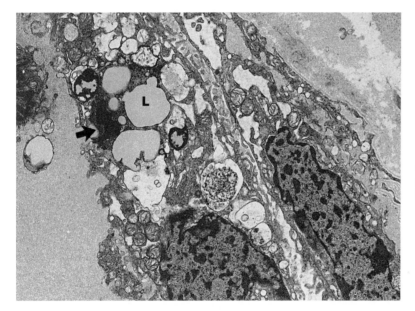

Figure 3-12

AMIODARONE TOXICITY

Higher magnification of figure 3-11 shows prominent lysosomes (arrow) with lipid (L) accumulation in the cytoplasm. A macrophage in the colloid is noted on the left (X6,000).

are partially explained by increased levels of thyroglobulin. There is no clinically significant change in the size of the thyroid gland during pregnancy in normal women receiving adequate amounts of iodine, but with iodine deficiency, a goiter can develop more easily than in the normal gland because of the increased demand for thyroid hormone. Clinical thyrotoxicosis can develop in patients with hydatidiform moles or choriocarcinoma because of an increase in T3 and T4 (54).

Neonates and the Aged. There is a TSH surge in neonates within the first 30 minutes of extrauterine life. Reverse T3 levels increase during the first 24 hours and then decrease by 10 days after birth. Serum T3 levels are slightly higher in the first year of life but gradually fall to the normal adult range (60).

Serum T3 concentrations remain in the normal range into the seventh and eighth decades of life (50).

Postpartum Thyroiditis. Transient thyrotoxicities may develop 3 to 12 months after delivery. They are often followed by a period of hypothyroidism which may last for several months before an eventual return to the euthyroid state. This occurs in about 10 percent of women in the general population and in more than 30 percent of women with a positive test for thyroid peroxidase autoantibodies (41).

HEREDITARY AND DEVELOPMENTAL DISORDERS

Transcription Factor Deficiencies

Transcription factors are proteins produced by specific cell types which regulate gene activity by interacting with nuclear DNA. They affect developmental differentiation and the regulation of specific genes in adults. The activity of transcription factors is considered the principal switch that regulates gene expression (73). There are several transcription factors that are specific for development and regulation of thyroid follicular cells. These include thyroid transcription factor (TTF)-1, TTF-2, and PAX8 (69, 71–73,76, 77,79). These genes regulate the transcription of thyroglobulin and thyroid peroxidase genes and influence the expression of the TSH receptor (66,78). Deficiency of TTF-1 has been associated with congenital goiter. Other deficiencies or decreased expression of transcription factors that lead to thyroid disease will be reported in the future as knowledge about existing thyroid transcription factors increases and more thyroid-specific transcription factors are described.

Genetic Disorders of the Thyrotropin Receptor Gene

Genetic alterations in the thyrotropin receptor gene can lead to nonautoimmune hyperthyroidism. Various families with hyperthyroidism due to genetic alterations in the thyrotropin receptor gene have been identified (67,68,70,73,75).

The thyrotropin receptor is encoded by 10 exons on chromosome 14 and is 58 kb in length. A number of splice variants of the receptor have been described (74). The receptor is coupled to the alpha subunit of the guanine-nucleotide–binding protein stimulatory subunit (Gs α) which activates adenylate cyclase and increases the accumulation of cyclic adenosine monophosphate (AMP).

There have been isolated case reports of congenital hyperthyroidism due to mutations in the thyrotropin receptor gene (75). In one report, four families had loss of function mutations of the TSH receptor gene (74). In all the patients the plasma TSH concentration was increased while T3 and T4 concentrations were normal. The TSH levels were normal in the heterozygous parents, indicating the recessive nature of these TSH receptor mutations.

Aplasia and Hypoplasia

These conditions denote a total or partial absence of the thyroid gland. Aplasia and hypoplasia are the most common causes of congenital hypothyroidism. In North America, permanent abnormalities leading to hypothyroidism occur in 1 in 3,000 to 4,000 live births (80b). Some infants may have hemiagenesis or aplasia of one lobe of the thyroid gland; this is seen more commonly in the left lobe and is not associated with functional defects. Patients with DiGeorge's syndrome in which there is arrested development of the parathyroid glands and thymus associated with the third and fourth branchial pouches also have arrested thyroid C-cell development (80,80a).

Aberrant (Ectopic) Thyroid Tissue

Thyroid tissue may be located in an abnormal location along the thyroglossal duct tract or at another site. Along the thyroglossal tract it may be localized in a lingual, sublingual, supralymphoid, or intrathyroid location (fig. 3-13). Ectopic thyroid has been reported in the pericardium, heart, chest wall, vagina, inguinal region, and porta hepatis (82,83,85,93,95,96,98).

Lingual thyroid tissue results from failure of the medial anlage to descend from the pharynx so that it remains at the base of the tongue (figs. 3-14, 3-15). This may be the only thyroid tissue in some patients and surgical excision can lead to hypothyroidism.

The presence of normal-appearing thyroid tissue in lymph nodes most commonly represents metastatic papillary carcinoma to lymph nodes (81,89,91,92), especially if the thyroid tissue is present within the nodes lateral to the jugular vein (89). Some authors have suggested that normal-appearing thyroid tissue in lymph nodes may represent ectopic thyroid rather than metastatic carcinoma (91): a recent report using molecular techniques suggested that ectopic thyroid tissue in the tongue and bilateral neck nodes represents normal thyroid tissue because of a polyclonal pattern on clinical analysis (88), but this finding is extremely uncommon.

Thyroglossal Duct Cysts

Definition. The persistence of the thyroglossal duct leading to the development of cysts or fistulas.

Clinical Features. The connection between the median anlage of the thyroid gland, the foramen cecum, and the descended thyroid gland is the thyroglossal duct. Thyroglossal duct cysts can occur at any age. They are located at or below the thyroid lobe in the anterior midline of the neck (fig. 3-16). If the cysts become infected a fistula may develop (86,87,97,99).

Macroscopic Findings. Cysts can vary greatly in size, but most are between 1 and 4 cm in diameter (fig. 3-17). Fistulas may develop secondary to infection and may open into the pharynx or skin, with subsequent spontaneous or surgically-induced drainage.

Microscopic Findings. The cysts are lined by ciliated respiratory epithelium which often undergoes squamous metaplasia (fig. 3-18). Thyroid follicles may be seen in the cyst wall on careful sectioning. With chronic infection and inflammation the epithelial lining may be lost and granulation tissue and fibrosis may be seen microscopically. With the appropriate clinical setting, a diagnosis of inflamed, fibrotic thyroglossal duct cyst can be made even in the absence of an epithelial lining.

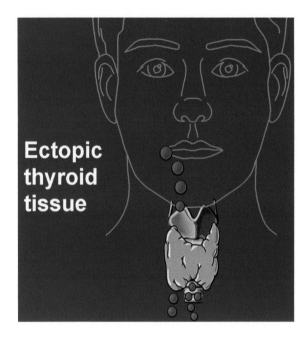

Figure 3-13

ECTOPIC THYROID

Diagrammatic illustration of sites of potential ectopic thyroid tissue in adults.

Figure 3-14

LINGUAL THYROID TISSUE

An iodine-131 scan localized thyroid tissue in the posterior portion of the tongue. Intense iodine uptake is seen in the anterior and left lateral views.

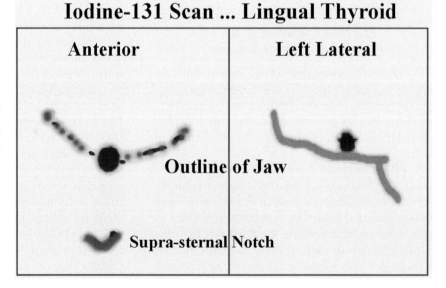

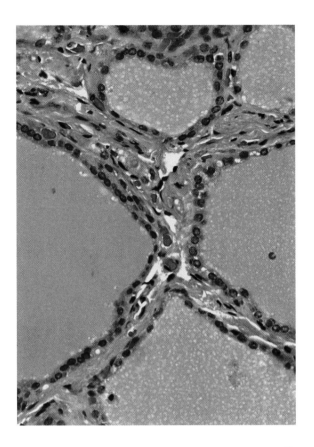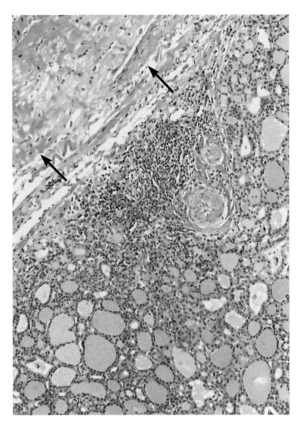

Figure 3-15

ECTOPIC THYROID TISSUE

Left: Ectopic thyroid tissue from the posterior tongue shows colloid follicles with cuboidal epithelium. This tissue may be mistaken for metastatic thyroid carcinoma; however, the cytologic features are benign.

Right: Ectopic thyroid tissue from the right ventricle. Myocardial muscle is present in the upper left (arrow).

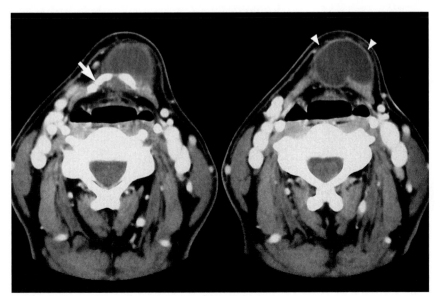

Figure 3-16

THYROGLOSSAL DUCT CYST

Left: This cyst is intimately associated with the hyoid bone (arrow) and characteristic of a thyroglossal duct cyst.

Right: Contrast-enhanced CT scans show a fluid density structure in the soft tissues of the anterior neck (arrowheads).

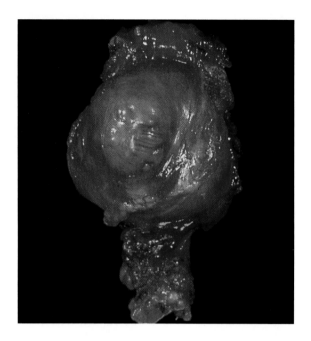
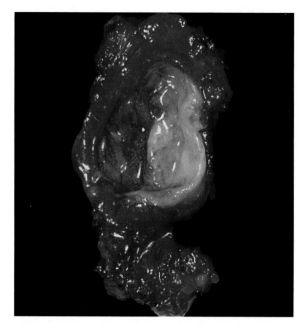

Figure 3-17

THYROGLOSSAL DUCT CYST

Left: Gross appearance of a thyroglossal duct cyst with a fluid-filled tense external surface.
Right: Cut surface shows the viscous brown fluid in the cyst lumen.

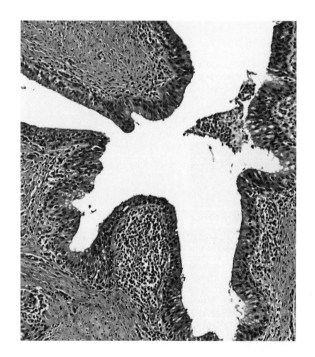
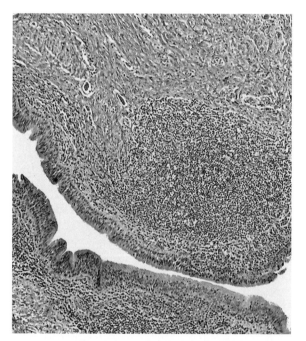

Figure 3-18

THYROGLOSSAL DUCT CYST

Left: Histologic section shows the cyst lined by epithelium and lymphoid follicles in the cyst wall.
Right: Ciliated respiratory epithelium and lymphoid aggregates.

Differential Diagnosis. Other benign cysts such as epidermoid cysts may be present in the thyroid gland. These cysts are lined by squamous epithelium and are filled with keratin, and the cell mass is not surrounded by lymphoid follicles (fig. 3-19). Cystic degeneration of colloid nodules may also be seen with adjacent multinodular goiters. In thyroglossal duct cysts, the midline location and distinct lining with lymphoid follicles are helpful in establishing the diagnosis.

Treatment and Prognosis. The treatment of thyroglossal duct cyst is surgical excision of the entire tract of the duct extending to the foramen cecum to prevent recurrence.

One complication of these cysts is the development of thyroid carcinoma. Most carcinomas that develop from thyroglossal ducts are papillary carcinomas, although Hurthle's cell and anaplastic thyroid tumors have been reported (90,94). Medullary thyroid carcinomas have not been reported because of the absence of C cells in this midline structure. Thyroglossal duct cancers constitute less than 1 percent of all thyroid cancers. Most occur in adults, although they have developed in a few children under age 10 (90). These tumors may metastasize to lymph nodes, as with other thyroid papillary carcinomas. Surgical treatment consists of removal of the middle portion of the thyroid gland, including the suprathyroid tract up to the foramen cecum, to prevent recurrences.

Parasitic Nodule

Definition. A parasitic nodule is a thyroid nodule in the neck that is anatomically separate from the main thyroid gland which is usually multinodular.

Clinical Features. This is an infrequently reported condition, although it may be seen in different clinical settings (102,105). Conditions labeled as aberrant lateral thyroid and some cases diagnosed as metastatic thyroid carcinoma usually represent parasitic nodules. The parasitic nodule probably results from a colloid or hyperplastic nodule located outside the thyroid gland. It becomes enlarged and migrates laterally in the neck. In some cases it is connected to the thyroid gland by a thin fibrous strand of vascular tissue, while in other cases it may be completely separate and obtain its blood supply from the surrounding tissues.

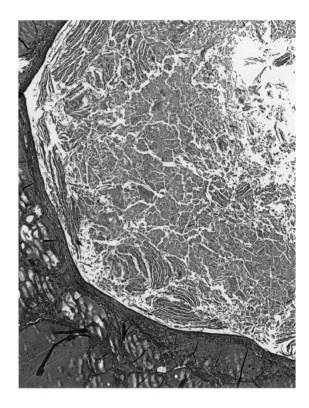

Figure 3-19

EPIDERMOID CYST

A midline epidermoid cyst of the thyroid gland is lined by squamous epithelium, with keratin debris in the lumen.

Macroscopic Findings. The nodule may vary from 1 to over 4 cm in size. A connection to the thyroid by a fibrovascular pedicle is often apparent at surgery with careful dissection (fig. 3-20).

Microscopic Findings. The histologic appearance of parasitic nodule is usually that of normal thyroid tissue with dilated colloid-filled and/or hyperplastic follicles (fig. 3-21). Comparison to the orthotopic thyroid gland shows similar histologic features.

In some cases in which there is also Hashimoto's thyroiditis, the presence of many lymphoid cells may simulate a lymph node, especially in a small biopsy specimen. The pseudoground glass nuclei that are sometimes seen in Hashimoto's thyroiditis can simulate papillary carcinoma and this can be a pitfall in the histologic evaluation of parasitic nodules. In a recent case report, a 67-year-old Japanese woman with Graves' disease had a 1.5 cm parasitic nodule with a dense lymphocytic infiltrate that simulated a

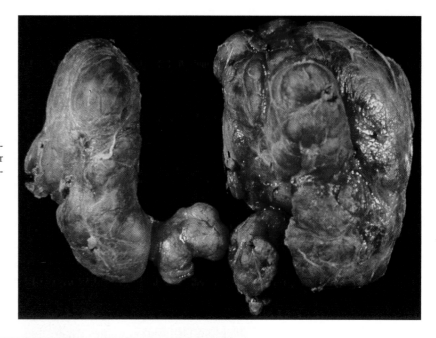

Figure 3-20

PARASITIC NODULE

Multinodular goiter with sequestered nodules is attached to the lower poles of the gland by a thin fibrovascular pedicle.

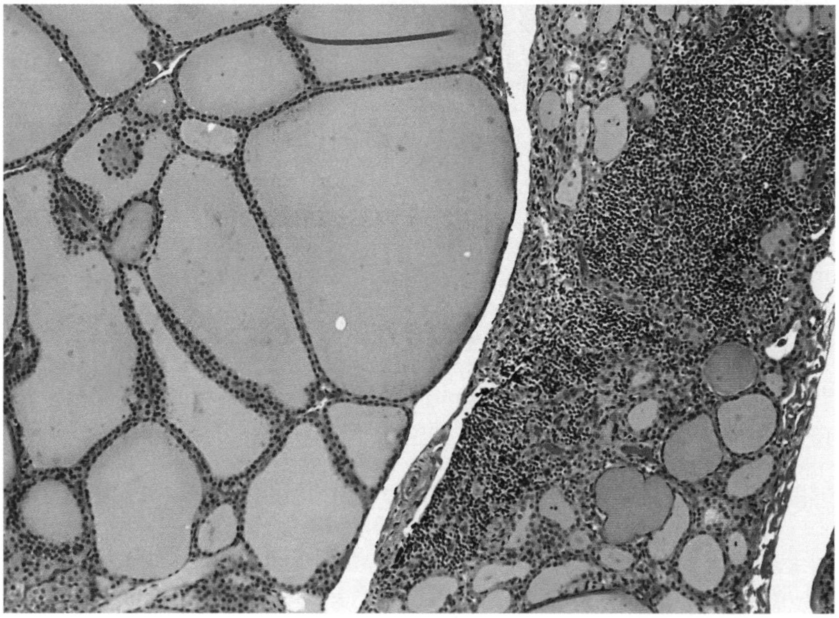

Figure 3-21

PARASITIC NODULE

Parasitic nodule composed of dilated, colloid-filled follicles lined by flattened epithelium. If lymphocytes are present in the background, these lesions can be mistaken for carcinoma metastatic to lymph nodes because of the physical separation from the thyroid gland. The histologic and cytologic features are those of benign thyroid tissue.

lymph node (104). Parasitic nodules may also simulate a carotid body tumor (100).

The differential diagnosis of parasitic nodule includes metastatic papillary and follicular carcinomas. It also includes mechanical implantation of thyroid tissue into the soft tissues of the neck from previous surgery or accidental trauma. The presence of suture material along with fibrosis may be a clue to previous surgery (101,103). This condition may be similar to the parathyromatosis that may occur after surgical implantation of parathyroid tissue in the neck.

Radiation Changes

Radiation changes in the thyroid gland are dependent on the dose and type of administration of the radioactive isotope (106–108, 110,111). A dose of radiation less than 15 Grenz can lead to nodular hyperplasia of the thyroid. These changes are seen in thyroid tissue after the

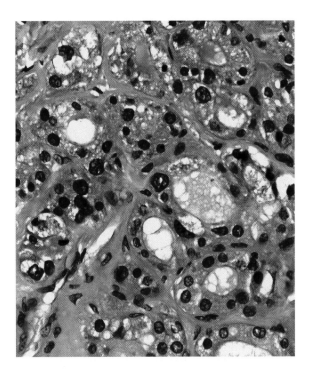 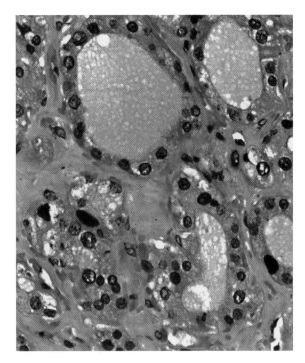

Figure 3-22

RADIATION CHANGES

Thyroid tissue from a patient treated with iodine 131 for Graves' disease before surgery.
Left: There is marked nuclear pleomorphism. The stroma shows moderate fibrosis with pleomorphic follicular epithelial cells.
Right: Higher magnification shows the marked nuclear pleomorphism.

radiation of tonsils or other structures adjacent to the thyroid gland. Acute changes in the thyroid gland include follicular disruption, focal hemorrhagic necrosis, and neutrophilic infiltration (110). In one study there was a decrease in radioactive uptake and serum thyroxine levels between 2 days and 2 months after thyroid radiation (106).

Patients irradiated as treatment for lymphomas have striking changes in the thyroid that include hypercellularity, cytologic atypia with hyperchromasia, increased nodule size and pleomorphism, fibrosis, and chronic thyroiditis (106). Patients receiving radioactive iodine may have variable changes in the thyroid: the cytologic atypia and hypercellularity seen with external irradiation may occur or the changes may be more subtle (fig. 3-22) (107,111).

Although it is well documented that external radiation can lead to an increased incidence of thyroid cancer (109,112), the relationship between treatment with radioactive iodine and thyroid tumor development is less certain.

MISCELLANEOUS CONDITIONS

Langerhans' Cell Granulomatosis (Histiocytosis X or Eosinophilic Granuloma)

Exceptional cases of Langerhans' cell granulomatosis involving the thyroid gland have been reported (114,117). The disease may be associated with papillary thyroid carcinoma (116). The histologic picture of Langerhans' cells with the appropriate background of eosinophils and other benign cells is diagnostic, as is immunohistochemical staining for CD1a and the finding of Birbeck granules by ultrastructural studies (114,116,117).

Sinus Histiocytosis with Massive Lymphadenopathy

Rare cases of sinus histiocytosis with massive lymphadenopathy have been reported in the thyroid gland (113,115,116). When the thyroid is involved it may represent an extension from adjacent lymph nodes. In one reported case, the clinical picture was similar to subacute thyroiditis (115).

The microscopic appearance of the thyroid gland is similar to that in other extranodal sites, with numerous histiocytes with large vesicular nuclei and abundant clear cytoplasm; some histiocytes show emperipolesis.

Plasma Cell Granuloma

This tumor-like condition affecting the thyroid gland consists of inflammatory infiltrates of mainly mature plasma cells with Russell's bodies and other inflammatory cells including lymphocytes (118,119). Immunohistochemical stains or in situ hybridization analysis shows that the plasma cells are polyclonal and express both kappa and lambda light chains.

Scleroderma

Patients with progressive systemic sclerosis or scleroderma may have involvement of the thyroid gland (120–122). Thyroid involvement is manifested by thyroid dysfunction with abnormal thyroid tests. Microscopic examination of the gland shows fibrosis and a chronic lymphocytic infiltrate. Rare cases of scleroderma developing in patients with Graves' disease have been reported (122).

METABOLIC DISEASES

Metabolic diseases involving the thyroid gland are uncommon and only a few reports are well documented in the literature (123–125).

Glycogenosis

Glycogen storage diseases have been reported in the thyroid gland in a few cases (124). Patients with Pompe's disease (type IIA glycogenesis) have lysosomal accumulation of glycogen in many tissues due to a deficiency of the lysosomal enzyme acid alpha-1-4-glucosidase. The disease is associated with muscle weakness, cardiomegaly, respiratory failure, and death. One study (124) reported accumulation of glycogen in the thyroid gland of patients with Pompe's disease.

Cystinosis

This disease is inherited as an autosomal recessive condition and is characterized by intracellular deposits of cystine (123). In some cases it is associated with hypothyroidism (125). It is possible that the cystine crystals produce follicular atrophy which leads to the clinically observed hypothyroidism.

The presence of pituitary thyrotroph hyperplasia indicates that the thyroid condition is primary with secondary hyperplasia of pituitary cells (123). Microscopically, the gland shows follicular atrophy with fibrosis and decreased amounts of colloid. These are focal areas of papillary hyperplasia with dilated follicles and focal acute inflammation (123). Frozen section examination of the thyroid tissue usually shows cystine crystals, but these are usually not seen in fixed tissue sections.

Lipidoses

This group of diseases, known historically as *amaurotic familial idiocy,* is associated with severe mental retardation. Lipofuscin-like pigment accumulates in neurons, autonomic ganglia, muscle, and other cells. The thyroid gland has been reported to be involved in some cases (126–128).

Follicular epithelial cells have yellow, autofluorescent pigmented granules which represent lipofuscin. Ultrastructural examination of the thyroid shows the osmophilic characteristic deposits in the cytoplasm of follicular cells as is seen in the brain, muscle, and other tissues.

Some patients with Batten-Speilmeyer-Vogt disease have hypothyroidism and there is decreased or absent thyroid peroxidase activity (126).

Iron Pigment Accumulation

Disorders of iron metabolism, including cases in which trauma is associated with degeneration and hemorrhage, can lead to iron deposition in thyroid follicular cells. Most cases are not associated with thyroid dysfunction. However, with severe pituitary involvement secondary to iron overload, secondary hypothyroidism may develop (129,130).

The gland may appear dark brown to rust colored due to significant iron accumulation. Golden brown granular pigments are seen in follicular epithelial cells. Occasionally, increased fibrosis may be present.

Minocycline–Associated Changes

Definition. Accumulation of a dark brown to black pigment in the thyroid gland occurs

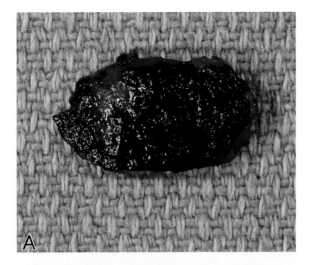

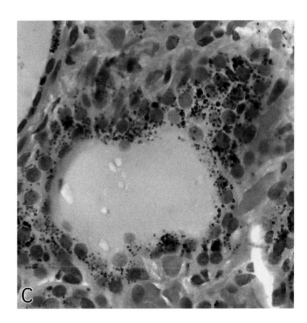

Figure 3-23

MINOCYCLINE-ASSOCIATED CHANGES

This patient was treated with minocycline for acne.

A: Gross photograph showing darkly pigmented thyroid gland.

B: The thyroid follicular cells show a dark brown cytoplasmic pigment which is thought to be lipofuscin with other associated chemicals.

C: Higher magnification shows the irregular cytoplasmic pigment.

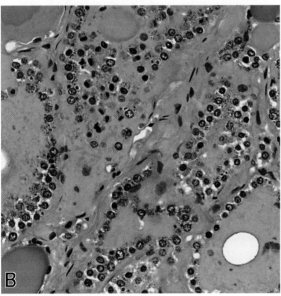

secondarily to the administration of minocycline and related tetracyclines.

General Remarks. The striking changes in the thyroid gland that occur with this condition have led to the designation "black thyroid." This was first observed in animals given minocycline and has been well documented in humans (131–133,135–137,139).

Patients who were given minocycline for acne, pyelonephritis, and pulmonary or other infectious conditions have been frequently involved. The minocycline-associated pigmentation is thought to be lipofuscin as well as other associated unknown compounds (135). Ultrastructural studies have shown that there is an accumulation of pigments in the lysosomes resulting from a lipid-drug complex. The impaired lysosomal function leads to pigment accumulation (131,136). In most reported series, thyroid function is usually unchanged.

Macroscopic Findings. The thyroid gland is normal in size and has a dark brown to black color. Cut sections show minimal fibrosis.

Microscopic Findings. The follicular epithelial cells contain a granular brown-black pigment in the apical portion of the epithelium (fig. 3-23), which may be present in the colloid as well. Follicular cell hyperplasia and hypertrophy have been reported in experimental animals given minocycline, but not

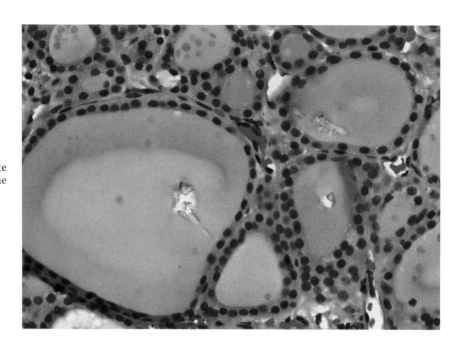

Figure 3-24

CALCIUM OXALATE
IN COLLOID

Refractile calcium oxalate crystals are readily found in the colloid of thyroid tissues.

in humans. Ultrastructural studies show prominent lysosomes which are associated with electron dense pigment with lipid.

Treatment and Prognosis. No treatment is necessary since most individuals have normal thyroid function. There is no reported increased risk of neoplastic development or thyroid dysfunction.

Crystal Deposits in the Thyroid

Calcium oxalate crystals are frequently found in normal thyroid tissue (fig. 3-24) (134, 137,138,140,141), usually within the colloid. One report indicated that oxalate crystals were almost always present at autopsy (detected in 77 of 80 cases) in patients who had received hemodialysis for renal failure (134). In these patients the crystals were also noted predominantly in the colloid within the follicles. Scully et al. (142) have used the presence of calcium oxalate crystals in struma ovarii as one of the features for identifying thyroid tissues.

The anisotropic crystals commonly seen in older patients with normal thyroid glands, but only rarely in hyperplastic glands, are probably calcium oxalate crystals (138,140,141). Reid et al. (140) reported anisotropic oxalate crystals in 79 percent of autopsies; the crystals were more common in older patients.

Teflon (Polytef) in Thyroid

Several authors have described Teflon (polytef) as a crystal-like material in the thyroid and cervical tissues (143,143a,144). Polytef is injected into the larynx in patients with unilateral vocal cord paralysis. It produces a granulomatous foreign body–type reaction with fibrosis. The inflammatory response to polytef injection results in improved phonation in these patients.

INFECTIONS AND GRANULOMATOUS DISEASES

Acute Thyroiditis

Definition. This is an acute inflammation of the thyroid gland with polymorphonuclear leukocyte infiltration.

General Remarks. Acute thyroiditis may be caused by many different organisms including Gram-positive bacteria (*Staphylococcus, Streptococcus*), and Gram-negative bacteria especially in the setting of neck trauma (156,157). Fungal organisms including *Aspergillus, Cryptococcus, Candida,* and *Coccidioides* have also been reported in acute thyroiditis (145,147,148,150, 152,153,155,158). Viral infections such as rubella (151) and cytomegalovirus (146) have been documented. The latter is usually seen in the setting of immunosuppression such as in patients with human immunodeficiency virus (HIV) or acquired immunodeficiency syndrome (AIDS).

Clinical Features. Most cases of acute thyroiditis secondarily involve the thyroid gland, spreading from general infections or from adjacent infected structures in the neck, such as from pharyngitis (145,148,158). Patients usually have chills, fever, malaise, and a painful swollen neck often aggravated by movement. Some patients may have dysphagia or hoarseness. On physical examination the thyroid is variably enlarged and this may be unilateral in some cases. The thyroid tests are usually within normal limits although some patients may have hypothyroidism or hyperthyroidism (148,158).

Macroscopic Findings. The gland may appear normal or slightly enlarged often because suppuration causes focally or diffusely soft and purulent areas.

Microscopic Findings. Infiltration with neutrophils, areas of microabscesses, necrotic foci, and vasculitis may be present. Careful search of the H&E-stained sections may show clusters of bacteria or fungal organisms. Special stains are very helpful for identifying the etiologic organism. Viral infections may be identified by intranuclear or cytoplasmic inclusions, or by specific cytopathic changes. Immunohistochemical or in situ hybridization studies are important when a viral etiology is suspected. In immunosuppressed individuals multiple infectious organisms may be present with a paucity of inflammatory cells.

Differential Diagnosis. The differential diagnosis includes other conditions with neutrophilic infiltrates such as subacute thyroiditis (discussed in next section) and ischemic necrosis.

Treatment and Prognosis. After the diagnosis is made by serologic tests, histologic examination, special stains, and culture, treatment with the appropriate agents, such as antibiotics, antifungal or antiviral agents, is indicated.

Most patients with bacterial thyroiditis recover from the infection and the thyroid function stabilizes unless there is overwhelming sepsis or other underlying conditions. Surgical incision and drainage may be needed if there is suppurative inflammation and abscess formation. With appropriate management mortality from bacterial thyroiditis is rare (149,154,156).

Fungal thyroiditis is very uncommon, and is most frequently seen as an autopsy finding in immunosuppressed patients with systemic fungal infections. When it is diagnosed from surgical biopsy or resection specimens of the thyroid, systemic treatment with antifungal agents is often effective.

Granulomatous Thyroiditis

Definition. Granulomatous thyroiditis is an inflammatory disease of the thyroid gland in which granulomas form. Synonyms include *subacute thyroiditis, nonsuppurative thyroiditis, giant cell thyroiditis, pseudotuberculous thyroiditis,* and *de Quervain's thyroiditis.*

General Remarks. The etiology of granulomatous thyroiditis is usually thought to be a systemic viral infection. There has been an association of subacute thyroiditis with certain viral epidemics including mumps, Coxsackie adenovirus, measles, and influenza (160,161, 177). Antibodies to different viruses have been detected in some patients.

Clinical Features. Granulomatous thyroiditis occurs predominantly in women, in a ratio of about 5 to 1 (162,167,170). Several studies have proposed a genetic predisposition for the development of this disease with linkage to human leukocyte antigen (HLA) Bw35 (172,173). Patients usually present with fever, malaise, neck pain, elevated erythrocyte sedimentation rate, and abnormal thyroid function tests (166,178–180).

Clinically, three phases of the disease are recognized: a hyperthyroid, a hypothyroid, and a recovery phase (159,160). In the hyperthyroid phase there is destruction of the follicles by the inflammatory process, leading to hyperthyroidism. Iodine uptake is usually low in this phase. The phase of hypothyroidism occurs after a significant portion of the gland is destroyed and there is decreased capacity to synthesize thyroid hormone. Antithyroid antibodies may be detected in the serum during this phase (178, 179). After several weeks to months, patients usually recover and become euthyroid. Permanent hypothyroidism is very uncommon in granulomatous thyroiditis (163).

A few patients with subacute thyroiditis present without pain, and there may be confusion with silent or painless thyroiditis in such cases (178) (see Silent Thyroiditis). Some patients with painless subacute thyroiditis may present with thyromegaly associated with fever

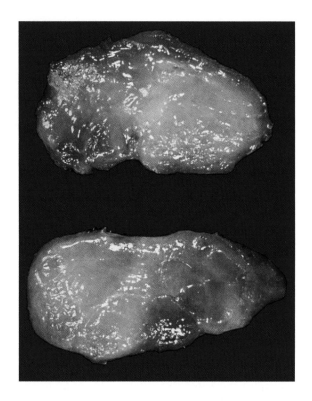

Figure 3-25

SUBACUTE THYROIDITIS

The macroscopic appearance of the thyroid is that of an enlarged, somewhat firm, tan gland. On cut section, the gland may be slightly nodular.

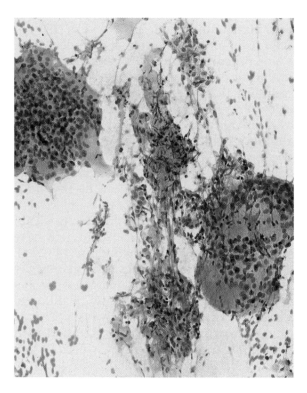

Figure 3-26

SUBACUTE THYROIDITIS

Cytologic examination shows sheets of follicular epithelioid cells, neutrophils, lymphocytes, and multinucleated gland cells.

and weight loss. Laboratory studies usually show an elevated erythrocyte sedimentation rate and low radioiodine uptake (163,173).

Macroscopic Findings. The thyroid gland is usually asymmetrically enlarged and firm, but is not as hard as with some carcinomas. Cut sections show a firm, tan gland with variable-sized nodules ranging from a few millimeters to a few centimeters in size (fig. 3-25).

Cytologic Findings. Cytologic features include follicular cells admixed with neutrophils, lymphocytes, histiocytes, and multinucleated giant cells; foamy cytoplasm; and up to 50 nuclei per cell (fig. 3-26). The follicular cells may be in sheets, nests, or isolated. Colloid may be present within acini or as an isolated finding.

Microscopic Findings. The histologic features that may be detected by needle biopsy, fine needle aspiration, or resection include multinucleated giant cells, lymphocytes, plasma cells,

histiocytes, areas of acute inflammation, and a variable degree of fibrosis. During the early or hyperthyroid phase there is disruption of the follicular cells and depletion of colloid, which correlate with clinical hyperthyroidism from the contribution of the escaping colloid and thyroid hormone. There may be acute inflammation with microabscess formation. A few multinucleated giant cells may be present at this stage. In the hypothyroid phase the follicular epithelium may disappear. There is a mixed inflammatory infiltrate of macrophages, multinucleated giant cells, lymphocytes, and plasma cells. The multinucleated giant cells often contain engulfed colloid (fig. 3-27). During the recovery phase, there is regeneration of follicles and a central fibrotic reaction (182,183).

Treatment and Prognosis. The disease may smolder for up to a few months, but usually subsides with a return to normal thyroid function.

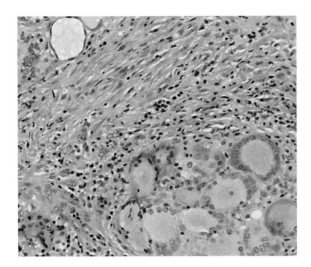 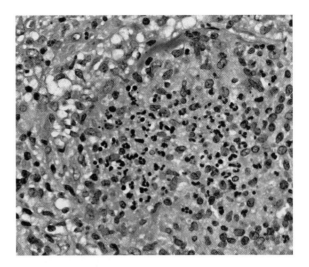

Figure 3-27

SUBACUTE THYROIDITIS

Left: Prominent multinucleated giant cells are present in the disrupted follicles.
Right: There is an intense focal neutrophilic infiltrate with lymphocytes and macrophages in the background.

Aspirin is adequate treatment in mild cases. In more severe cases, treatment with prednisone is usually effective. Beta-adrenergic blocking agents such as propranolol and arterolol may be used to treat the symptoms of thyrotoxicosis if they develop (175). General recovery is almost universal and less than 1 percent of patients become permanently hypothyroid (178).

Other Granulomatous Infections

Tuberculous Thyroiditis. This infection is associated with caseating granulomas as are seen at other sites of tuberculous infection (169, 174). When present in the thyroid gland they are more commonly associated with disseminated tuberculosis. Immunosuppressed patients are more susceptible to the development of tuberculous thyroiditis.

Fungal Thyroiditis. Most cases of fungal thyroiditis are associated with an acute necrotizing reaction or very little reaction. Occasionally, granulomatous inflammation occurs with the fungal reaction (164).

Postoperative Necrotizing Granulomas. Postoperative necrotizing granulomas of the thyroid gland have been reported in isolated cases (168). These are similar to the postoperative granulomas seen in other organs such as bladder and prostate. The clinical history and

absence of organisms by special stains or culture help support the diagnosis.

Granulomatous Vasculitis. Rare cases of systemic vasculitis with secondary involvement of the thyroid gland have been reported. Hypersensitivity vasculitis can occur as a reaction to phenytoin (184).

Sarcoidosis. Sarcoidosis with noncaseating granulomas may be present in the thyroid gland (fig. 3-28) (165,171,175,181). The granulomas are usually in an interstitial location which allows distinction from subacute thyroiditis and palpation thyroiditis (discussed below). If there is no history of sarcoidosis, special stains for fungi and acid fast organisms should be performed to exclude infection.

Palpation Thyroiditis. Palpation thyroiditis is an iatrogenic condition caused by vigorous palpation of the thyroid gland. This distinct histologic change in the thyroid gland was first described by Carney et al. (186). It is also designated as *multifocal granulomatous folliculitis*. Because the condition was more commonly seen in surgically excised thyroid glands with nodules (more than 83 percent) compared to glands examined at autopsy (10 to 40 percent) at the Mayo Clinic, the authors concluded that it was caused by preoperative injury or rupture of isolated follicles caused by palpation of the gland. They were able

113

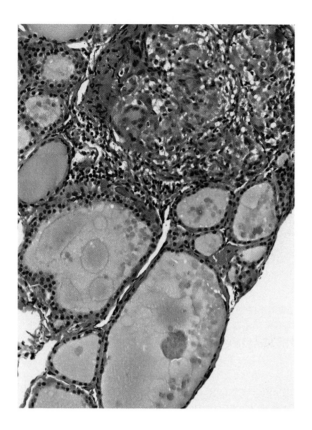 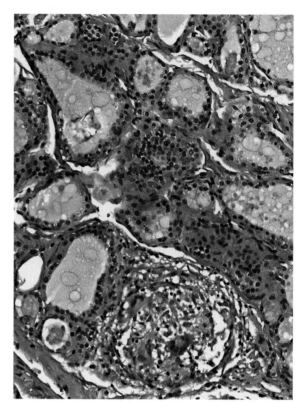

Figure 3-28

SARCOIDOSIS

Left: Tight clusters of noncaseating granulomas are located in the interstitium of the thyroid parenchyma.
Right: The granulomas do not involve the colloid. Thyroid sarcoidosis is usually associated with pulmonary or systemic disease.

to produce an identical histologic picture experimentally by vigorously squeezing the thyroid glands of dogs for 3 days before sacrificing them. Helling had reported a related condition termed colloidopathy (187), which was not associated with destruction of the follicular epithelium. Others investigators have analyzed the serum thyroglobulin levels of patients with palpation thyroiditis and have not found an increase (185,188), indicating that the release of thyroglobulin into the serum is probably not significant. Fine needle aspiration biopsy also has been reported to produce an increase in serum thyroglobulin levels (188).

Occasionally, gross areas of hemorrhage may be present, but there are usually no other gross changes noted. Focal or patchy folliculitis is present with inflammatory cells consisting of histiocytes, lymphocytes, and multi-nucleated giant cells. The inflammatory reaction is usually within the follicles (fig. 3-29) or adjacent to ruptured follicles.

Palpation thyroiditis may be confused with sarcoidosis or granulomatous inflammation. However, in sarcoidosis, the granulomas are usually interstitial. The unique appearance of palpation thyroiditis and the absence of necrosis allow distinction from granulomatous infectious diseases such as tuberculous or fungal thyroiditis. The acute inflammatory cells seen in subacute thyroiditis, along with the granulomas, allows distinction from palpation thyroiditis which is not associated with acute inflammation.

The condition is so common that a pathologic diagnosis is usually not made when palpation thyroiditis is recognized histologically. This is a self-limited condition, so no specific treatment is needed.

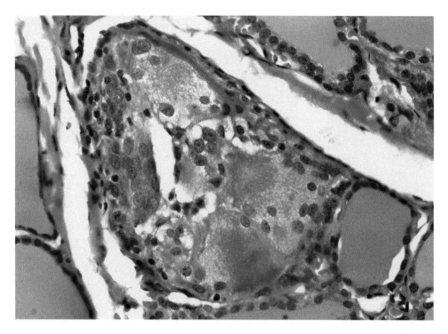

Figure 3-29

PALPATION THYROIDITIS
There is granulomatous folliculitis with multinucleated giant cells, macrophages, and histiocytes within the colloid.

Alterations Following Fine Needle Aspiration Biopsy. Fine needle aspiration (FNA) of the thyroid is a common diagnostic procedure. One of the complications of this procedure is histologic alteration and distortion of the thyroid tissue, so one may have difficulty analyzing a lesion after FNA (fig. 3-30). In some cases, benign lesions are mistakenly interpreted as malignant (190–192). A history of previous FNA or histologic clues suggesting previous FNA, such as infarction, hemorrhage, inflammation, and early fibrosis, should lead to a cautious interpretation of unusual histologic features.

AUTOIMMUNE THYROID DISEASE

Autoimmune thyroiditis defines a broad spectrum of non-neoplastic thyroid diseases that have an immunologic etiology and a predisposition to be associated with certain HLA susceptibility haplotypes. The latter are commonly circulating antibodies against thyroid cellular antigens. The two most common autoimmune thyroid conditions are Graves' disease and Hashimoto's thyroiditis, but other conditions such as atrophic autoimmune thyroiditis (primary myxedema) and Riedel's thyroiditis are also included in this category.

Hashimoto's Disease

Definition. This is an autoimmune disease characterized by goiter and elevated circulating thyroid antibodies including thyroid peroxidase and thyroglobulin autoantibodies. Synonyms include *struma lymphomatosa, Hashimoto's struma,* and *lymphadenoid goiter.*

General Remarks. This disease occurs most frequently in middle-aged women (210, 219). It is also the most common cause of sporadic goiter in children. The two principal autoantibodies are the antithyroglobulin antibody, detected by the tanned red cell agglutination test, and antithyroid peroxidase antibody (previously known as antimicrosomal antibody), detected by immunofluorescence, complement fixation, or enzyme-linked immunosorbent assay. Hashimoto's thyroiditis may coexist with other autoimmune diseases including Sjogren's syndrome, pernicious anemia, chronic active hepatitis, adrenal insufficiency, diabetes mellitus, and Graves' disease. An association of HLA-DR3 and HLA-DR5 with the atrophic and goitrous forms of Hashimoto's disease has been reported (202).

There is good evidence for a familial association of Hashimoto's disease, since up to 5 percent of first-degree relatives of patients with chronic autoimmune thyroiditis have antithyroid antibodies, which are inherited as a dominant trait (196,197,202). Patients from Japan with HLA-DR2 and HLA-DQ1 have a protective effect against autoimmune thyroid disease (196, 212). There is a high prevalence of autoimmune

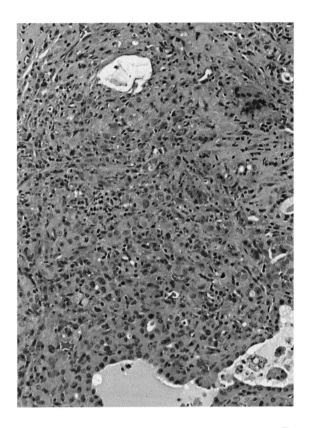 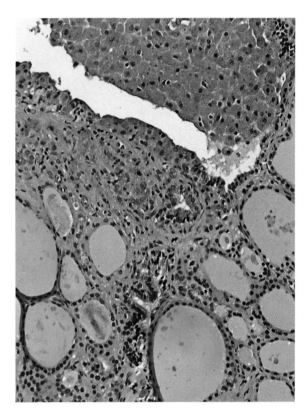

Figure 3-30

FINE NEEDLE ASPIRATION BIOPSY CHANGES

Left: Fine needle aspiration biopsy changes in a thyroid gland include chronic inflammation and fibrosis.
Right: Areas of old hemorrhage with macrophages and lymphocytes. These changes may simulate some of the changes seen in the fibrous variant of Hashimoto's thyroiditis or in thyroid carcinoma.

thyroid disease in patients with Down's syndrome, familial Alzheimer's disease, and Turner's syndrome (203,205,216,236).

Certain chemicals can lead to an increased incidence of autoimmune thyroiditis. High intake of iodine is associated with autoimmune thyroiditis (219) as well as with lymphocytic thyroiditis (208). As discussed earlier, amiodarone treatment can lead to iodine-induced hypothyroidism because of its high iodine content and long half-life (243). Lithium is another chemical that is associated with elevated levels of antithyroid antibodies and hypothyroidism (220). Treatment of patients with interferon-alpha for malignancies or chronic viral hepatitis may lead to the development of autoantibodies and hypothyroidism (196,237).

Chronic autoimmune thyroiditis is a common condition. At autopsy, about 45 percent of women and 20 percent of men in the United States and the United Kingdom have focal thyroiditis (1 to 10 foci/cm^2) and 5 to 15 percent of women and 1 to 5 percent of men have severe thyroiditis (more than 40 foci/cm^2) (230,247). The prevalence of elevated titers of autoantibodies for thyroid disease increases with age and may reach as high as 33 percent in women after age 70 (194,231).

Pathogenesis. The pathogenesis of autoimmune thyroiditis involves activation of the CD4 or helper T cells targeted at thyroid antigen (246). Activation may occur by infection with bacteria or viruses that have a protein similar to a thyroid protein, resulting in molecular mimicry (199,242,244). Serologic evidence of recent viral and bacterial infections has been reported (242,244), but the link between the infection and initiation of the autoimmune disease has not been conclusively documented.

An alternative hypothesis is that thyroid epithelial antigen proteins which are normally sequestered are exposed to CD4+ cells. This view is supported by the observation that thyroid cells in patients with autoimmune thyroiditis, in contrast to normal thyroid cells, express HLA-DR, HLA-DPd, and HLA-DQ proteins which are required for CD4 antigen presentation (207,222,241). Interferon-gamma can induce the expression of major histocompatibility (MHC) class II molecules by thyroid cells when these molecules are released from activated CD4 cells; these molecules further stimulate thyrocytes and lead to an autoimmune reaction (200,223). Adhesion molecules such as intercellular adhesion molecule (ICAM) have been identified on the thyroid epithelial cells from patients with Hashimoto's thyroiditis (204).

Once the helper T cells are activated, they stimulate B cells which are recruited into the thyroid and produce antibodies (223). The principal antigen targets are thyroglobulin, thyroid microsomal antigen, thyroid peroxidase, and thyrotropin receptor. The autoantibodies that have been identified include antibodies to the TSH receptor or thyroid-stimulating immunoglobulin (TSI) which stimulates thyroid function. This is more common in patients with Graves' disease (200). Thyroid growth-stimulating immunoglobulins, which are also directed against the TSH receptor, stimulate proliferation of thyrocytes and lead to goiter development. TSH binding-inhibitor immunoglobulins prevent TSH from binding to its receptors in thyroid epithelial cells. Some of these antibodies stimulate while others inhibit thyrocyte function.

Clinical and Radiologic Findings. Patients with autoimmune thyroiditis can present with a goiter, hypothyroidism, or both. The sex ratio is high in favor of women with a 5 to 7 times higher incidence than men. The mean overall age at diagnosis is 59 years for women and 58 years for men (194,203,245). Children rarely develop autoimmune thyroiditis before age 5 years, however, autoimmune thyroiditis may account for about 40 percent of goiters in adolescents (233). Patients often have a goiter, but compression of the trachea or recurrent laryngeal nerves is uncommon. Thyroid tenderness and pain are uncommon, but a feeling of tightness in the neck is frequently noted. Typically, the thyroid is symmetrically enlarged and has a firm bosselated surface. The thyroid may be asymmetric on physical examination and the gland may sometimes be mistaken for a solitary nodule or multinodular goiter, especially in glands with fibrosis.

Thyroid imaging is usually not necessary in patients with autoimmune thyroiditis. However, if it is done for an unusual case, the radioiodine scan can be very misleading because the uptake pattern may be similar to that of Grave's disease and multinodular goiter: a hot or cold nodule (234). The uptake of radioiodine is usually normal or elevated in patients with autoimmune thyroiditis with goiter, even when the patient is hypothyroid (fig. 3-31); in contrast, patients with subacute thyroiditis or silent thyroiditis usually have a low radioiodine uptake (201). Ultrasonographic studies show a enlarged gland with a hypoechogenic pattern in the majority of patients (228,238).

Laboratory Findings. Laboratory tests show thyroid-specific autoantibodies in the serum. Antithyroglobulin antibodies are present in about 60 percent of patients with diffuse goiter, hypothyroidism, or both, and antithyroid microsomal antibodies in 95 percent (193). The titers tend to be higher in patients with the atrophic form of autoimmune thyroiditis. A positive test for antithyroid peroxidase antibodies is a slightly more sensitive indicator of chronic autoimmune thyroiditis than a positive test for antithyroid microsomal antibodies.

Macroscopic Findings. The thyroid gland is diffusely enlarged and firm, and the surface is bosselated or irregular (fig. 3-32). The gland may be very fibrotic, especially in older patients, suggesting malignancy on examination. The thyroid is usually two to three times normal weight or about 40 g, but it may occasionally weigh more than 200 g. Patients with atrophic autoimmune thyroiditis have small thyroid glands with no evidence of a goiter.

In Hashimoto's thyroiditis the enlargement is usually symmetric, but the midline pyramidal lobe may be prominent. Cut sections often reveal accentuated lobulation with increased fibrosis (fig. 3-33). The gland is tan-yellow rather than the usual red-brown because of the abundant lymphoid tissue.

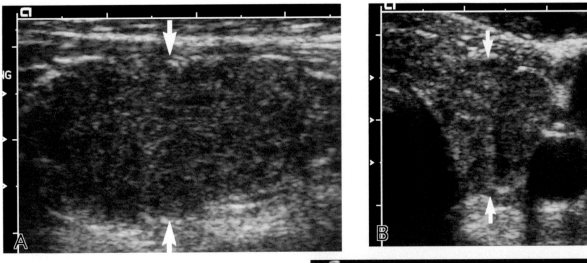

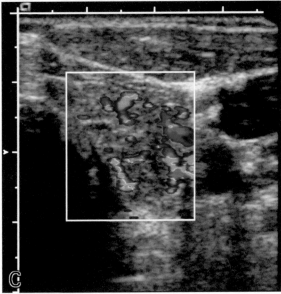

Figure 3-31

HASHIMOTO'S THYROIDITIS

Longitudinal (A) and transverse (B) ultrasound images of the thyroid show a diffusely enlarged gland with a heterogeneous nodular appearance. The color Doppler image (C) shows diffusely increased blood flow to the gland.

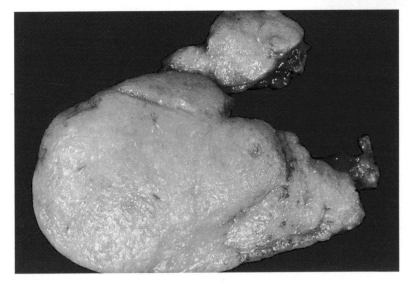

Figure 3-32

HASHIMOTO'S THYROIDITIS

The cut surface of the gland is tan-yellow because of the abundant lymphoid tissue. The gland is also slightly nodular.

Figure 3-33

HASHIMOTO'S THYROIDITIS

A,B: Cytologic examination shows clusters of follicular and Hurthle cells in a background of lymphocytes and occasional plasma cells.

C: Higher magnification shows the Hurthle cells to have a granular cytoplasm with a background of lymphocytes. (Courtesy of Dr. J. R. Goellner, Rochester, MN.)

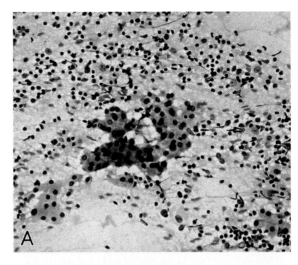

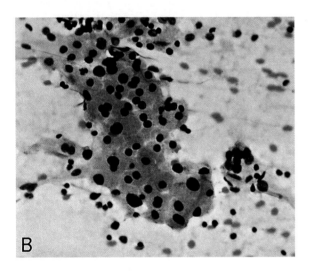

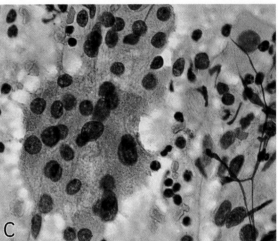

Cytologic Findings. The aspiration biopsy is usually cellular and consists of Hurthle cells and lymphocytes (fig. 3-34). Hurthle cells are larger than follicular cells, contain more granular cytoplasm, and usually appear as sheets or small groups of cells or as single cells. Lymphocytes are usually abundant. Plasma cells, neutrophils, and macrophages may also be seen.

Microscopic Findings. Histologic examination shows a thyroid gland with sheets of lymphocytes and plasma cells, often with prominent germinal centers (fig. 3-35). The thyroid follicles are atrophic, and there is usually fibrosis in the background. Squamous metaplasia of the follicular cells may be present (fig. 3-36). Another diagnostic feature is the presence of large metaplastic follicular cells with abundant granular eosinophilic cytoplasm.

These cells are often referred to as Hurthle, oxyphilic, or Askanazy cells. They usually have large nuclei and prominent nucleoli. On rare occasions, a few multinucleated giant cells may be present in the thyroid gland, but they do not occur in the same histologic background as with subacute thyroiditis. The inflammatory cells may extend to the adjacent skeletal muscle, especially if there is preexisting intermingling of skeletal muscle and thyroid follicles, resulting in adherence of the gland to the neck during surgery. The perithyroid lymph nodes are usually enlarged and show follicular hyperplasia on microscopic examination.

Immunohistochemical Findings. Immunohistochemical staining with B- and T-cell antibodies shows a mixture of B and T cells (fig. 3-37). The plasma cells show a spectrum of

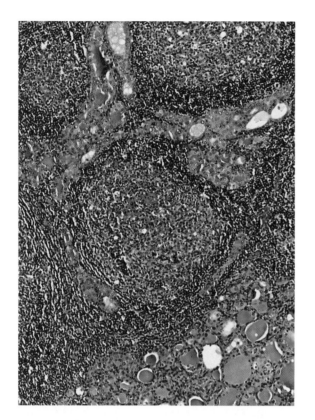 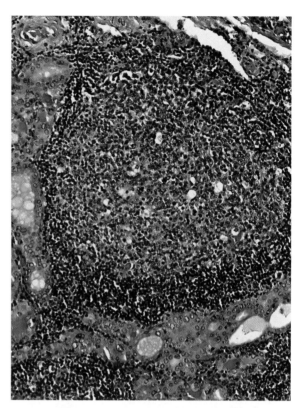

Figure 3-34

HASHIMOTO'S THYROIDITIS

Lymphoid follicles with prominent germinal centers and a background of lymphocytes and plasma cells.

immunoreactivity for heavy chains (IgG, IgM, IgA) as well as polyclonal kappa and lambda light chains. Many of the T cells are CD4+ helper cells with HLA-DR II expression suggesting activated T cells (202,222). The CD4+ cells are widely distributed in the thyroid and are present between follicles, around blood vessels, and in lymphoid tissue. CD8+ suppressor/cytotoxic T cells are admixed with the CD4+ and B cells in the follicles (202). Some of the CD8+ T cells may be present in the extracellular spaces formed by invaginations of the epithelial cell membranes (202). The suppressor T cells have cytolytic activity in vitro, so they may contribute to the damage to the follicle seen in Hashimoto's disease.

Ultrastructural Findings. Ultrastructural studies have characterized the Hurthle cells as containing many large mitochondria with decreased volumes of other organelles including rough endoplasmic reticulum and Golgi complexes (fig. 3-38) (235). The T cells can be ob-served between epithelial cells. Duplication and rupture of the follicular basement membrane have also been noted (195,210,217).

Variants of Hashimoto's Thyroiditis. *Fibrous Variant.* This variant was first recognized by Hashimoto in his original description (210); Katz and Vickery redefined this lesion many decades later (215). The fibrous variant of Hashimoto's thyroiditis constitutes about 10 percent of cases. It occurs in a slightly older age group, and the patients present with marked hypothyroidism and a large symptomatic goiter. The disorder usually requires surgical treatment to relieve the local symptoms of dysphagia or dyspnea. Laboratory studies usually show a markedly elevated antithyroglobulin antibody titer, and the patients are hypothyroid with elevated serum TSH levels.

The gland is usually larger and more fibrotic than the usual Hashimoto's gland. Histologic examination shows preservation of the

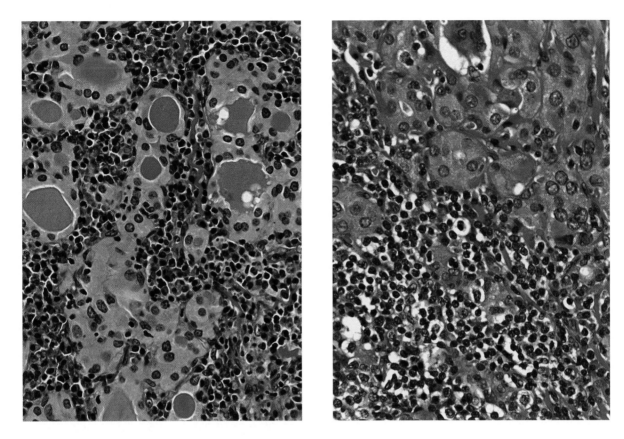

Figure 3-35

HASHIMOTO'S THYROIDITIS

Hurthle's cell (oxyphil cell) metaplasia is prominent.

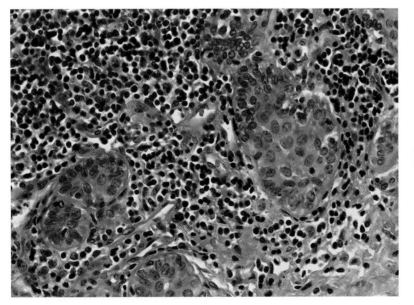

Figure 3-36

HASHIMOTO'S THYROIDITIS

Prominent squamous metaplasia of the follicular cells is seen with longstanding Hashimoto's thyroiditis.

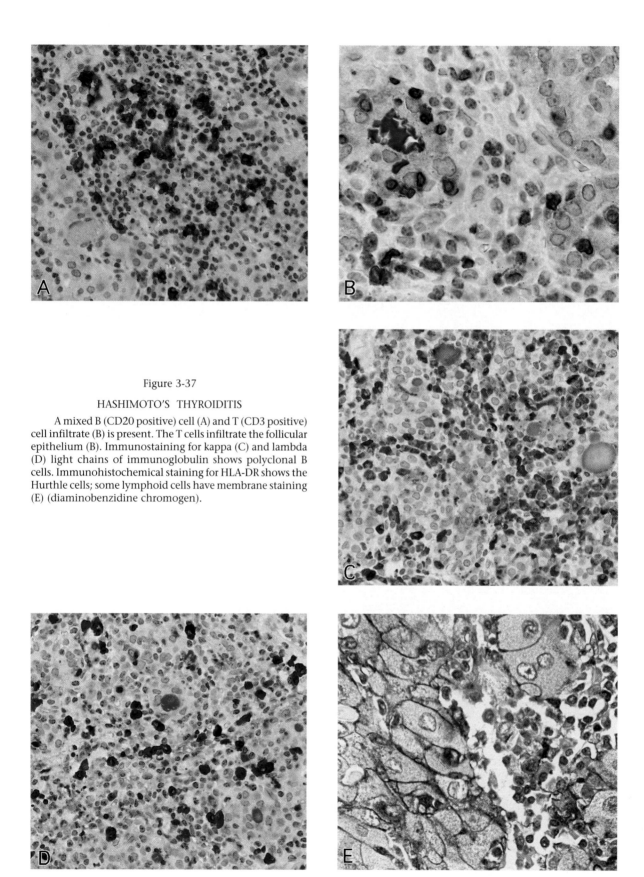

Figure 3-37

HASHIMOTO'S THYROIDITIS

A mixed B (CD20 positive) cell (A) and T (CD3 positive) cell infiltrate (B) is present. The T cells infiltrate the follicular epithelium (B). Immunostaining for kappa (C) and lambda (D) light chains of immunoglobulin shows polyclonal B cells. Immunohistochemical staining for HLA-DR shows the Hurthle cells; some lymphoid cells have membrane staining (E) (diaminobenzidine chromogen).

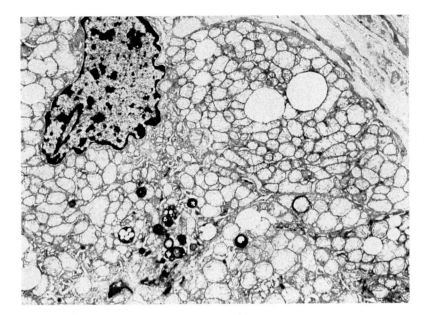

Figure 3-38

HASHIMOTO'S THYROIDITIS

Ultrastructural view of metaplastic Hurthle's cell shows prominent cytoplasmic mitochondria which occupy most of the cytoplasm (X4,000).

lobulated pattern of the normal thyroid gland. Atrophic follicular cells with degenerative changes and broad areas of fibrosis are present (fig. 3-39). The features of the usual Hashimoto's thyroiditis with Hurthle cells and lymphoplasmacytic infiltrates with prominent germinal centers are readily seen. In addition, there is more extensive squamous metaplasia. The pathogenesis of this variant is unknown, but Katz and Vickery (215) suggested that the fibrous variant may develop by progression from the usual type of Hashimoto's thyroiditis.

Fibrous Atrophy Variant. Some patients with or without a history of Hashimoto's thyroiditis present with a small fibrotic gland associated with hypothyroidism or "idiopathic myxedema." The gland is very small and weighs between 1 and 6 g. Histologically, there is extensive destruction of the thyroid parenchyma with minimal preservation of the follicular architecture (fig. 3-40). Extensive fibrosis and lymphoplasmacytic infiltrates are features reminiscent of the fibrous variant of Hashimoto's thyroiditis. These patients, who are usually elderly, often have high titers of antithyroid antibodies and severe hypothyroidism (198). The histologic features in fibrous atrophy are similar to those of the fibrosis variant (215), but the thyroid gland is much smaller.

Juvenile Variant. The juvenile variant is a poorly defined form of chronic lymphocytic thyroiditis that has been described in younger

patients (232,248). Some patients present with hyperthyroidism that progresses to hypothyroidism with time. The glands contain a lymphoplasmacytic infiltrate of Hurthle cells along with squamous cell metaplasia. Follicular atrophy is uncommon.

Cystic Variant. Two cases of multiple bronchial cleft–like cysts in patients with Hashimoto's thyroiditis have been reported (224). The cysts are thought to be derived from developmental rests, lined by squamous and columnar epithelium, and surrounded by follicular lymphoid tissue and a fibrous capsule. Both patients were females, 46 and 47 years of age. The thyroid gland in both cases had marked atrophy, Hurthle cell change, lymphocytic infiltrates, and follicle formation diagnostic of Hashimoto's thyroiditis, but fibrosis was minimal. It is uncertain whether these cases represent a fortuitous occurrence of the same condition or a separate disorder. However, microscopic cysts with squamous epithelial lining in patients with Hashimoto's thyroiditis have been previously reported (225).

Differential Diagnosis. The differential diagnosis of Hashimoto's thyroiditis includes thyroid carcinoma, lymphoma of the thyroid, Riedel's thyroiditis, Graves' disease, and "hashitoxicosis" or "hyperthyroiditis" (248). The extensive fibrosis that can be seen in some cases of Hashimoto's thyroiditis, especially in the fibrous variant which may be adherent to

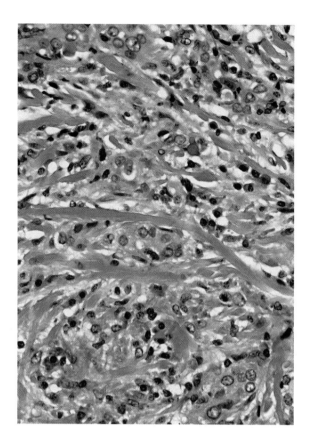 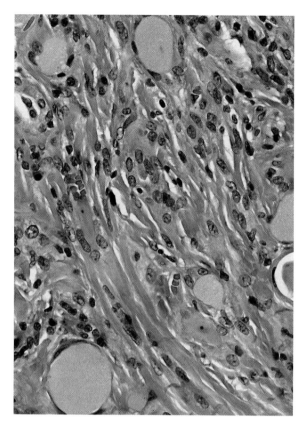

Figure 3-39

FIBROUS VARIANT OF HASHIMOTO'S THYROIDITIS

Left: There is a marked fibrotic reaction admixed with lymphocytes and plasma cells in the background.

Right: The fibrotic reaction compresses and traps some of the Hurthle cells. The gland may be mistaken for a carcinoma at the time of clinical examination.

Figure 3-40

HASHIMOTO'S THYROIDITIS

Fibrous atrophy in chronic Hashimoto's thyroiditis. There is extensive fibrosis, and atrophic follicles are entrapped in the fibrotic areas.

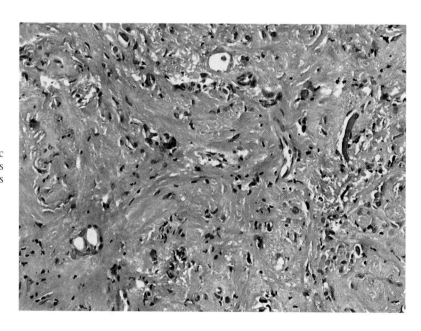

the thyroid at surgery, may suggest a carcinoma. The histologic preservation of the normal lobulated architecture, the lack of architectural and cytologic features of papillary or other carcinomas, and the histologic features of Hashimoto's thyroiditis allow distinction. Although it has been suggested that Hashimoto's thyroiditis may be premalignant or associated with an increased incidence of carcinoma, there is no strong evidence for this.

Fine needle aspiration biopsy of the thyroid gland before surgical excision of a lobe leads to hemorrhage, chronic inflammation, and fibrosis, features that simulate carcinoma or the fibrous variant of Hashimoto's thyroiditis (see fig. 3-30) (195).

A condition described as peritumor thyroiditis may be confused with Hashimoto's thyroiditis, especially in small biopsy specimens. In this condition there are lymphocytic and mixed lymphocytic-plasmacytic infiltrates at the periphery of a thyroid neoplasm, especially an infiltrative papillary carcinoma (221). Adequate sampling of the lesion should lead to the correct diagnosis.

Hashimoto's thyroiditis, especially the fibrosis variant, may be difficult to distinguish from Riedel's thyroiditis (discussed below). The adherence of the thyroid to neck structures and the extensive fibrosis of the gland contribute to this confusion. Riedel's thyroiditis is associated with more extreme fibrosis in which fibrous tissue extends into nerve, fat, and muscle as well as the parathyroid glands, and is often associated with vasculitis with internal proliferation and destruction of the media, features not commonly seen in Hashimoto's thyroiditis.

The dense lymphoplasmacytic infiltrate in Hashimoto's thyroiditis may simulate a lymphoma. This situation is made more difficult by the fact that most thyroid lymphomas arise in a setting of Hashimoto's thyroiditis (211,214). The mixed lymphoplasmacytic infiltrate seen in the latter may also be present in thyroid lymphoma. The absence of sheets of atypical lymphoid cells allows distinction between these two conditions. Immunophenotyping for B- and T-cell markers, and clonality and gene rearrangement studies can readily allow distinction between lymphoid hyperplasia of Hashimoto's thyroiditis and the monoclonal B-cell prolifera-

tion of most thyroid lymphomas. Woolner et al. (248,249) previously described a lymphoma-like thyroiditis that may be challenging for the pathologist to distinguish from thyroid lymphoma. Some of these cases undoubtedly represent mucosa-associated lymphoid tissue (MALT) lymphomas of the thyroid as described by Isaacson (213) and later by other investigators (250). Hashimoto's thyroiditis may share some histologic features with Graves' disease, and a condition with features of both Graves' disease and Hashimoto's thyroiditis has been described (206). These patients have glands with lymphoplastic infiltrates, Hurthle cell changes, and follicular atrophy or hyperplasia, features that show the overlap of these two conditions. Clinical and laboratory studies along with the usual histologic features allow separation of classic Hashimoto's thyroiditis and Graves' disease.

Treatment and Prognosis. Patients with overt hypothyroidism are treated with thyroxine, with the dose adjusted to normalize the serum TSH. Up to 24 percent of patients with hypothyroidism due to chronic autoimmune thyroiditis who are treated with thyroxine for more than 1 year remain euthyroid when the drug is withdrawn (226). This may be related to the disappearance of TSH-blocking antibodies (226,240).

Various complications can develop in patients with Hashimoto's thyroiditis. If hypothyroidism occurs, Graves' disease can develop (218), indicating that gland destruction is not always irreversible. Thyroid lymphoma is a serious complication of Hashimoto's thyroiditis. In one study of women in Japan followed for an average of 8 years, 0.1 percent developed thyroid lymphoma, a prevalence rate that was 80-fold higher than expected (214).

Lymphomas arising in patients with Hashimoto's thyroiditis are usually of B-cell phenotype and are usually confined to the thyroid gland (227). Treatment with radiotherapy alone or with chemotherapy leads to 5-year survival rates of 13 to 92 percent, depending on the grade of the tumor (229).

In pregnant women the most common thyroid complication is postpartum thyroiditis which develops 2 to 6 months after delivery. It is diagnosed by hypothyroidism, hyperthyroidism followed by hypothyroidism, or hyperthyroidism with a low 24-hour radioiodine uptake. The disorder usually resolves spontaneously within 1 year (239).

Graves' Disease

Definition. Graves' disease is an autoimmune condition characterized by diffuse goiter, thyrotoxicosis, infiltrative orbitopathy, and occasionally, infiltrative dermopathy.

General Remarks. The prevalence of Graves' disease is unknown in the United States. One study from England showed a prevalence of 2.7 percent in women and 0.3 percent in men (287). Graves' disease is the most common cause of spontaneous hyperthyroidism in patients younger than age 40 (266). Patients have serum antibodies against thyroid peroxidase or microsomal antigen, thyroglobulin, and TSH receptor (280). An increased incidence of Graves' disease occurs among family members of affected individuals, and the incidence in monozygotic twins may be as high as 60 percent. The development of Graves' disease is strongly associated with HLA-B8 and HLA-DR3.

Patients with Graves' disease have antibodies to the TSH receptor (thyroid-stimulating immunoglobulin [TSI]). This antibody is relatively specific for Graves' disease since autoantibodies to thyroid peroxidase and thyroglobulin are frequently found in patients with other autoimmune types of thyroiditis such as Hashimoto's disease. Thyroid growth-stimulating immunoglobulin is also directed against the TSH receptor but is associated with thyrocyte proliferation (251). TSH-binding immunoglobulins are anti-TSH receptor antibodies and prevent TSH from binding to its receptor and thyroid cells. Some forms of TSH-binding immunoglobulins inhibit TSH activity while others stimulate TSH activity.

Pathogenesis. Patients with Graves' disease have reduced levels of circulatory suppressor/cytotoxic or CD8+ cells, suggesting that a lack of suppressor/cytotoxic T cells may be responsible for the breakdown of immune tolerance in Graves' disease (251,282). A possible etiologic factor is infection, which induces MHC class II expression in experimental animals. Specific viral infections can lead to autoimmune thyroid disease (252,285). Various forms of stress have been suggested as etiologic stimuli

in Graves' disease. Some research suggests that stress results in general immune suppression because of the effects of glucocorticoids and corticotropin-releasing hormone on the immune system (267,291); the immune system overcompensates for the stress, leading to autoimmune disease. This may be why Graves' disease develops 3 to 9 months after delivery (266).

The role of gonadal steroid hormones in the initiation of Graves' disease has been suggested because of the higher incidence in women (approximately 8 to 1), and the development of the disease in times of changes in gonadal steroid hormone production such as puberty, pregnancy, and menopause. In men, Graves' disease occurs at a later age, is more severe, and is frequently associated with ophthalmopathy (266).

Ophthalmopathy and Dermopathy. The pathogenesis of changes in the eye and skin have not been completely elucidated. Some of the muscle fibers in the orbit have been shown to express HLA class II antigens as is seen with the thyroid gland, and in vitro studies have shown that activated T cells react with retro-orbital tissue (260). TSH receptor mRNA has been detected in retro-orbital fibroblasts, suggesting that the TSH receptor may be involved in the ophthalmopathy (266). This would fit with the empirical observation that patients with severe eye disease have the highest titers of antibodies to the TSH receptor.

Although the most likely explanation for the eye and skin changes is that there are antigens common to the thyroid gland and these tissues that are recognized by T cells, the specific antigens have not been characterized as yet. Preliminary studies suggest that retro-orbital and dermal fibroblasts are the most likely sources of these antigens (289).

Clinical and Radiologic Findings. Graves' disease is seen most commonly in the third or fourth decade of life. Although it develops in adolescents, it is rare before age 10. The ratio of women to men is about 8 to 1. Patients have a diffuse goiter with thyrotoxicosis, eye disease, and possible skin manifestations. The most common symptoms include nervousness, increased sweating, hypersensitivity to heat, palpitations, fatigue, tachycardia, muscle wasting, and weight loss (fig. 3-41, right). On physical examination, patients usually have a diffuse goiter, tachycardia, tremors, warm moist skin, and eye signs.

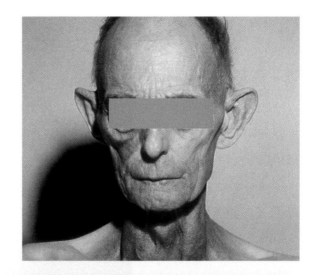

Figure 3-41

GRAVES' DISEASE

Right: A 76-year-old man with advanced Graves' disease. Muscle wasting and goiter are demonstrated.

Below: Pertechnetate portable images show an enlarged thyroid with a diffuse increase in thyroid uptake, including the pyramidal lobe.

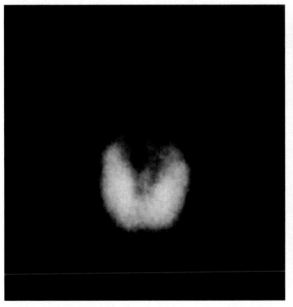 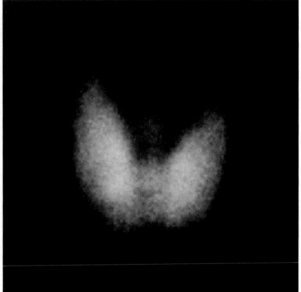

Men tend to develop Graves' disease at an older age than women, and the degree of thyroid hyperfunction is often more severe, but symptoms may also be less severe. Muscle weakness and eye disease are more likely to develop in men (266).

Imaging studies with radioactive iodine show a diffuse increase in tracer uptake in the thyroid gland (fig. 3-41, below) (277,278). This increase is not unique to Graves' disease, since other conditions including Hashimoto's thyroiditis can lead to a similar imaging pattern (277,278).

Laboratory Findings. The serum T3 and T4 levels are elevated (Table 3-1) while the TSH level is very low. Serum T3 concentration is usually more elevated than T4. The presence of TSH receptor antibodies of the stimulating subtype in the serum is diagnostic of Graves' disease (266), but this does not always correlate with the clinical state. The thyroid radioactive iodine uptake values (RAIU) are invariably increased in patients with Graves' disease. The RAIU is measured 24 hours after the isotope is given, since it usually reaches a plateau at this time. However, in Graves' disease the RAIU usually peaks early, and therefore, this test is not as diagnostically accurate as others, such as determination of TSH and free T4 levels (266).

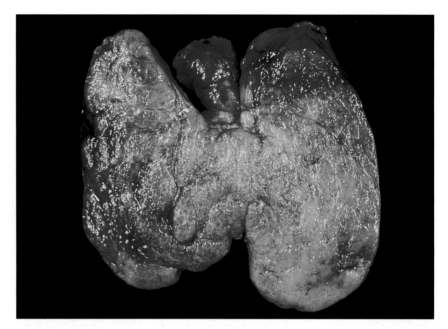

Figure 3-42

GRAVES' DISEASE

There is diffuse symmetrical enlargement of the gland and a beefy deep red parenchyma.

Table 3-1

NORMAL VALUES FOR THYROID FUNCTION TESTS[a]

Test	SI[b]	Conventional
Calcitonin, plasma	<19 ng/L	<19 pg/ml
Free thyroxine	9–26 pmol/L	0.7–2.0 ng/dL
Radioactive iodine uptake, 24 hr	0.05–0.30	5–30%
Resin T3 uptake serum	0.25–0.35	23–35%
Reverse triiodothyronine (rT3), serum	0.15–0.61 nmol/L	10–40 ng/dL
Thyroid hormone-binding ratio (THBR)	0.85–1.10	85–110%
Thyrotropin (TSH), serum	0.5–5.0 mU/L	0.5–5.0 µU/ml
Thyroxine (T4), serum	64–154 nmol/L	5–12 µg/dL
Triiodothyronine (T3), serum	1.1–2.9 nmol/L	70–90 ng/dL

[a]Wilson JD, Foster DW, Kronengberg HM, Larsen PR. Williams textbook of endocrinology, 9th ed. Philadelphia: W.B. Saunders, 1998:back cover.

[b]SI – System of international units.

Macroscopic Findings. The gland is usually diffusely enlarged and symmetric, and weighs between 50 to 150 g. It glistens and has a prominent vascular pattern. The cut surface shows a beefy, deep red parenchyma (fig. 3-42).

Cytologic Findings. Cytologic examination shows sheets of follicular cells (fig. 3-43), with rings that are formed by the peripherally situated basal nuclei, and marginal vacuoles of variable sizes with discrete vacuoles adjacent to the nuclei. These vacuoles can also be found in aspirates from patients without hyperthyroidism.

Microscopic Findings. Microscopic examination shows preservation of the normal lobular architecture. The stromal vessels are usually prominent, and there is hyperplasia of tall columnar cells in the follicle (fig. 3-44). Colloid is decreased in the untreated gland and, when present, there is a decreased follicular lumen and prominent "scalloping" or vacuoles in the colloid adjacent to the apex of the follicular cells. The "scalloping" is a fixation artifact due to decreased amounts of colloid and marked shrinkage during tissue processing. Papillae with fibrovascular cores may be present, suggesting a diagnosis of papillary carcinoma. Lymphocytes are commonly seen in the stroma around follicles. Mixed B and T cells are often present with B cells in the germinal centers and T cells in a perifollicular location. Dendritic cells, which are antigen-producing cells, are usually increased in number (257,265). The dendritic cells and thyrocytes often express adhesion molecules such as CD54, while the mononuclear cells express other adhesion molecules such as CD11a/CD18 (257).

In cases of treated Graves' disease, a different histologic picture is seen depending on the type of treatment. Treatment with iodine before surgery leads to a decrease in the vascularity of the gland and involution of the follicular epithelium, which becomes cuboidal rather than columnar. There is also an increase in colloid storage in some areas of the gland (253). If radioactive iodine treatment is subsequently followed by surgery, the histologic changes may be a variable, depending on the period of iodine therapy. The histologic picture can vary from slight changes with nuclear pleomorphism to extensive follicle cell destruction, fibrosis, and oncocytic metaplasia with marked nuclear pleomorphism (256,262). Treatment with drugs that interfere with thyroid hormone synthesis, such as propylthiouracil, leads to increased hyperplastic changes while treatment with beta-adrenergic blockers such as propranolol, does not have any predictable morphologic effect on the thyroid gland (268,283).

Psammoma bodies may occasionally be seen in Graves' disease without associated papillary carcinoma (276). Some studies have reported an increased incidence of thyroid cancer in patients with Graves' disease (281).

Ultrastructural Findings. Ultrastructural examination of the thyroid in patients with Graves' disease shows increased activity of the follicular cells: prominent rough endoplasmic reticulum and Golgi complexes as well as well-developed nucleoli in the enlarged nuclei (284). Other studies have reported immune complex deposits in the basement membrane of thyroid tissues (263).

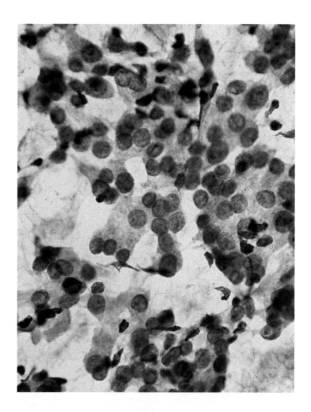

Figure 3-43

GRAVES' DISEASE

Cytologic examination shows sheets of tall follicular cells with basal nuclei.

Immunohistochemical Findings. Immunohistochemical staining for HLA-DR is positive on the thyrocytes as well as the lymphoid cells in Graves' disease (fig. 3-45) (269). Studies of the lymphocytes in the thyroid have shown changes in the T cells, with increases in the CD4+ cells (275). Differences in the ratio of B and T cells in the thyroid compared to the peripheral blood have been reported by immunophenotyping studies (270,273).

The changes of Graves' orbitopathy or ophthalmopathy include increases in the volume of the orbital tissue resulting in increased mass of the extraocular muscles, an increase in the retrobulbar connective tissue secondary to edema, and accumulation of hyaluronic acid and chondroitin sulfates leading to proptosis (fig. 3-46, top). Histologically, the muscles are swollen and edematous with loss of striation, fragmentation of fibers, and a diffuse lymphocytic infiltration (fig. 3-46, bottom) (258,290).

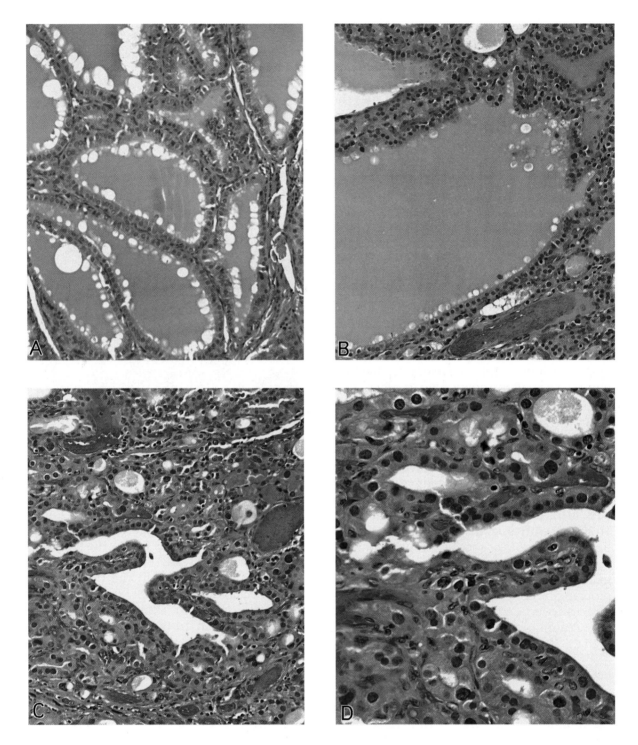

Figure 3-44

GRAVES' DISEASE

A: The follicles are lined by tall cells in some areas. The prominent "scalloping" formed by vacuoles in the colloid adjacent to the follicle cell apex is a fixation artifact.

B: Some dilated follicles with flatter epithelium are present from treatment before surgery.

C: Areas of papillary hyperplasia remain in spite of treatment.

D: Higher magnification shows that the papillary areas can have fibrovascular cores as in papillary carcinomas.

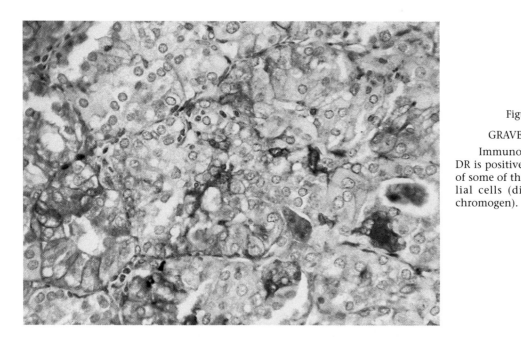

Figure 3-45

GRAVES' DISEASE

Immunostaining for HLA-DR is positive in the cytoplasm of some of the follicular epithelial cells (diaminobenzidine chromogen).

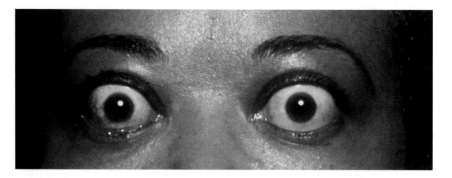

Figure 3-46

GRAVES' ORBITOPATHY

Top: Graves' orbitopathy with proptosis and stare.

Bottom: Periorbital fibro-adipose tissue with a lympho-plasmacytic infiltrate.

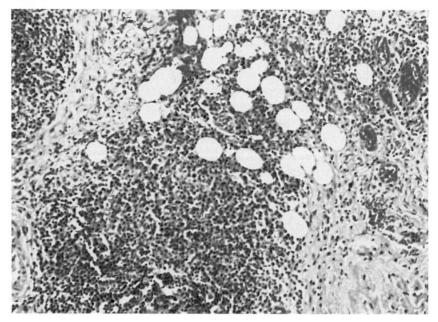

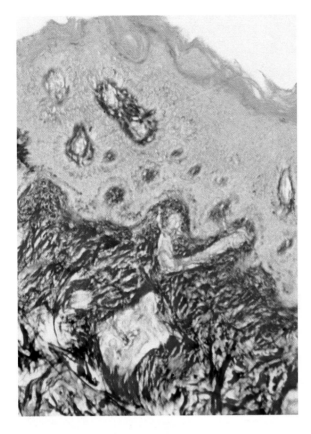

Figure 3-47

GRAVES' DERMOPATHY

The epithelium shows hyperkeratosis. There is a deposit of acid mucopolysaccharides in the dermis in this area of localized myxedema.

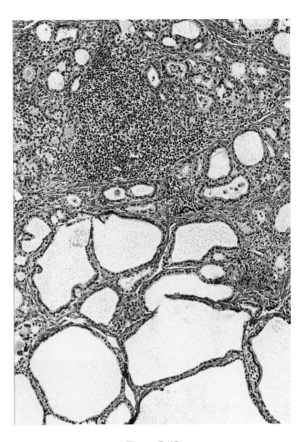

Figure 3-48

HASHITOXICOSIS

Features of Graves' disease and Hashimoto's thyroiditis with lymphoid follicles and germinal centers are present. This illustrates the continuum between these two autoimmune diseases.

These changes in the muscle and connective tissues lead to the exophthalmus that is present in many patients.

The dermal changes of pretibial myxedema consist of deposits of mucopolysaccharides in the dermis and thickening of the skin in these areas (fig. 3-47) (274). This develops in 5 to 10 percent of patients with Graves' disease.

Differential Diagnosis. The histologic differentiation of Graves' disease from papillary thyroid carcinoma can be difficult, since papillae with fibrovascular cores and psammoma bodies can be seen in Graves' disease. In addition, the diffuse hyperplasia in Graves' disease may involve the skeletal muscle adjacent to the thyroid gland, simulating an invasive papillary carcinoma. However, the absence of enlarged overlapping nuclei, nuclear grooves, and cyto-plasmic invaginations into the nucleus helps to make the distinction.

Many other thyroid conditions can lead to hyperthyroidism and may be a problem clinically, but these can be readily distinguished histologically. Hashitoxicosis or hyperthyroiditis (fig. 3-48) is a disease in which patients have thyrotoxicosis along with a histologic picture of epithelial hyperplasia admixed with the changes seen in Hashimoto's thyroiditis (257), including lymphocytic infiltration with germinal centers, Hurthle cell changes, and variable follicular atrophy. The clinical and pathologic features distinguish these cases from typical Graves' disease.

Neoplasms, including hyperfunctioning follicular adenomas and primary and metastatic follicular carcinomas, can be associated with

thyrotoxicosis (261,271,286,288). The histologic appearance of the hyperfunctioning neoplasms is similar to that of nonfunctioning ones, so it is usually easy to distinguish these lesions from Graves' disease.

Toxic nodular goiters are frequently associated with hyperthyroidism (264). Grossly, there is a multinodular gland rather than the diffuse hyperplasia of Graves' disease. Microscopically, focal areas of toxic goiter are seen in some of the nodules rather than diffusely as in Graves' disease. Retrogressive changes are common in multinodular goiters including fibrosis, recent and old hemorrhage, and calcification, while these changes are uncommon in diffuse hyperplasia.

Other conditions associated with hyperthyroidism but which are usually not a problem in the histologic differential diagnosis are gestational trophoblastic disease (272); iodine-induced hyperthyroidism (259); struma ovarii with hyperthyroidism (265); rapidly growing tumors of the thyroid gland including lymphomas, anaplastic carcinomas, and metastatic tumors to the thyroid; ectopic production of TSH; thyrotropin-releasing hormone (TRH) resistance to thyroid hormone (255,279) usually secondary to pituitary resistance (254); and factitious or exogenous thyroid hormone intake (292) including accidental overdose from consumption of contaminated food (263).

Treatment and Prognosis. There are multiple approaches to the treatment of Graves' disease including medical, radioactive, and surgical. Medical treatment includes using drugs that inhibit iodine transport such as thioisocyanate and perchlorate, and iodine and iodine-containing agents that inhibit increased glandular storage of organic iodine and retard the rate of secretion of thyroxine (266). Other drugs such as lithium, dexamethasone, and beta-adrenergic blocking agents such as propranolol can also be used to treat Graves' disease.

The use of radioiodine to cause ablation of the thyroid gland is another method of treatment, but an expected outcome is the high frequency of late hypothyroidism. The incidence of postradioiodine hypothyroidism is 30 percent at 5 years and 40 percent at 10 years (266). There is no documented increase in thyroid cancer with this therapeutic approach (266).

The surgical treatment of Graves' disease is bilateral subtotal thyroidectomy. The frequency of recurrent hyperthyroidism is usually less than 5 percent, but the incidence of permanent hypothyroidism can range from 4 to 30 percent (266).

Postpartum Thyroiditis

Definition. This autoimmune thyroid dysfunction occurs in the first year after delivery.

General Remarks. Postpartum thyroiditis is associated with painless enlargement of the thyroid gland, transient thyrotoxicosis, low thyroid radioactive iodine uptake, and a late hypothyroid phase which may last for a few years (293–296).

The immunologic findings are similar to those in chronic lymphocytic thyroiditis. There is a relative increase in B cells in the thyroid compared to the peripheral blood and a relative decrease in suppressor T cells, leading to an increase in the ratio of helper to suppressor T cells (293, 294). Antimicrosomal antibodies are present in postpartum thyroiditis patients after recovery. The hyperthyroidism in this disorder is probably related to destruction of thyroid follicular cells resulting in immunologic reactivity to thyroglobulin as a sequestered antigen. The hypothyroid phase is probably related to the destruction of follicles resulting in decreased thyroid hormone production. Regeneration of follicles and restoration of normal thyroid function are associated with recovery and a return to a euthyroid stage.

Macroscopic Findings. The thyroid may be slightly enlarged diffusely without localized nodules.

Microscopic Findings. There is usually a lymphocytic infiltration of the gland, variable disruption of follicular cells, and slight follicular hyperplasia (296).

Differential Diagnosis. The differential diagnosis includes Hashimoto's disease. However, the Hurthle cell metaplasia and minimal fibrosis of Hashimoto's disease are not seen in postpartum thyroiditis. The histologic features of postpartum thyroiditis are similar to those of silent thyroiditis: lymphocytic infiltrates without significant Hurthle cell metaplasia.

Treatment and Prognosis. This disease is often self-limited, with a transient hypothyroid state that is related to depletion of thyroglobulin as

well as destruction of the follicular cells. Recurrence is relatively common. In a recent series, 15.6 percent of 605 healthy women developed permanent hypothyroidism (294).

Silent Thyroiditis

Definition. This transient form of hyperthyroidism is characterized by a painless nontender thyroid gland, elevated blood levels of T4 and T3, a low radioactive iodine uptake, and spontaneously resolving hyperthyroidism. Synonyms include *painless thyroiditis, transient hyperthyroidism with lymphocytic thyroiditis, atypical subacute thyroiditis,* and *chronic lymphocytic thyroiditis.*

General Remarks. Several reports of this uncommon form of thyroiditis have been published (297–299).

The etiology of the condition is uncertain. A viral etiology has been sought, but not confirmed. Most patients are female, although the disease also occurs in males. Many investigators think that an autoimmune mechanism is invalid. One group of investigators reported a relative accumulation of B cells and a relative decrease of CD8-positive suppressor-cytotoxic T cells in the thyroid tissue of patients with this disease (298). The thyrotoxicosis observed probably results from destruction of thyroid follicles.

Macroscopic Findings. A diffuse goiter in a slightly enlarged thyroid gland is usually present.

Microscopic Findings. The thyroid gland shows a variable lymphocytic infiltrate with preservation of the normal lobular pattern. There may be focal or diffuse thyroiditis. Oxyphilic change is uncommon, but may be seen focally. Fibrosis is usually absent, and when present is usually only focal. Follicular destruction is present in all cases and is a useful diagnostic feature. The degree of follicular destruction is variable and lymphoid follicles are present in about half the cases. During the late recovery phase, there is usually focal thyroiditis but no follicular destruction, oxyphilic changes, or fibrosis.

Immunohistochemical Findings. The studies of Mizukami et al. (297) showed T cells concentrated in the paracortex, with a small percentage in the germinal center, while B cells predominated in the germinal centers. The lymphoid cells infiltrating between follicles were predominantly T cells (298).

Differential Diagnosis. The main differential diagnosis is postpartum thyroiditis which has many clinical histologic similarities to silent thyroiditis. The principal difference is the anteceding pregnancy in the former and its absence in males. Chronic thyroiditis is another consideration, but the extensive follicular destruction is usually not seen. Subacute thyroiditis differs from silent thyroiditis clinically and by the presence of multinucleated giant cells.

Treatment and Prognosis. The disease is often self-limited, and treatment is usually not necessary. Adrenergic beta-blockers may be used in the hyperthyroid phase and temporary thyroxine replacement in the hypothyroid phase. About half of the patients return to a euthyroid phase and remain well for some time. Permanent hypothyroidism may develop years later (299).

Focal Lymphocytic Thyroiditis

Definition. This disorder is usually discovered incidentally in surgically excised thyroid glands or at autopsy. Focal lymphocytic thyroiditis is characterized by dense collections of lymphocytes in the interlobular or intralobular fibrous tissue of the thyroid. Synonyms include *nonspecific thyroiditis* and *focal autoimmune thyroiditis.*

General Remarks. Focal lymphocytic thyroiditis is found in 5 to 20 percent of adult autopsies and is most common in elderly women (300–303). Some studies have suggested that it may be related to the addition of iodine to water supplies and to salt in the United States. The lesions are commonly present in older patients who are asymptomatic for thyroid disease and who have low levels of antithyroid antibodies.

Macroscopic Findings. There are no specific gross findings. The thyroid is usually of normal size. Occasionally, nodules may be present in the thyroid.

Microscopic Findings. Focal aggregates of lymphocytes in the interlobular or intralobular fibrous tissue are present (fig. 3-49). Rarely, there is germinal center formation. The infiltrate usually spares any adenomatous nodules present. Follicular atrophy or disruption does not usually occur. In surgical specimens this disorder may be seen in association with nontoxic nodular goiters, adenomas, and carcinomas, as well as in glands resected for Graves' disease.

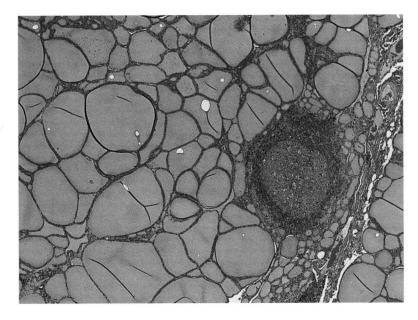

Figure 3-49

FOCAL NONSPECIFIC THYROIDITIS

A thyroid colloid nodule shows focal nonspecific thyroiditis with lymphoid infiltrates, some with germinal centers. The significance of these findings is unknown.

Prognosis and Treatment. Focal thyroiditis is an incidental finding that does not represent a progressive condition. It is most likely not an early form of diffuse autoimmune thyroiditis.

Riedel's Thyroiditis

Definition. Riedel's thyroiditis is a densely sclerotic inflammatory process involving the thyroid gland and adjacent neck tissue.

General Remarks. This is a very rare disorder and constituted 0.05 percent of 42,000 thyroidectomies in an early Mayo Clinic series (306). Early reports emphasized the involvement of the thyroid gland, although other tissues in the neck as well as in other locations may be involved in the inflammatory process. It occurs mainly in adults and has a slight female predominance (306). Thyroid function is normal in the majority of patients, although hypothyroidism or hyperthyroidism may be present (306). Most patients present with a painless goiter. They may have stridor or vocal cord paralysis on occasion.

An autoimmune basis for Riedel's thyroiditis is suggested but not proven. The concomitant development of multifocal sclerosing processes such as idiopathic retroperitoneal fibrosis or sclerosing mediastinitis supports the autoimmune nature of Riedel's thyroiditis. Recent immunohistochemical studies have shown a predominance of lambda light chains, while IgA heavy chains were the main constituent of plasma cells (307). Other studies have shown circulating antithyroid antibodies in the majority of patients with Riedel's thyroiditis, with immunohistochemical studies showing a mixture of B and T cells (in a ratio similar to that of Hashimoto's thyroiditis) (305,308).

A recent study of 16 patients with Riedel's thyroiditis by Heufelder et al. (304) showed a striking tissue eosinophilia and abundant extracellular deposition of major basic proteins derived from the eosinophils. This was not seen in patients with Hashimoto's thyroiditis or Graves' disease.

Macroscopic Findings. There is a goiter with extensive fibrosis involving part or the entire thyroid gland (fig. 3-50). The gland is very hard, and the fibrosis often extends to the adjacent muscle and soft tissues of the neck. The cut surface is tan-gray, woody, and avascular, without the normal lobulation of the gland being apparent.

Microscopic Findings. The normal lobular pattern is obliterated by dense sclerotic fibrous tissue (fig. 3-51). Thyroid follicles are completely obliterated and shrunken by the fibrosis. Oxyphilic cells are not present, but there is an infiltrate of inflammatory cells consisting of lymphocytes, plasma cells, a few neutrophils, and eosinophils. Occasional giant cells may be present. The fibrous tissue may also

Figure 3-50

RIEDEL'S THYROIDITIS

A goiter with extensive fibrosis involves the entire thyroid gland. The cut section shows a tan-gray, woody, relatively avascular surface without the normal thyroid lobulation.

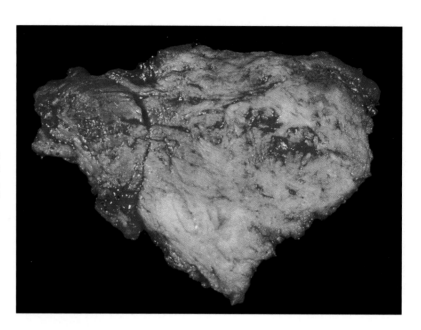

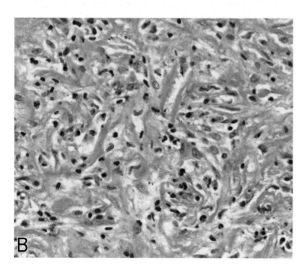

Figure 3-51

RIEDEL'S THYROIDITIS

The normal lobular pattern is obliterated. A few residual follicles may be seen in the fibro-inflammatory background. The infiltrate of lymphocytes and plasma cells along with the sclerosis extends beyond the thyroid gland to the adjacent skeletal muscle (C).

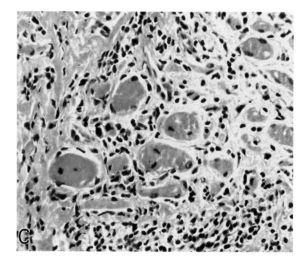

involve the parathyroid glands. Occasionally, there is a vasculitis with intimal proliferation and thrombosis. Some reported cases of Riedel's thyroiditis are associated with a follicular adenoma in the areas of fibrosis (306).

Immunohistochemical Findings. Staining of the plasma cells reveals a predominance of lambda light chains and IgA heavy chains in contrast to Hashimoto's thyroiditis which usually has kappa light chains and IgG heavy chains (307). Analysis of B and T cells shows a similar proportion of CD4+ helper and CD8+ suppressor cells, as is seen in Hashimoto's thyroiditis (308). Immunofluorescence studies of proteins in human eosinophilic granules show extracellular deposition of major basic protein in Riedel's but not in Hashimoto's thyroiditis (304).

Differential Diagnosis. The fibrous variant of Hashimoto's thyroiditis is most often confused with Riedel's thyroiditis. Clinical features such as the absence of very high antibody titers and histologic features including fibrosis extending beyond the thyroid to the neck muscle, loss of the lobular architecture, absence of oxyphil cells, and a limited lymphocytic infiltrate are helpful distinguishing features of Riedel's thyroiditis. Rapidly growing tumors such as anaplastic thyroid carcinoma and thyroid lymphoma may be confused clinically with Riedel's thyroiditis. However, histologic examination allows distinction. The parvicellular variant of undifferentiated thyroid carcinoma may also be confused with Riedel's thyroiditis, especially in small biopsy specimens. The presence of marked cellular pleomorphism and atypical mitoses in the parvicellular population should suggest this diagnosis. An unusual type of fibroinflammatory lesion of the head and neck that can simulate Riedel's thyroiditis has been reported (309).

Treatment and Prognosis. Surgery may be required in some patients to preserve tracheal and esophageal function (306). Patients with hypothyroidism usually require thyroid hormone therapy. Associated conditions in these patients include retroperitoneal fibrosis, mediastinal fibrosis, orbital and lacrimal sclerosis, sclerosing cholangitis, and pituitary and testicular fibrosis which forms part of the spectrum of systemic idiopathic fibrosis or idiopathic multifocal fibrosclerosis.

SIMPLE, MULTINODULAR, DYSHORMONOGENETIC, AND DIFFUSE TOXIC GOITERS

The term goiter is nonspecific and refers simply to an enlargement of the thyroid gland. Goiters have a variety of etiologies ranging from inflammatory diseases, non-neoplastic enlargements, and neoplasms. The presence of a goiter does not reflect the functional activity of the gland which can range from euthyroid to hyperthyroid and hypothyroid states. Thyroid hyperplasia often results from disturbances of the feedback system in which decreased production of thyroid hormone can lead to increased production of thyrotropin-releasing hormone (TRH) from the hypothalamus and thyroid stimulating hormone (TSH) from the pituitary. TSH stimulates hyperplasia of the thyroid gland, leading to enlargement of the gland.

Simple and Multinodular Nontoxic Goiter

Definition. These are diffuse enlargements of the thyroid gland with varying degrees of nodularity not associated with hyperthyroidism or hypothyroidism and which do not result from inflammation or neoplasms.

General Remarks. About 10 percent of thyroid glands seen at autopsy contain gross evidence of nodules, but microscopic nodularity is much more common (311,327). Most simple and multinodular goiters are associated with a euthyroid state, although hyperthyroidism may occur (see Toxic Multinodular Goiter below).

Simple goiters usually weigh more than 40 g, although this may vary with the patient's geographic location. In the pathogenesis of simple and multinodular goiters, it is assumed that there is initially diffuse hyperplasia which becomes nodular with increasing size, fibrosis, and distortion of the vascular supply of the thyroid gland (fig. 3-52).

The etiologic stimuli for goiter development can be quite variable. Chemically-induced goiters may result from excessive consumption of goitrogenic foods including thiocyanates and perchlorates, which affect the iodine-trapping mechanisms in the thyroid. The thiocarbamides and aniline derivatives which inhibit the organification of iodine can also lead to simple goiter. Elements such as iodine and lithium can interfere with the breakdown of thyroglobulin and the release of thyroid hormone.

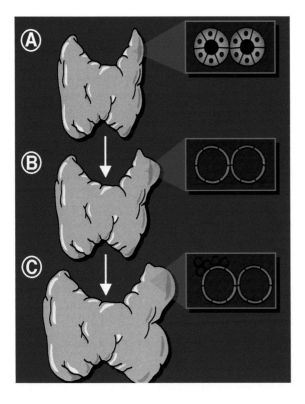

Figure 3-52

MULTINODULAR GOITER

Schematic diagram of the development of a simple goiter and progression to a multinodular goiter. The normal thyroid (A) enlarges and develops a few colloid nodules with dilated follicles (B). Histologic examination shows dilated follicles with flattened epithelium. Progression to a multinodular goiter occurs with continued stimulation or failure to correct the intrinsic defect for normal thyroid hormone synthesis. This results in variable-sized follicles with some areas of follicular hyperplasia due to focal increased stimulation and degenerative changes including fibrosis, hemorrhage, and dystrophic calcification (C).

Drug-induced goiters from compounds such as sulfonamides, phenylbutazones, and phenindione act by inhibiting organification of iodine. Excessive intake of iodine-containing medications such as amiodarone may lead to goiters by interfering with thyroglobulin proteolysis, as discussed above. Some natural goitrogens that occur in foods, such as members of the Brassica family, lead to goiters by releasing of isothiocyanates, thiocyanates, and thiouracil-like compounds (314,317,333).

The pathogenesis of simple and multinodular nontoxic goiter is probably related to factors that impair hormone synthesis (315, 318). This impairment leads to hypersecretion of TSH which stimulates thyroid growth, and increased thyroid hormone biosynthesis to compensate for the prior impairment. This homeostatic compensation results from the increase in thyroid mass and a greater capacity to produce the required amount of thyroid hormone. Another theory about the development of simple and multinodular goiters without hyperthyroidism is that the thyroid is stimulated by thyroid growth immunoglobulins (TGI) which do not stimulate thyroid adenylate cyclase activity (as TSH autoantibodies do) so that there is no concomitant hyperthyroidism (316,319,339,342). The nodularity of the gland in progression from simple to multinodular goiter would be explained by the "marine cycle" in which hyperstimulation of the thyroid by TSH (because of prior decreased hormone production and hypothyroidism) leads to homeostasis; further stimulation leads to focal nodular hyperplasia and this is followed by involutional changes with fibrosis, hemorrhagic changes in blood flow, and dystrophic calcification, leading to more retrogressive changes (fig. 3-52) (332,340).

Molecular genetic analyses have provided some insight into the pathogenesis of adenoma and adenomatous nodules in multinodular goiters. The principle of the Lyon hypothesis is used in these studies which assumes that during embryonic development in females one of the two sets of X chromosomes is inactivated, with different X chromosomes inactivated in different cells. There is a random distribution of cells with X inactivation throughout the body (330,331). Many X-linked genes have been used in these studies in which the subject must be a female. One assumes that in a true neoplasm clonal cells will all express the active X-chromosome marker. A comparison between the normal cells and tumor tissues or nodules shows two bands in the normal tissue and inactivation of one allele in the clonal nodule or tumor. Although the results from different studies have been variable (310, 326,329,341), when careful morphological studies are correlated with the molecular biological studies, some nodules within multinodular goiters are indeed monoclonal and represent true adenomas. More recent clonality studies have used the androgen receptor on the X

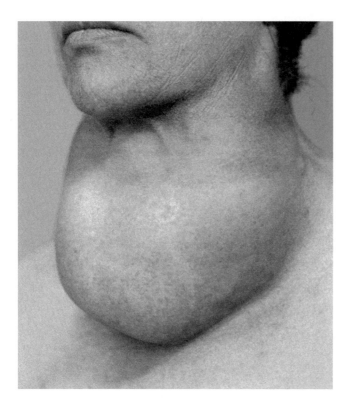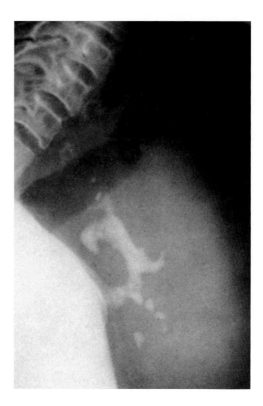

Figure 3-53

MULTINODULAR GOITER

Left: A 52-year-old woman with a huge colloid goiter. The goiter was first noticed at age 14 and it slowly enlarged. She finally sought medical care because of compressive symptoms and hyperthyroidism. A 1,023 g gland was removed at surgery.

Right: This X-ray view of a large nodular goiter shows central calcifications secondary to regressive changes. (Figure 24 from Fascicle 4, 2nd Series.)

chromosome. This technique is more sensitive than earlier X chromosome targets and has the potential to analyze greater than 90 percent of the target female population rather than the 25 percent in earlier studies (312,320).

Studies in a few families have implicated a role of heredity in the development of nontoxic goiters (325,334).

Clinical and Radiologic Findings. Patients present with thyroid enlargement or goiter. About 70 percent of patients with nontoxic goiters have neck discomfort. Large goiters (fig. 3-53, left) may displace or compress the esophagus or trachea with associated dysphagia or inspiratory stridor.

Occasionally, venous engorgement from narrowing of the thoracic inlet may occur. Vocal cord paralysis may occasionally result from a large multinodular goiter, although this sign is usually more diagnostic of a thyroid carcinoma.

Nontoxic goiters have a female predominance of about 8 to 1. They tend to develop more frequently during adolescence and pregnancy (323). Scintigraphic thyroid scanning with radioactive iodine in patients with diffuse or nodular simple goiter often shows a heterogeneous picture (328). Evidence of degenerative changes and calcification may be seen on X ray (fig. 3-53, right). The radioactive iodine uptake is usually normal but may be increased due to mild iodine deficiency or other defects. T3 and T4 concentrations are usually normal, although the proportion of T3 to T4 may be increased secondary to defective iodination of thyroglobulin (337). Serum thyroglobulin levels are often elevated.

Macroscopic Findings. Simple goiters are firm and diffusely enlarged, with the normal thyroid gland weighing up to 40 g. The cut surface shows a uniform amber color with a translucent appearance. Multinodular goiters are of varying

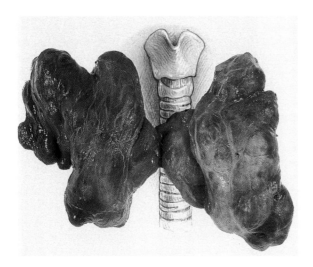 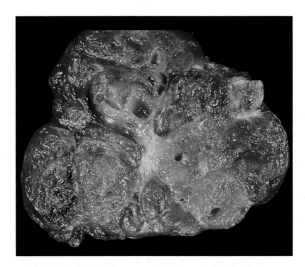

Figure 3-54

MULTINODULAR GOITER

Left: Early multinodular goiter shows enlarged thyroid gland with nodules involving both lobes.
Right: A cut section shows a slightly nodular tan surface with focal areas of scarring.

sizes and often weigh from 60 to 1,000 g or more (figs. 3-54, 3-55). The gland has a distorted shape and is nodular. Some nodules may be partially or completely separated from the gland, constituting sequestered or parasitic nodules. Cut sections of the multinodular goiter show areas of nodularity, fibrosis, old and recent hemorrhage, and calcification. The nodules can be quite variable in size and number and may be cystic. Some nodules contain a thickened fibrous connective tissue capsule and have the general appearance of follicular neoplasms. Some multinodular goiters may descend into the anterior mediastinum as substernal or plunging goiters (fig. 3-56). Extensive hemorrhage in these goiters as part of the degenerative or retrogressive process may lead to tracheal compression and present as a surgical emergency.

Cytologic Findings. There is colloid and a mixed cell population, with relatively few cells in the aspirate, which can include follicular cells, inflammatory cells, and Hurthle cells. Follicular cells are present in sheets of 15 to 100 monolayers with uniform nuclei (fig. 3-57). Colloid is present on large globules or as discrete rounded or hexagonal droplets. Hypercellular foci within a multinodular goiter may simulate a follicular neoplasm.

Microscopic Findings. The histologic appearance of simple diffuse goiters consists of follicles of varying size that may be as large as a few millimeters in diameter. The follicles are lined by flattened epithelium with involutional changes. Smaller follicles are lined by epithelial cells that are more columnar (suggestive of more active binding of organic iodine and synthesis of thyroglobulin). These smaller follicles correlate with autoradiographic studies showing more active iodine binding.

The histology of multinodular goiter parallels the macroscopic features, with nodules consisting of irregularly enlarged follicles of variable size with distended colloid and flattened epithelium adjacent to smaller follicles with a taller, more active epithelium (fig. 3-58). The larger nodules compress the adjacent parenchyma. Large distended follicles often coalesce to create cystic areas which may be several millimeters in diameter. Focal areas of papillary hyperplasia with "Sanderson polster" or a cluster of small follicles protruding into large dilated follicles may be seen (fig. 3-59). The polster is usually made up of taller, more columnar epithelium since the colloid in the cytoplasm adjacent to the follicular cells contains reabsorption vacuoles. There may be evidence of old and

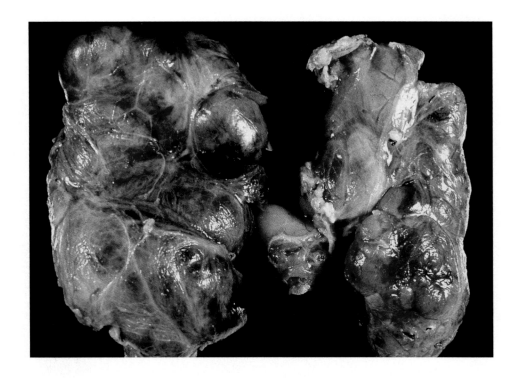

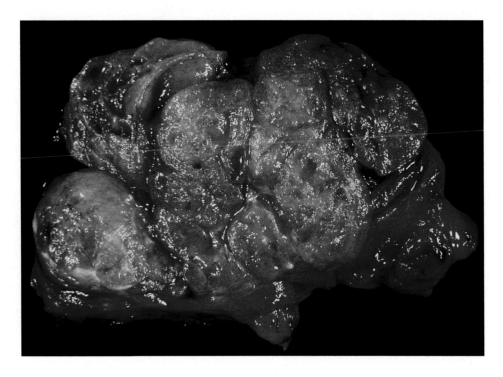

Figure 3-55

MULTINODULAR GOITER

Top: Markedly enlarged goiter with multiple nodules. Many large nodules are present on the surface of the gland.
Bottom: The cut surface of this large goiter shows nodules of variable size with fibrosis and cystic degeneration.

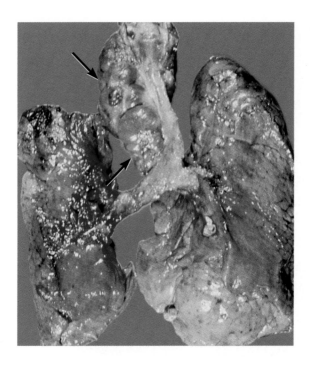

Figure 3-56

MULTINODULAR GOITER

The mediastinal or substernal goiter was discovered at autopsy. The goiter extends to the level of the carina. Acute hemorrhage in the goiter could lead to tracheal compression and respiratory difficulties. (Courtesy of Dr. Lee Weatherbee, Ann Arbor, MI.)

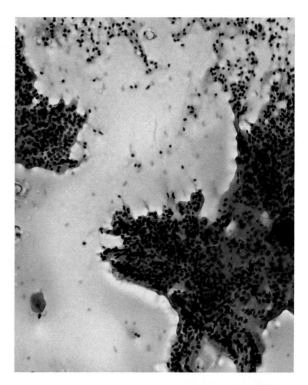

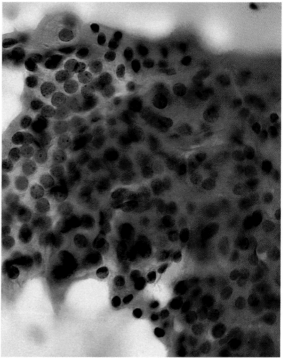

Figure 3-57

MULTINODULAR GOITER

Sheets of follicular cells with abundant colloid in the background are noted. The follicular cells have uniform nuclei.

recent hemorrhage with hemosiderin-laden macrophages, and ischemic necrosis with lipid-laden macrophages. Cholesterol clefts are usually evident along with extensive irregular fibrosis, variable dystrophic calcification, and ossification. Hyperplastic nodules with variable degrees of encapsulation are often seen. Some of these nodules may be completely encapsulated and look like adenomas. They are often referred to as adenomatous or adenomatoid nodules and the goiter as adenomatous goiter. Colloid nodules usually refer to the dilated follicles lined by flattened epithelium.

It may be difficult to distinguish on a morphological basis an adenomatous nodule in multinodular goiter and a true follicular neoplasm arising in this setting. Clonality studies with X-chromosome inactivation have shown that some of these adenomatous nodules are monoclonal (312,326,329). It has been postulated that the hyperplastic process with more rapidly proliferating cells may lead to somatic mutations

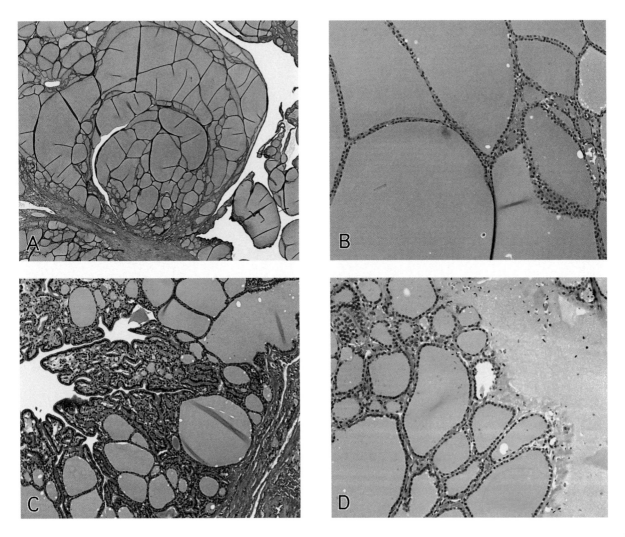

Figure 3-58

MULTINODULAR GOITER

Multiple colloid nodules of variable size (A) and dilated follicles lined by flattened epithelium (B) are present. Other areas show hyperplastic smaller follicles, papillary hyperplasia (C), and retrogressive changes including fibrosis and cystic degeneration (D).

and neoplastic development in these multinodular goiters (312).

Differential Diagnosis. The differential diagnosis includes other causes of multinodular goiter and neoplasms arising in multinodular goiter. Multinodular goiters can be confused with dyshormonogenetic goiters, which are caused by thyroid hyperplasia secondary to enzyme defects in thyroid hormone biosynthesis. The cellular appearance of dyshormonogenetic goiter is similar to that of multinodular goiter, but the increased cellularity of the latter is usu-

ally focal as opposed to the diffuse involvement in dyshormonogenetic goiter (321).

Follicular neoplasms arising in a multinodular goiter may be difficult to distinguish from a hyperplastic nodule if there is a completely thickened capsule (Table 3-2). The diagnosis of a follicular carcinoma should only be made in the presence of vascular invasion of the capsule or beyond (343). However, rare cases of multinodular goiter may also show vascular invasion at the periphery of the nodules, so this finding must be interpreted cautiously (336). Although

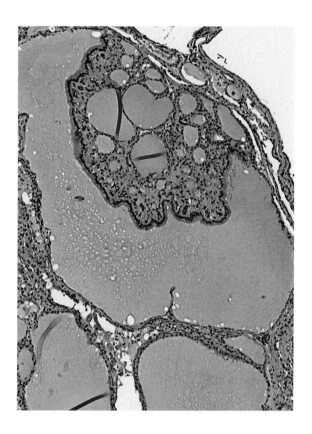 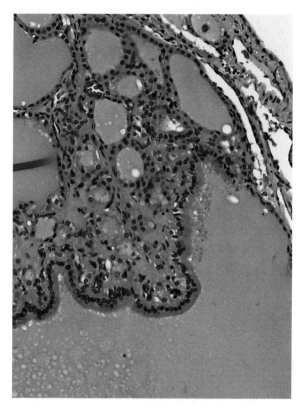

Figure 3-59

MULTINODULAR GOITER

Left: Sanderson polster formed by a cluster of small follicles protruding into a large dilated follicle.
Right: Higher magnification shows that the polster is lined by more columnar epithelium.

nontoxic goiter may look similar to toxic multinodular goiter, clinicopathological correlation enables one to make the distinction.

Treatment and Prognosis. Treatment with thyroxine is an effective way of reducing the size of diffuse simple goiters, although this is less effective with multinodular goiters (324, 338). Radioactive iodine treatment of nontoxic multinodular goiter is usually effective and safe (335). One complication, especially in younger patients, is the increasing incidence of hypothyroidism in a time-dependent manner (322). Surgery is probably the most definitive method of treating multinodular nontoxic goiter in symptomatic patients, although they recur in 10 to 20 percent of patients by 10 years (314). The rate of postoperative hypothyroidism depends on the extent of the surgical resection.

Dyshormonogenetic Goiter

Definition. These familial goiters develop because of a defect in the metabolism of thyroid hormone secondary to an inherited disorder.

General Remarks. Dyshormonogenetic goiters are rare, with a prevalence of 1 in 30,000 to 50,000 live births in Europe and North America (346). It is the second most frequent cause of permanent congenital hypothyroidism after thyroid dysgenesis, including aplastic and hypoplastic thyroid disorders (344,349). There are five major biochemical defects which lead to decreased thyroid hormone synthesis. The resultant alterations in thyroid gland homeostasis, disturbance of the feedback system, and chronic TSH stimulation lead to enlarged thyroid glands or goiters (Table 3-3).

Table 3-2

DIAGNOSTIC FEATURES DISTINGUISHING HYPERPLASTIC NODULES FROM ADENOMAS

Hyperplastic Nodule	Adenoma
Multiple lesions	Solitary lesion
Variable degree of encapsulation	Well-developed capsule
Variable cells in nodules without compression and similar to those outside nodule	Uniform lesion with compression of adjacent dissimilar thyroid
Polyclonal cell population	Monoclonal cell population

Table 3-3

DEFECTS CAUSING DYSHORMONOGENETIC GOITERS

Iodine transport

Peroxide organification

Iodotyrosinase coupling

Iodotyrosinase cholagenase

Thyroglobulin synthesis with formation and synthesis of abnormal iodoprotein

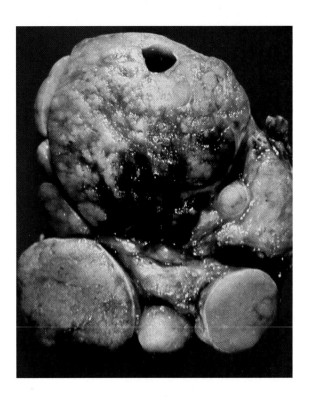

Figure 3-60

DYSHORMONOGENETIC GOITER

Cut surface of a thyroid gland from a patient with a dyshormonogenetic goiter. Nodular hyperplastic and retrogressive changes including hemorrhage and fibrosis are present. (Plate XLIB from Fascicle 5, 3rd Series.)

The defect is usually transmitted as an autosomal recessive trait and is a cause of cretinism and hypothyroidism. The goiter is usually not present at birth but appears later in life.

Clinical and Radiologic Findings. In a recent study of 56 patients with dyshormonogenetic goiter, ages ranged from neonates to 52 years, with a median of 16 years (347). Most goiters (75 percent) developed before age 24 years. Patients usually present with clinical evidence of a goiter, although sometimes the diagnosis is made at autopsy. Of the 56 cases described above, there were 34 females and 22 males; a family history of goiter or hypothyroidism was present in 11 cases (20 percent). Only one patient had *Pendred's syndrome* which is a dyshormonogenetic goiter associated with nerve deafness (345,350).

Macroscopic Findings. The thyroid gland is enlarged asymmetrically and may weigh up to 600 g. As with other multinodular goiters, areas of cystic change, fibrosis, and old and recent hemorrhage are present (fig. 3-60). The cut surface is firm and tan with nodules of varying size, which may be up to a few centimeters in diameter.

Microscopic Findings. The nodules are hypercellular and often have a trabecular pattern with pale-staining colloid. Prominent papillary hyperplasia may be present in the nodules. Some authors have described a characteristic microcystic pattern in dyshormonogenetic goiters associated with a thyroglobulin synthetic defect (348). Myxoid change may also

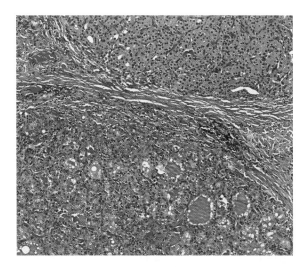 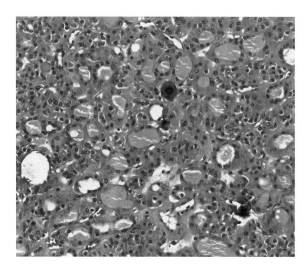

Figure 3-61

DYSHORMONOGENETIC GOITER

Hypercellular areas with fibrosis (left) and dystrophic calcification (right) are present.

be seen. The most common patterns in the nodules are solid and microfollicular (fig. 3-61). The extensive fibrosis in the internodular tissue may simulate true capsular invasion. Nuclear abnormalities consist of enlarged, irregularly shaped, hyperchromatic nuclei and vesicular nuclei (347). There may be focal areas with clear cytoplasmic change.

Immunohistochemical studies show positive staining for thyroglobulin and negative staining for calcitonin (347). Ultrastructural studies show cells with abundant mitochondria, rough endoplasmic reticulum with dilated cisternae, and tall follicular cells with numerous microvilli (347).

Differential Diagnosis. The two most significant differential diagnoses include distinguishing dyshormonogenetic goiter from thyroid carcinoma and from other multinodular goiters. Because of the hypercellularity, these lesions may be misdiagnosed as carcinomas. However, to make a diagnosis of carcinoma, there must be convincing vascular invasion, massive extrathyroidal extension, distant metastasis, or the architectural and cytologic features of papillary carcinomas (347).

Distinction of dyshormonogenetic goiter from endemic multinodular goiter may be difficult, since both lesions may have extensive hyperplasia (351). In dyshormonogenetic goiter there is a marked decrease in colloid, fewer degenerative changes, and absence of normal internodular tissue. Marked nuclear atypia may be present in both conditions, but in dyshormonogenetic goiter, the atypia is present only in the nodules while in endemic goiter it is present inside and outside the nodules.

Treatment and Prognosis. Treatment is usually symptomatic and the approach is the same as that used for multinodular goiter, including medical and surgical therapies.

Toxic Multinodular Goiter

Definition. This is a condition in which hyperthyroidism arises in a multinodular goiter, usually of longstanding duration.

General Remarks. Some investigators separate multinodular goiter from *toxic adenoma* or *Plummer's disease* in which an adenoma in a relatively normal thyroid is hyperfunctioning (354). The term *toxic nodular goiter* usually includes both toxic multinodular goiter and toxic adenoma or Plummer's disease (353,355).

The pathogenesis of toxic multinodular goiter is uncertain (352,354). Although in toxic adenomas a mutation in the TSH receptor gene has been demonstrated, this has not been shown in toxic multinodular goiter (356).

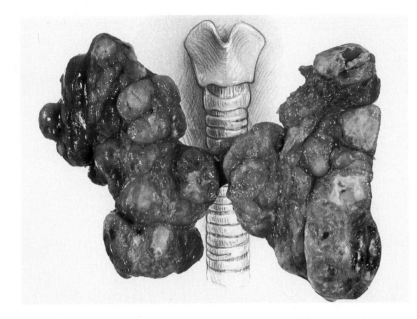

Figure 3-62

PLUMMER'S DISEASE

Multinodular goiter involving both thyroid lobes in a patient with a toxic goiter.

In some toxic goiters, hyperthyroidism may develop abruptly after exposure to increased amounts of iodine; the iodine allows autonomous foci to increase thyroid hormone secretion to high levels, exacerbating chronic mild hyperthyroidism (354).

Clinical and Radiologic Findings. The overproduction of thyroid hormone in toxic multinodular goiter is usually less than in Graves' disease. The serum T3 and T4 concentrations may be only slightly increased while suppressed TSH may be the only early manifestation of this condition (356). The incidence of toxic multinodular goiter is unknown. It usually occurs after age 50 in patients with a history of chronic nontoxic multinodular goiter. It is more common in women than men and is rarely associated with eye disease. The principal clinical manifestation is cardiovascular, with atrial fibrillation or tachycardia. Weakness and muscle wasting are also common (356).

The radioactive iodine uptake is not helpful in establishing the diagnosis because thyrotoxicosis may exist in association with values that are normal or only slightly increased. Imaging studies with radioiodine show localization in one or more discrete nodules of the multinodular gland while iodine accumulation in the remainder of the gland is usually suppressed. TSH administration stimulates iodine uptake in the inactive areas, confirming that the suppression is due to a lack of TSH.

Macroscopic Findings. The thyroid gland is enlarged, with multiple nodules showing fibrosis, old and recent hemorrhage, and dystrophic calcification (figs. 3-62, 3-63).

Microscopic Findings. The nodules are variable in appearance. Hyperactive nodules are well demarcated with a discrete fibrous capsule. They consist of follicles with tall columnar cells and papillary hyperplasia. The other nonfunctional nodules may appear inactive and have degenerative changes as seen in the usual multinodular goiter (fig. 3-64).

Differential Diagnosis. The histologic appearance of a toxic multinodular goiter and a nontoxic multinodular goiter overlap, so distinguishing these two entities without clinical correlation and imaging studies may be difficult. The increased cellularity of the toxic nodules looks similar to that of dyshormonogenetic goiters, but the changes are focal rather than diffuse. Distinguishing the hyperplastic nodules from follicular carcinoma relies on the presence of vascular invasion or invasion beyond the thyroid. Distinction from papillary carcinoma relies on cytological and architectural features. Grave's disease is distinguished by the uniformity of changes, with diffuse hyperplasia and absence of nodules in the diffusely enlarged thyroid gland.

Treatment and Prognosis. The treatment of choice is radioactive iodine. There is usually a variation in the sensitivity to radioiodine (354). Patients with obstructive syndromes are usually

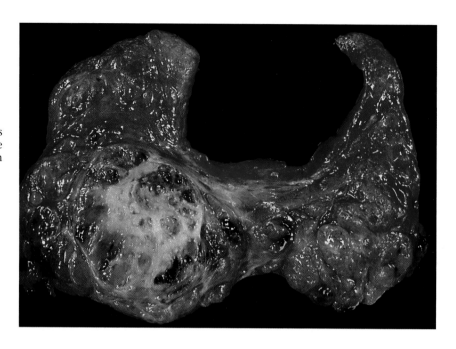

Figure 3-63

PLUMMER'S DISEASE

Multinodular goiter shows an area of retrogressive change with fibrosis and hemorrhage in a patient with a toxic goiter.

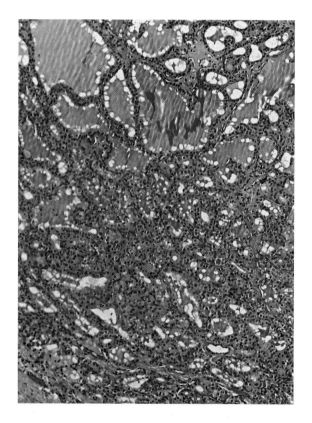
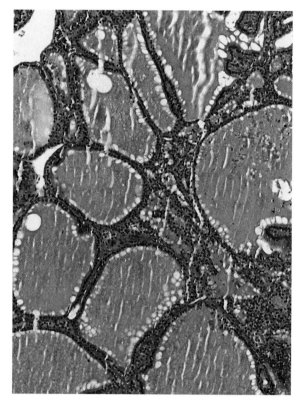

Figure 3-64

PLUMMER'S DISEASE

Left: Variably hypercellular areas with scalloping of the colloid.
Right: Other areas show dilated follicles, fibrosis, and old hemorrhage in a patient with a toxic goiter.

treated with surgery, especially when there is danger of further obstruction from the temporary thyroid enlargement that radioactive iodine treatment sometimes produces.

Endemic Goiters

Endemic goiters are those that develop in certain geographic regions, usually secondary to iodine deficiency. They are also termed *iodine deficiency disorder.*

Historically, endemic goiters have developed in geographic areas such as the Great Lakes Region in North America, the mountainous regions of South America, and Western Europe (362,363). The use of the term "iodine deficiency disorder" emphasizes the results of iodine deficiency on mental and physical development (358,359). The incidence of endemic goiter and cretinism decreases markedly when iodine is introduced into the diet as a supplement.

There are probably interactions between iodine deficiency and other factors that work permissively to lead to endemic goiters: there are reports that increased calcium and fluoride in the water of iodine-deficient regions contribute to goiter development (361). In some regions of the world, cassava ingestion can interact with iodine deficiency and lead to goiter development (357,364). Contamination of drinking water by sewage has been associated with goiter development in the Himalayas (360). Thus, the interaction of nutritional and environmental factors leading to endemic goiters appears more complex than simply iodine deficiency (357,364).

The macroscopic and microscopic findings in endemic goiters are similar to those of multinodular goiters, with multiple nodules in a background of degenerative changes including fibrosis, old and recent hemorrhage, and dystrophic calcification. The histologic picture is variable-sized follicles, with thin follicular cells in dilated colloid follicles admixed with smaller follicles lined by columnar epithelium.

Amyloid Goiter

Deposits of amyloid in the thyroid not associated with a neoplasm can lead to glandular enlargement or goiter. The amyloid in the thyroid is usually of the AA type, a type associated with chronic infection or inflammation, but AL amyloid, usually associated with plasma cell abnormalities, may also be present (367, 368). Amyloid goiters are extremely uncommon. Patients present with thyroid enlargement and may have dysfunction of other organs affected by amyloidosis. The thyroid gland is usually enlarged and has a solid white to tan appearance (fig. 3-65) (365,366). Microscopic examination shows sheets of amyloid surrounding thyroid follicles (fig. 3-65). Fat cells may be admixed with the nodules. Calcification and foreign body giant cells may be present.

The differential diagnosis includes medullary thyroid carcinoma in which the neoplastic cells should be present, amyloidosis associated with multiple myeloma or plasma cell disorders, and possibly hyalinizing trabecular adenomas.

The prognosis of patients with amyloid goiter depends on the underlying disease. Surgical treatment is performed if needed to relieve symptoms of mass effect.

C-CELL HYPERPLASIA

Definition. There is an increase in the total mass of C cells within the thyroid gland usually associated with multifocal proliferation of calcitonin-producing cells.

General Remarks. C cells are often difficult to identify on H&E-stained sections (fig. 3-66), so immunostaining is very important for their detection (fig. 3-67). Ultrastructural examination is also useful (fig. 3-68). The etiology of C-cell hyperplasia as well as the definition of this disorder can be quite variable (Table 3-4) (369–372,375,385–387). Historically, the finding of 50 C cells per low-power field (10X) has been used as the definition. A recent study using autopsy-obtained thyroid glands from 42 adults found that 33 percent (41 percent males and 15 percent females) have at least 50 C cells per three 10X fields (381), suggesting that C-cell hyperplasia may be more common than previously thought (369,370,380,381,391). C-cell hyperplasia occurs more often in men than in women in various studies (381,391).

Some investigators have divided C-cell hyperplasia into physiologic and neoplastic types (392,397). Physiologic hyperplasia is observed in neonatal and elderly patients and is associated with various conditions as shown in Table 3-3. Neoplastic hyperplasia is associated with

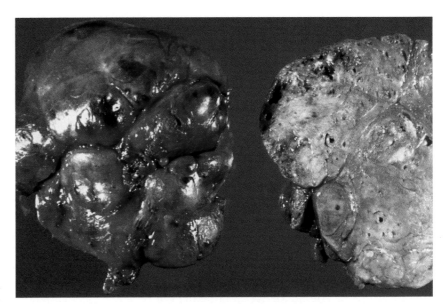

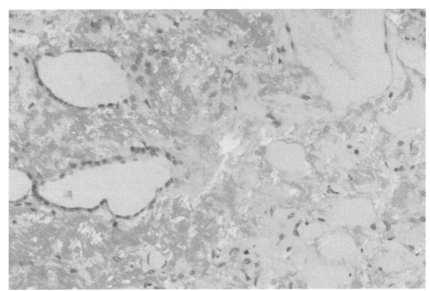

Figure 3-65

AMYLOIDOSIS OF THE THYROID

Top: The outer aspect and cut surface of localized amyloidosis of the thyroid (amyloid tumor) shows an enlarged gland with a salmon color on cross section.

Bottom: Apple-green birefringence after Congo red staining of the amyloid under polarized light. (Plate VLII A and B, Fascicle 5, 3rd Series.)

multiple endocrine neoplasia (MEN) 2a and 2b. It has been suggested that physiologic hyperplasia may be associated with over-stimulation by thyroid-stimulating hormone (369,370).

The pathogenesis of neoplastic C-cell hyperplasia in patients with MEN 2a and 2b has been reported by DeLellis et al. and by others (374,375,390,393,400,401). In their model of neoplastic C-cell hyperplasia, the C cell undergoes hypertrophy, focal and diffuse hyperplasia, and then progresses to nodular hyperplasia and medullary thyroid carcinoma (374,375).

The RET proto-oncogene, which encodes a member of the tyrosine kinase family of transmembrane receptors, is frequently associated with germ-line mutations in familial medullary thyroid carcinoma (MTC) and in some sporadic cases of MTC (377,378, 383,388). Recent studies have shown that RET immunoreactivity is associated with RET codon 918 or codon 803 mutations in patients with sporadic MTC (378). However, RET mutations and results of immunostaining in hyperplastic C-cell hyperplasia have not been examined. Another gene

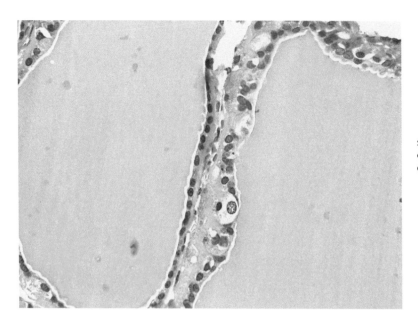

Figure 3-66

NORMAL C CELL

Hematoxylin and eosin-stained section of a normal C cell with clear cytoplasm located within the follicular epithelial basement membrane.

Table 3-4

DISORDERS ASSOCIATED WITH C-CELL HYPERPLASIA

Physiologic
Neonates and elderly
Hemithyroidectomy
Hashimoto's thyroiditis
Follicular neoplasm
Non-Hodgkin's lymphoma
Hyperparathyroidism
Hypergastrinemia

Neoplastic
Multiple endocrine neoplasia type 2a
Multiple endocrine neoplasia type 2b
Idiopathic

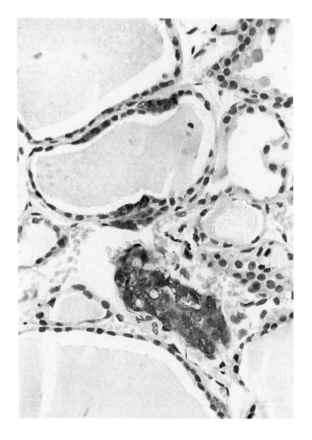

Figure 3-67

NORMAL C CELLS

Immunohistochemical staining with anticalcitonin shows C cells in an adult. Some of the C cells are present in small clusters (diaminobenzidine chromogen).

involved in the pathogenesis of MTC is the trk family neurotropin receptor. Of the three members of the trk family, trkB was consistently expressed in C-cell hyperplasia while in normal C cells only a subset expressed trk receptors (389). TrkB was also reduced in MTC while trkC was increased in these tumors, suggesting that expression of some members of the neurotropin receptor family is turned off or on at various stages in C-cell disease progression (389).

Macroscopic Findings. There is usually no obvious striking changes associated with C-cell

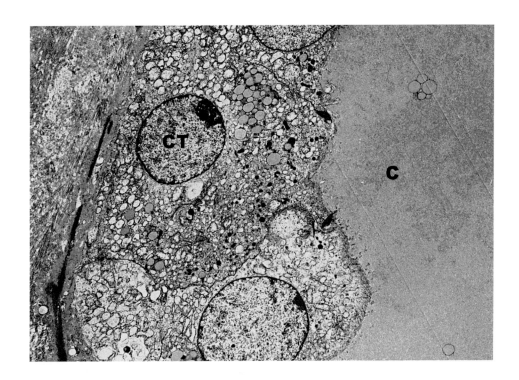

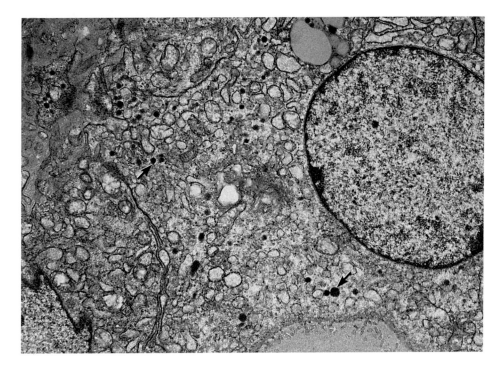

Figure 3-68

NORMAL C CELLS

Top: Ultrastructural view of C cells (CT) located within the follicular epithelium basement membrane adjacent to the luminal colloid (C) (X2,300).

Bottom: Higher magnification shows scattered dense core secretory granules (arrows) in the cytoplasm. The secretory granules contain calcitonin and other hormones (X5,000).

hyperplasia. Careful sectioning may show small 1 to 2 mm foci in the middle to upper portions of both lobes.

Microscopic Findings. C-cell hyperplasia is commonly associated with an increased number of C cells in the middle and upper regions of the thyroid lobes compared to age- and sex-matched controls. The recommended number of C cells to make this diagnosis is 50 per low-power (10X) field. The hyperplasia may be diffuse or nodular. The proliferation of C cells within the follicle may be extensive enough to replace or mask the follicular cells that are commonly seen in nodular C-cell hyperplasia.

Immunohistochemical staining is positive for calcitonin, chromogranin A, calcitonin gene-related peptide, and many other peptides in the C cells (figs. 3-69, 3-70) (393). Ultrastructural studies show a proliferation of C cells within the basement membrane of the follicles, and these are separated from the interstitium by the follicular basal lamina (374,396). There are two types of secretory granules: smaller type II granules, 130 nm in diameter, and larger type I granules, 280 mm. The secretory granules of normal C cells and hyperplastic C cells are similar while MTC cells have a smaller number of secretory granules. Other distinctive ultrastructural features include a prominent rough endoplasmic reticulum and Golgi response.

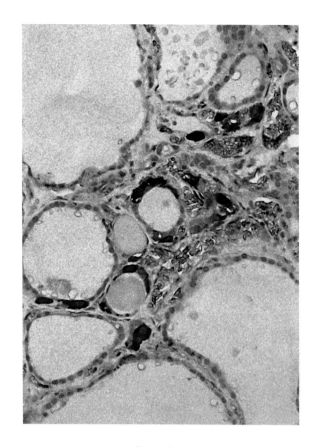

Figure 3-69

C-CELL HYPERPLASIA

Physiological C-cell hyperplasia showing increased numbers of calcitonin-positive C cells (diaminobenzidine chromogen).

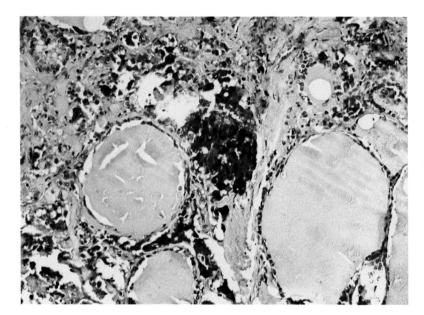

Figure 3-70

C-CELL HYPERPLASIA

C-cell hyperplasia and microscopic medullary thyroid carcinoma in a patient with multiple endocrine neoplasia type 2b. After calcitonin immunostaining, the increased numbers of C cells are readily appreciated.

Differential Diagnosis. One of the most difficult problems is to distinguish between physiologic and neoplastic hyperplasia. Demographic data and patient history should help in this distinction. Gross and microscopic findings such as the presence of a follicular neoplasm, hyperparathyroidism, or hypergastrinemia suggest a diagnosis of physiologic hyperplasia. Patients with a family history of MEN type 2a or 2b most likely have neoplastic C-cell hyperplasia (fig. 3-70). Histologic features of C-cell hyperplasia associated with MEN 2a or MEN 2b are cytologic atypia of the C cells, hyperplasia adjacent to the MTC, and bilateral involvement; these features are not seen with physiologic hyperplasia (392). It is not known at this time if analysis of the RET proto-oncogene by molecular or immunohistochemical methods would separate physiologic and preneoplastic C-cell hyperplasia.

In the differential diagnosis of nodular C-cell hyperplasia, it is important to distinguish C-cell nodules from solid cell nests, squamous metaplasia, parathyroid tissue, and thyroid tissue. Solid cell nests represent remnants of the ultimobranchial bodies embedded in the thyroid (402). The usually stain for keratin and polyclonal carcinoembryonic antigen (CEA), and may be positive for calcitonin, which makes the distinction even more difficult. The ultrastructural findings of intermediate filaments and cytoplasmic projections that lack dense core secretory granules allow a diagnosis of solid cell nests in difficult cases.

Squamous metaplasia usually occurs with inflammatory conditions such as Hashimoto's thyroiditis, including the fibrous variant. These cell nests are more reminiscent of solid cell nests (398). Parathyroid nests and thymic remnants can usually be distinguished from C cell nests by histologic findings such as distinct and prominent cell membranes in parathyroid cells, the lymphoid elements associated with thymic

cells, or by immunostaining for calcitonin and parathyroid hormone.

Occasionally, nests of thyroid follicular cells may look like foci of nodular C-cell hyperplasia. The nuclear features of neuroendocrine cells are absent in the follicular nests and the cytoplasm does not have the clear to granular basophilic appearance seen in C cells. Staining for calcitonin and thyroglobulin assists in making the distinction.

Treatment and Prognosis. Total thyroidectomy is the usual treatment of patients with C-cell hyperplasia, especially for those with a family history of MEN 2a or 2b or a positive test for the RET proto-oncogene mutation (376,379,382, 384,399) since C-cell hyperplasia will progress to MTC in these patients (fig. 3-71). Of 75 patients with RET mutations and clinically asymptomatic thyroid C-cell disease who underwent total thyroidectomy, 46 had MTC while C-cell hyperplasia only was seen in 29 (376). Calcitonin levels were not useful for differentiating between C-cell hyperplasia and MTC. The investigators recommended that prophylactic total thyroidectomy be performed by 6 years of age.

In another study in which patients had elevated calcitonin levels, routine screening of 30 patients who underwent total thyroidectomy showed C-cell hyperplasia, defined as 50 C-cells/low-power field, in both lobes, including 6 of 16 patients with sporadic MTC (382). Interestingly, of the 30 patients with MTC, none of the 14 females had early C-cell hyperplasia while 11 males had C-cell hyperplasia only, indicating that C-cell hyperplasia may be more common in males.

Once a patient develops MTC (fig. 3-72), the 5-year survival rate varies from 60 to 70 percent, and the 10-year survival rate ranges from 40 to 50 percent (394). The prognosis is much better for those with disease confined to the thyroid gland than for those who develop lymph node or other metastases.

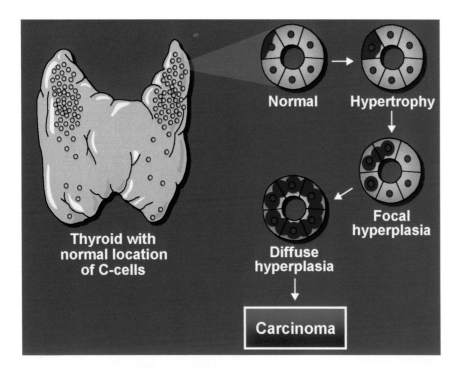

Figure 3-71

DIAGRAM OF C-CELL DISEASE PROGRESSION

Progression from normal to hyperplastic C cells and to invasive medullary thyroid carcinoma in patients with multiple endocrine neoplasia type 2a or 2b. The hyperplastic C cells invade through the follicular basement membrane when they become malignant. Based on the studies of DeLellis et al. (Figure 20 from DeLellis RA, Wolfe HJ. The pathobiology of the human calcitonin (C) cell: a review. Pathol Annu 1981;16:25–52.)

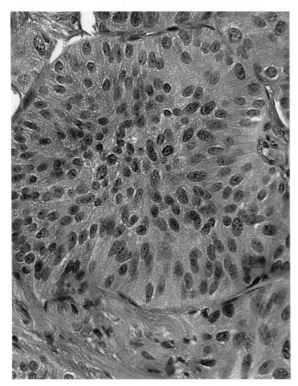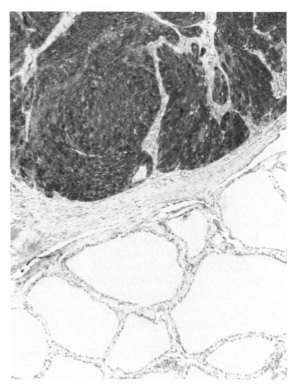

Figure 3-72

MEDULLARY THYROID CARCINOMA

Left: Medullary thyroid carcinoma composed of spindle and epithelioid cells.
Right: Calcitonin immunostain is strong in the tumor cells on the left.

REFERENCES

Embryology, Anatomy, and Histology

1. Bergé-Lefranc JL, Cartuozou G, DeMicco C, Fragu P, Lissitzky S. Quantification of thyroglobulin messenger RNA by in situ hybridization in differentiated thyroid cancers. Differences between well-differentiated and moderately differentiated histologic types. Cancer 1985;56:345–50.

2. Brown RA, Al-Moussa M, Beck JS. Histometry of normal thyroid in man. J Clin Pathol 1986;39:475–82.

3. Buley ID, Gatter KC, Heryet A, Mason DR. Expression of intermediate filament proteins in normal and diseased thyroid glands. J Clin Pathol 1987;40:136–42.

4. DeLellis RA, May L, Tashjian AH Jr, Wolfe HJ. C-cell granule heterogeneity in man. An ultrastructural immunohistochemical study. Lab Invest 1978;38:263–9

5. DeLellis RA, Wolfe HJ. The pathobiology of the human calcitonin (C)-cell: a review. Pathol Annu 1981;16(2):25–52.

6. Dockhorn-Dworniczak B, Franke WW, Schroeder S, Czernobilsky B, Gould VE, Bocker W. Pattern of expression of cytoskeletal proteins in human thyroid gland and thyroid carcinomas. Differentiation 1987;35:53–71.

7. Eales JG. The influence of nutritional state on thyroid function in various vertebrates. Am Zool 1988;20:351–62.

8. Gould VE, Johannesser JV, Sobrinho-Simoes M. The thyroid gland. In: Johannessen JV, ed. Electron microscopy in human medicine, vol. 10. Endocrine organs. New York: McGraw-Hill, 1981:29–107.

9. Hankin RC, Lloyd RV. Detection of messenger RNA in routinely processed tissue sections with biotinylated oligonucleotide probes. Am J Clin Pathol 1989;92:166–71.

10. Hanson GA, Komorowski RA, Cerletty JM, Wilson SD. Thyroid gland morphology in young adults: normal subjects versus those with prior low-dose neck irradiation in childhood. Surgery 1983;94:984–8.

11. Harach HR. Solid cell nests of the thyroid. J Pathol 1988;155:191–200.

12. Hegedus L, Karstrup S, Rasmussen N. Evidence of cyclic alterations of thyroid size during the menstrual cycle in healthy women. Am J Obstet Gynecol 1986;155:142–5.

13. Hegedus L, Perrild H, Poulsen LR, et al. The determination of thyroid volume by ultrasound and its relationship to body weight, age, and sex in normal subjects. J Clin Endocrinol Metab 1983;56:260–3.

14. Janzer RC, Weber E, Hedinger C. The relation between solid cell nests and C-cells of the thyroid gland: an immunohistochemical and morphometric investigation. Cell Tissue Res 1979;197:295–312.

15. Klinck GH, Oertel JE, Winship T. Ultrastructure of normal thyroid. Lab Invest 1970;22:2–22.

16. Kurata A, Ohta K, Mine M, et al. Monoclonal antihuman thyroglobulin antibodies. J Clin Endocrinol Metab 1984;59:573–9.

17. LeDouarin N, Fontaine J, LeLievre C. New studies on the neural crest origin of the avian ultimobranchial glandular cells—interspecies combinations and cytochemical characterization of C-cells based on the uptake of biogenic amine precursors. Histochemistry 1974;38:297–305.

18. LiVolsi VA. Surgical pathology of the thyroid. Major problems in pathology series, vol. 22. Philadelphia: WB Saunders Co., 1990.

19. Nadig J, Weber E, Hedinger CH. C-cell in vestiges of the ultimobranchial body in human thyroid glands. Virchows Arch [Cell Pathol] 1978;27:189–91.

20. Noris EH. The early morphogenesis of the human thyroid gland. Am J Anat 1918;24:443–65.

21. Papotti M, Negro F, Carney JA, Bussolati G, Lloyd RV. Mixed medullary-follicular carcinoma of the thyroid. A morphological, immunohistochemical, and in situ hybridization analysis of 11 cases. Virchows Arch 1997;430:397–405.

22. Pearse AG, Polak JM. Cytochemical evidence for the neural crest origin of mammalian ultimobranchial C-cells. Histochemistry 1971;27:96–102.

23. Reid JD, Choi CH, Oldroyd NO. Calcium oxalate crystals in the thyroid. Their identification, prevalence, origin, and possible significance. Am J Clin Pathol 1987;87:443–54.

24. Rosai J, Carcangiu ML, DeLellis RA. Tumors of the thyroid gland. Atlas of Tumor Pathology, 3rd Series, Fascicle 5. Washington, DC: Armed Forces Institute of Pathology, 1992.

25. Scopsi L, Ferrari C, Pilotti S, et al. Immunocytochemical localization and identification of prosomatostatin gene products in medullary carcinoma of human thyroid gland. Hum Pathol 1990;21:820–30.

26. Stanta G, Carcangiu ML, Rosai J. The biochemical and immunohistochemical profile of thyroid neoplasia. Pathol Annu 1988;23:129–57.

27. Tice LW, Creveling CR. Electron microscopic identification of adrenergic nerve endings on thyroid epithelial cells. Endocrinology 1975;97: 1123–9.

28. Weller GL. Development of the thyroid, parathyroid, and thyroid glands in man. Contrib Embryol Carney Institute 1933;141:93–140.

29. Williams ED, Toyn CE, Harach HR. The ultimobranchial gland and congenital thyroid abnormalities in man. J Pathol 1989;159:135–41.

30. Wolfe HJ, DeLellis RA, Voelkel EF, Tashjian AH Jr. Distribution of calcitonin-containing cells in the normal neonatal human thyroid gland: a correlation of morphology with peptide context. J Clin Endocrinol Metab 1975;41:1076–81.

31. Zajac JD, Penshow J, Mason T, Tregear G, Coghlan J, Martin TJ. Identification of calcitonin and calcitonin gene-related peptide messenger ribonucleic acid in medullary thyroid carcinomas by hybridization histochemistry. J Clin Endocrinol Metab 1986;62:1037–43.

32. Zannini M, Francis-Lang H, Plachov D, DiLauro R. Pax 8, a paired domain containing protein binds to a sequence overlapping the recognition site of a homeodomain and activates transcription from two thyroid-specific promoters. Mol Cell Biol 1992;12:4230–41.

Physiology

33. Abrams GM, Larsen PR. Triiodothyronine and thyroxine in the serum and thyroid glands of iodine-deficient rats. J Clin Invest 1973;52: 2522–31.

34. Austin LA, Heath H. Calcitonin: physiology and pathophysiology. N Engl J Med 1981;304:269–78.

35. Bocchetta A, Bernardi F, Pedditzi M, et al. Thyroid abnormalities during lithium treatment. Acta Psychiatr Scand 1991;83:193–8.

36. Boyages SC. Clinical review 49: iodine deficiency disorders. J Clin Endocrinol Metab 1993;77:587–91.

37. Boyages SC, Halpern JP. Endemic criticism: toward a unifying hypothesis. Thyroid 1993;3:59–69.

38. Brent GA, Hershman JM. Thyroxine therapy in patients with severe nonthyroidal illnesses and low serum thyroxine concentration. J Clin Endocrinol Metab 1986;63:1–8.

39. Burrow GH. Thyroid status in normal pregnancy. J Clin Endocrinol Metab 1990;71:274–5.

40. DiLaino R, Obici S, Condliffe D, et al. The sequence of 967 amino acids at the carboxyl end of rat thyroglobulin: location and surroundings of two thyroxine-forming sites. Eur J Biochem 1985;148:7–11.

41. Ermans AM. Goitrogens of vegetable origin as possible aetiological factors in endemic goiter. Ann Endocrinol 1981;42:435–8.

42. Freeman R, Rosen H, Thysen B. Incidence of thyroid dysfunction in an unselected postpartum population. Arch Intern Med 1986;146:1361–4.

43. Gammage MD, Franklyn JA. Amiodarone and the thyroid. Q J Med 1987;238:83-6.

44. Green WI. The physiology of the thyroid gland and its hormone. In: Green WI, ed. The thyroid. New York: Elsevier, 1987:1–46.

45. Guillaume J, Schussler GG, Goldman J. Components of the total serum thyroid hormone concentrations during pregnancy: high free thyroxine and blunted thyrotropin (TSH) response to TSH-releasing hormone in the first trimester. J Clin Endocrinol Metab 1985;60:678–84.

46. Hawthorne GC, Campbell NP, Geddes JS, et al. Amiodarone-induced hypothyroidism. Arch Intern Med 1985;145:1016–9.

47. Ishii H, Inada M, Tanaka K, Mishio Y, Naito K, Nishikawa M. Induction of outer and inner ring monodeiodinases in human thyroid gland by thyrotropin. J Clin Endocrinol Metab 1983;57:500–5.

48. Laresen PR, Davies TF, Hay ID. The thyroid gland. In: Wilson JD, Foster DW, Kronenberg HM, Larsen PR, eds. Williams textbook of endocrinology, 9th ed. Philadelphia: WB Saunders, 1998:389–515.

49. Kuiper JJ. Lymphocytic thyroiditis possibly induced by diphenylhydantoin. JAMA 1969;210: 2370–2.

50. Mariotti S, Franceschi C, Cossarizza A, Pinchera A. The aging thyroid. Endocr Rev 1995;16:686–715.

51. Martino E, Safran N, Aghini-Lombardi F, Rajatanarin R, Lenziardi M, Fay M. Environmental iodine intake and thyroid dysfunction during chronic amiodarone therapy. Ann Intern Med 1984;101:28–34.

52. Michalkiewicz M, Huffman LJ, Connors JM, Hedge GA. Alterations in thyroid blood flow induced by varying levels of iodine intake in the rat. Endocrinology 1989;125:54–60.

53. Modholm-Hansen J, Skovsted L, Lauridsen VB, et al. The effects of diphenylhydantoin on thyroid function. J Clin Endocrinol Metab 1974;39:785–9.

54. Norman RJ, Green-Thompson RW, Jialal I, Soutter WP, Pillay NL, Joubert SM. Hyperthyroidism in gestational trophoblastic neoplasia. Clin Endocrinol 1981;15:395–401.

55. Oppenheimer JH, Tavernetti RR. Displacement of thyroxine from human thyroxine binding globulin by analogues of hydantoin. J Clin Invest 1962;41:2213–20.

56. Pittman JA Jr. Thyrotropin-releasing hormone. Adv Intern Med 1974;19:303–25.

57. Sinclair AJ, Lonigro R, Civitareale D, Ghibelli L, Di Lauro R. The tissue-specific expression of the thyroglobulin gene requires interaction between thyroid-specific and ubiquitous factors. Eur J Biochem 1990;193:311–18.

58. Smyrk TC, Goellner JR, Brennan MD, Carney JA. Pathology of the thyroid in amiodarone-associated thyrotoxicosis. Am J Surg Pathol 1987;11:197–204.

59. Spaulding SW, Burrow GN, Bermudez F, Himmelhoch JM. The inhibitory effect of lithium on thyroid hormone release in both euthyroid and thyrotoxic patients. J Clin Endocrinol Metab 1972;35:905–11.

60. Thorpe-Beeston JG, Nicolaides KH, Felton CV, Butler J, McGregor AM. Maturation of the secretion of thyroid hormone and thyroid-stimulatory hormone in the fetus. N Engl J Med 1991;324:532–6.

61. Wiersinga WM, Trip MD. Amiodarone and thyroid hormone metabolism. Postgrad Med J 1986;62:909–14.

62. Wartofsky L, Burman KD. Alterations in thyroid function in patients with systemic illness: the "euthyroid sick syndrome." Endocr Rev 1982;3:164–217.

63. Wilber JF. Thyrotropin-releasing hormone: secretion and actions. Ann Rev Med 1973;24:353–64.

64. Wolff J, Chaikoff IL. Plasma inorganic iodide as a homeostatic regulator of thyroid function. J Biol Chem 1948;174:555–62.

65. Yamada M, Radovick S, Wondisford FE, Nakayama Y, Weintraub BO, Wilber JF. Cloning and structure of human genomic DNA and hypothalamic cDNA encoding human preprothyrotropin-releasing hormone. Mol Endocrinol 1990;4:551–6.

65a. Zannini M, Francis-Lang H, Plachov D, DiLauro R. Pax 8, a paired domain containing protein binds to a sequence overlapping the recognition site of a homeodomain and activates transcription from two thyroid-specific promoters. Mol Cell Biol 1992;12:4230–41.

Hereditary and Developmental Disorders

66. Acebron A, Aza-Blanc P, Rossi DL, Lamas L, Santisteban P. Congenital human thyroglobulin defect due to low expression of the thyroid-specific transcription factor TTF-1. J Clin Invest 1995;96:781–5.

67. DeRoux N, Misrahi M, Brauner R. Four families with loss of function mutations of the thyrotropin receptor. J Clin Endocrinol Metab 1996;81:4229–35.

68. Duprez L, Parma J, van Sande J, et al. Germline mutations in the thyrotropin receptor gene causes non-autoimmune autosomal-dominant hyperthyroidism. Nature Genet 1994;7:396–401.

69. Fabbro D, DiLoreto C, Beltram CA, Belfiore A, DiLauro R, Damante G. Expression of thyroid-specific transcription factors TTF-1 and PAX-8 in human thyroid neoplasms. Cancer Res 1994;54:4744–9.

70. Führer D, Holzapfel HP, Wonerow P, Scherbaum WA, Paschke R. Somatic mutations in the thyrotropin receptor gene and not in the Gs α protein gene in 31 toxic thyroid nodules. J Clin Endocrinol Metab 1997;82:3885–91.

71. Guazzi S, Price M, DeFelice M, Damante G, Mattein MG, DiLauro R. Thyroid nuclear factor 1 (TTF-1) contains a homeodomain and displays a novel DNA binding specificity. EMBO J 1990;9:3631–9.

72. Kopp P, van Sande J, Parma J, et al. Brief report: congenital hyperthyroidism caused by a mutation in the thyrotropin-receptor gene. N Engl J Med 1995;332:150–4.

73. Latchman DS. Transcription-factor mutations and disease. N Engl J Med 1996;334:28-33.

74. Mitchell PJ, Tijan R. Transcriptional regulation in mammalian cells by sequence-specific DNA binding proteins. Science 1989;245:371–8.

75. Paschke R, Ludgate M. The thyrotropin receptor in thyroid diseases. N Engl J Med 1997;337:1675–81.

76. Rossi DL, Acebron A, Santisteban P. Function of the homeo and paired domain proteins TTF-1 and Pax-8 in thyroid cell proliferation. J Biol Chem 1995;270:23139–42.

77. Shimura H, Shimura Y, Ohmuri M, Ikuyama S, Kohn LD. Single-strand DNA-binding proteins and thyroid transcription factor-1 conjointly regulate thyrotropin receptor gene expression. Mol Endocrinol 1995;9:527–39.

78. Sinclair AJ, Lonigro R, Civitareale D, Ghibelli L, DiLauro R. The tissue-specific expression of the thyroglobulin gene requires intervention between thyroid-specific and ubiquitous factors. Eur J Biochem 1990;193:311–8.

79. Zannini M, Francis-Lang H, Plachov D, Di Lauro R. Pax-8, a paired domain containing protein binds to a sequence overlapping the recognition site of a homeodomain and activates transcription from two thyroid-specific promoters. Mol Cell Biol 1992;12:4230–41.

Aplasia and Hypoplasia

80. Acebron A, Aza-Blanc P, Rossi DL, Lamas L, Santisteban P. Congenital human thyroglobulin defect due to low expression of the thyroid-specific transcription factor TTF-1. J Clin Invest 1995;96:781–5.

80a. Burke B, Wick M. Thyroid C cells in DiGeorge syndrome. Lab Invest 1986;54:2.

80b. Fisher DA, Klein AH. Thyroid development and disorders of thyroid function in the newborn. N Engl J Med 1981;304:702–12.

Ectopic Thyroid and Thyroglossal Duct

81. Asp A, Hasbargen J, Blue P, Kidd GS. Ectopic thyroid tissue on thallium technetium parathyroid scan. Arch Intern Med 1987;147:595–6.
82. Baughman RA. Lingual thyroid and lingual thyroglossal tract remnants. A clinical and histopathologic study with review of the literature. Oral Surg 1972;34:781–98.
83. Block MA, Wylie JH, Patton RB, Miller JM. Does benign thyroid tissue occur in the lateral part of the neck? Am J Surg 1966;112:476–81.
84. Burke B, Wick M. Thyroid C cells in DiGeorge syndrome. Lab Invest 1986;54:2.
85. deSouza FM, Smith PE. Retrosternal goiter. J Otolaryngol 1983;12:393–6.
86. Jain SN. Lingual thyroid. Int Surg 1969;52:320–5.
87. Jaques DA, Chambers RG, Oertel JE. Thyroglossal tract carcinoma. A review of the literature and addition of 18 cases. Am J Surg 1970;120:439–46.
88. Kakudo K, Shan L, Nakamura Y, Inoue D, Koshiyama H, Sato H. Clonal analysis helps to differentiate aberrant thyroid tissue from thyroid carcinoma. Hum Pathol 1998;29:187–90.
89. LiVolsi VA. Surgical pathology of the thyroid. Major problems in pathology series, vol 22. Philadelphia: WB Saunders Co., 1990.
90. LiVolsi VA, Perzin KH, Savetsky L. Carcinomas arising in median ectopic thyroid (including thyroglossal duct tissue). Cancer 1974;34:1303–15.
91. Meyer JS, Steinberg LS. Microscopically benign thyroid follicles in cervical lymph nodes. Cancer 1969;24:302–11.
92. Moses DC, Thompson NW, Nishiyama RH, Sisson JC. Ectopic thyroid tissue in the neck. Benign or malignant? Cancer 1976;38:361–5.
93. Neinas FW, Gorman CA, Devine KD, Woolner LB. Lingual thyroid. Clinical characteristics of 15 cases. Ann Intern Med 1973;79:205–10.
94. Nussbaum M, Buchwald RP, Ribner A, Mori K, Litwins J. Anaplastic carcinoma arising from median ectopic thyroid (thyroglossal duct remnant). Cancer 1981;48:2724–8.
95. Pollice L, Caruso G. Struma cordis. Ectopic thyroid goiter in the right ventricle. Arch Pathol Lab Med 1986;110:452–3.
96. Rahm J. An unusual heterotopic of thyroid gland tissue. Zbl Allg Pat 1959;99:80–6.
97. Sohn N, Gumport SL, Blum M. Thyroglossal duct carcinoma. NY State J Med 1974;74:2004–5.
98. Spinner RJ, Moore KL, Gottfried MR, Lowe JE, Sabiston DC Jr. Thoracic intrathymic thyroid. Ann Surg 1994;220:91–6.
99. Stanley DG, Robinson FW. Thyroid carcinoma in thyroglossal duct cysts. Am Surg 1970;36:581–2.

Parasitic Nodule

100. Assi A, Sironi M, Di Bella C, Declich P, Cozzi L, Pareschi R. Parasitic nodule of the right carotid triangle. Arch Otolaryngol Head Neck Surg 1996;122:1409–11.
101. Block MA, Wylie JH, Patton RB, Miller JM. Does benign thyroid tissue occur in the lateral part of the neck? Am J Surg 1966;112:476–81.
102. Hathong BM. Innocuous accessory thyroid nodules. Arch Surg 1965;90:222–7.
103. Klopp CT, Kirson SM. Therapeutic problems with ectopic non-cancerous follicular thyroid tissue in the neck: 18 case reports according to etiological factors. Ann Surg 1966;163:653–64.
104. Shimizu M, Hirokawa M, Manabe T. Parasitic nodule of the thyroid in a patient with Graves' disease. Virchows Arch 1999;434:241–4.
105. Sisson JC, Schmidt RW, Beierwaltes WH. Sequested nodular goiter. N Engl J Med 1964;270:927–32.

Radiation Changes

106. Carr RF, LiVolsi VA. Morphologic changes in the thyroid after irradiation for Hodgkin's and non-Hodgkin's lymphoma. Cancer 1989;64:825–9.
107. Droese M, Kempken K, Schneider ML, Hor G. Cytologic changes in aspiration biopsy smears from various conditions of the thyroid treated with radioiodine. Verh Dtsch Ges Pathol 1973;57:336–8.
108. Favus MJ, Schneider AB, Stachura ME, et al. Thyroid cancer occurring as a late consequence of head and neck irradiation. Evaluation of 1,056 patients. N Engl J Med 1976;294:1019–25.
109. Fogelfeld L, Wiviott MB, Shore-Freedman E, et al. Recurrence of thyroid nodules after surgical removal in patients irradiated in childhood for benign conditions. N Eng J Med 1989;320:835–40.
110. Holten I. Acute response of the thyroid to external radiation. Acta Pathol Microbiol Scand 1983;91(Suppl 283):1–111.
111. Kennedy JS, Thomson JA. The changes in the thyroid gland after irradiation with ^{131}I or partial thyroidectomy for thyrotoxicosis. J Pathol 1974;112:65–81.
112. Schneider AB, Recant W, Pinsky SM, Ryo UY, Bekerman C, Shore-Freedman E. Radiation-induced thyroid carcinoma. Clinical course and results of therapy in 296 patients. Ann Int Med 1986;105:405–12.

Langerhans' Cell Granulomatosis and Sinus Histiocytosis

113. Carpenter RJ III, Banks PM, McDonald TJ, Sanderson DR. Sinus histiocytosis with massive lymphadenopathy (Rosai-Dorfman disease): report of a case with respiratory involvement. Laryngoscope 1978;88:1963–9.
114. Coode PE, Shaikh MU. Histiocytosis X of the thyroid masquerading as thyroid carcinoma. Hum Pathol 1988;19:239–41.
115. Larkin DF, Dervan PA, Munnelly J, Finucane J. Sinus histiocytosis with massive lymphadenopathy simulating subacute thyroiditis. Hum Pathol 1986;17:321–4.
116. Schofield JB, Alsarjari NA, Davis J, MacLennan KA. Eosinophilic granuloma of lymph nodes associated with metastatic papillary carcinoma of the thyroid. Histopathology 1992;20:181–3.
117. Teja K, Sabio H, Langdon DR, Johanson AJ. Involvement of the thyroid gland in histiocytosis X. Hum Pathol 1981;12:1137–9.

Plasma Cell Granuloma

118. Holck S. Plasma cell granuloma of the thyroid. Cancer 1981;48:830–2.
119. Yapp R, Linder J, Schenken JR, Karrer FW. Plasma cell granuloma of the thyroid. Hum Pathol 1985;16:848–50.

Scleroderma

120. D'Angelo WA, Fries JF, Masi AT, Shulman LE. Pathologic observations in systemic sclerosis (scleroderma). Am J Med 1969;46:428–40.
121. Gordon MB, Klein I, Dekker A, Rodnan GP, Medsger TA Jr. Thyroid disease in progressive systemic sclerosis: increased frequency of glandular fibrosis and hypothyroidism. Ann Intern Med 1981;95:431–5.
122. Nelson DF, Reddy KV, O'Mara RE, Rubin P. Thyroid abnormalities following neck irradiation for Hodgkin's disease. Cancer 1978;42:2553–62.

Metabolic Diseases

123. Chan AM, Lynch MJ, Bailey JD, Ezrin C, Fraser D. Hypothyroidism in cystinosis. A clinical, endocrinologic and histologic study involving sixteen patients with cystinosis. Am J Med 1970;48:678–92.
124. Hui KS, Williams JC, Borit A, Rosenberg HS. The endocrine glands in Pompe's disease. Report of two cases. Arch Pathol Lab Med 1985;109:921–5.
125. Lucky AW, Howley PM, Megyesi K, Spielberg SP, Schulman JD. Endocrine studies in cystinosis. Compensated primary hypothyroidism. J Pediatr 1977;91:204–10.

Lipidosis

126. Armstrong D, Van Warner DE, Neville H, Dimmitt S, Clingan E. Thyroid peroxidase deficiency in Batten-Speilmeyer-Vogt disease. Arch Pathol 1975;99:430–5.
127. Dayan AD, Trickey RJ. Thyroid involvement in juvenile amaurotic family idiocy (Batten's disease). Lancet 1970;2:296–7.
128. Dolman CL, Chang E. Visceral lesions in amaurotic family idiocy with curvilinear bodies. Arch Pathol 1972;94:425–30.

Iron Deposition

129. Cappell DF, Hutchison HE, Jowett M. Transfusional siderosis. The effects of excessive iron deposits on the tissues. J Pathol Bacteriol 1957;74:245–9.
130. Oliver RA. Siderosis following transfusion of blood. J Pathol Bacteriol 1959;77:171–6.

Minocycline and Crystals

131. Alexander CB, Herrara GA, Jaffe K, Yu H. Black thyroid: clinical manifestations, ultrastructural findings and possible mechanisms. Hum Pathol 1985;16:72–8.
132. Benitz KF, Roberts GK, Yusa A. Morphologic effects of minocycline in laboratory animals. Toxicol Appl Pharmacol 1967;11:150–70.
133. Billano RA, Ward WQ, Little WP. Minocycline and black thyroid. JAMA 1983;249:1887.
134. Fayemi AO, Ali M, Braun EV. Oxalosis in hemodialysis patients. Arch Pathol Lab Med 1979;103:58–62.
135. Gordon G, Sparano BM, Kramer AW, Kelley RG, Iatropoulos MJ. Thyroid gland pigmentation and minocycline therapy. Am J Pathol 1984;117:98–109.
136. Kurosumi M, Fujita H. Fine structural aspects of the fate of rat black thyroids induced by minocycline. Virchows Arch [Cell Pathol] 1986;51;207–13.
137. LiVolsi VA. Surgical pathology of the thyroid. Major problems in pathology, vol 22. Philadelphia: WB Saunders, 1990:125–8.
138. MacMahon HE, Lee HY, Rivelis CF. Birefringent crystals in human thyroid. Acta Endocrinol 1968;58:172–6.
139. Matsubara F, Mizukami Y, Tanaka Y. Black thyroid. Morphological, biochemical and geriatric studies on the brown granules in the thyroid follicular cells. Acta Pathol Jpn 1982;32:13–22.
140. Reid JD, Choi CH, Oldroyd NO. Calcium oxalate crystals in the thyroid. Their identification, prevalence, origin and possible significance. Am J Clin Pathol 1987;87:443–54.

141. Richter MN, McCarty KS. Anisotropic crystals in the human thyroid gland. Am J Pathol 1954;30:545–53.

142. Scully RE, Young RH, Clement PB. Tumors of the ovary, maldeveloped gonads, fallopian tube, and broad ligament. Atlas of Tumor Pathology, 3rd Series, Fascicle 23. Washington, DC: Armed Forces Institute of Pathology, 1998:290.

Teflon in Thyroid

143. LiVolsi VA. Surgical pathology of the thyroid. Major problems in pathology, vol 22. Philadelphia: WB Saunders, 1990:125–8.

143a. Sanfilippo F, Shelburne J, Ingram P. Analysis of a polytef granuloma mimicking a cold thyroid nodule 17 months after laryngeal injection. Ultrastruct Pathol 1980;1:471–5.

144. Walsh FM, Castelli JB. Polytef granuloma clinically simulating carcinoma of the thyroid. Arch Otolaryngol 1975;101:262–3.

Infectious/Granulomatous Diseases

145. Berger SA, Zonszein J, Villamena P, Mittman N. Infectious diseases of the thyroid gland. Rev Infect Dis 1983;5:108–22.

146. Frank TS, LiVolsi VA, Connor AM. Cytomegalovirus infection of the thyroid in immunocompromised adults. Yale J Biol Med 1987;60:1–8.

147. Hagan AD, Goffinet J, Davis JW. Acute streptococcal thyroiditis. JAMA 1967;202:842–3.

148. Hazard JB. Thyroiditis: a review. Am J Clin Pathol 1955;25:289–98.

149. Larsen PP, Daves TI, Hay ID. The thyroid gland. In: Wilson JD, Foster DW, Kronenberg HM, Larson PR, eds. Williams textbook of endocrinology, 9th ed. Philadelphia: WB Saunders, 1990:479.

150. Loeb JM, Livermore BM, Wofsy D. Coccidioidomycosis of the thyroid. Ann Intern Med 1979;91:409–11.

151. Nieburg PI, Gardner LI. Thyroiditis and congenital rubella syndrome [Letter]. J Pediatr 1976;89:156.

152. Robinson MF, Forgan-Smith WR, Craswell PW. Candida thyroiditis treated with 5-fluorocytosine. Aust NZ J Med 1975;5:472–4.

153. Soksouk F, Salti IS. Acute suppurative thyroiditis caused by Escherichia coli. Br Med J 1977;2:23–4.

154. Thomas CG. Acute supperative thyroiditis: surgical treatment. In: Werner SC, Ingbar SH, eds. The thyroid. New York: Harper & Row, 1971:852.

155. Van Heerden JA, O'Connell P. Acute suppurative thyroiditis due to Salmonella enteritides. Vir Med Mon 1971;98:556–7.

156. Volpe R. Acute suppurative thyroiditis. In: Werner SC, Ingbar SH, eds. The thyroid. New York: Harper & Row, 1971:852.

157. Weissel M, Wolf A, Linkesch W. Acute suppurative thyroiditis caused by a Pseudomonas aeruginosa. Br Med J 1977;2:580.

158. Womack NA. Thyroiditis. Surgery 1944;16:777–82.

Granulomatous Thyroiditis

159. Benker G, Olbricht T, Windeck R, et al. The sonographic and functional sequelae of deQuervain's subacute thyroiditis. Acta Endocrinol 1988;117:435–41.

160. DePauw BE, deRooy HA. DeQuervain's subacute thyroiditis. A report of 14 cases and a review of the literature. Neth J Med 1975;18:70–8.

161. Eylan E, Zmucky R, Sheba C. Mumps virus and subacute thyroiditis—evidence of a causal association. Lancet 1957;1:1063–3.

162. Furszyfer J, McConahey WM, Wahner HW, Kurland LT. Subacute (granulomatous) thyroiditis in Olmsted County, Minnesota. Mayo Clinic Proc 1970;45:396–404.

163. Hay ID. Thyroiditis: a clinical update. Mayo Clinic Proc 1985;60:836–43.

164. Kakudo K, Kanokogi M, Mitsunobu M, et al. Acute mycotic thyroiditis. Acta Pathol Jpn 1983;33:147–51.

165. Karlish AJ, MacGregor GA. Sarcoidosis, thyroiditis and Addison's disease. Lancet 1970;2:330–3.

166. Larsen PR. Serum triiodothyronine, thyroxine and thyrotropin during hyperthyroid, hypothyroid and recovery phases of subacute nonsuppurative thyroiditis. Metabolism 1974;23:467–71.

167. Lindsay S, Dailey ME. Granulomatous or giant cell thyroiditis. Surg Gynecol Obstet 1954;98:197–212.

168. Manson CM, Cross P, De Sousa B. Postoperative necrotizing granulomas of the thyroid. Histopathology 1992;21:392–3.

169. Markowicz H, Shanon E. Tuberculosis of the thyroid gland. Ann Otol Rhinol Laryngol 1959;67:223–6.

170. Meachim G, Young MH. DeQuervain's subacute granulomatous thyroiditis: histological identification and incidence. J Clin Pathol 1963;16:189–99.

171. Mizukami V, Nomomura A, Michigishi T, Ohmura K, Matsubara S, Noguchi M. Sarcoidosis of the thyroid gland manifested initially as thyroid tumor. Pathol Res Pract 1994;190:1201–5.

172. Nyulassy S, Hnilica P, Buc M, Guman M, Hirschova V, Stefanovic J. Subacute (deQuervian's) thyroiditis: associated with HLA-BW35 antigen and abnormalities of the complement system, immunoglobulins and other serum proteins. J Clin Endocrinol Metab 1977;45:270–4.

173. Rotenberg Z, Weinberger I, Fuchs J, Maller S, Agmon J. Euthyroid atypical subacute thyroiditis simulating systemic or malignant disease. Arch Intern Med 1986;146:105–7.

174. Sachs MK, Dickinson G, Amazon K. Tuberculous adenitis of the thyroid mimicking subacute thyroiditis. Am J Med 1988;85:573–5.

175. Sasaki H, Harada T, Eimoto T, Matsuoka Y, Okumura M. Concomitant association of thyroid sarcoidosis and Hashimoto's thyroiditis. Am J Med Sci 1987;249:441–3.

176. Singer PA. Thyroiditis. Acute, subacute and chronic. Med Clin North Am 1991;75:61–77.

177. Swan NH. Acute thyroiditis. Five cases associated with adenovirus infection. Metabolism 1964;13:908–10.

178. Volpe R. The management of subacute (DeQuervain's) thyroiditis. Thyroid 1993;3:253–5.

179. Volpe R. Subacute (deQuervain's) thyroiditis. Clin Endocrinol Metab 1979;8:81–95.

180. Volpe R. Thyroiditis: current review of pathogens. Med Clin North Am 1975;59:1163–75.

181. Warshawsky ME, Shanies HM, Rozo A. Sarcoidosis involving the thyroid and pleura. Sarcoidosis, Vasc Diffuse Lung Dis 1997;14:165–8.

182. Woolner LB. Thyroiditis: classification and clinicopathologic correlation. In: Hazard JB, Smith DE, eds. The thyroid. Baltimore: Williams & Wilkins, 1964:23.

183. Woolner LB, McConahey WB, Beahrs OH. Granulomatous thyroiditis (deQuervain's thyroiditis). J Clin Endocrinol Metab 1957;17:1202–21.

184. Yermakov VM, Hitti IF, Sutton AL. Necrotizing vasculitis associated with diphenylhydantoin: two fatal cases. Hum Pathol 1983;14:182–4.

Palpation Thyroiditis

185. Buergi U, Gebel F, Maier E, Koening MP, Studer H. Palpation thyroiditis. Serum thyroglobulin before and after palpation of the thyroid. N Engl J Med 1983;308:777.

186. Carney JA, Moore SB, Northcutt RC, Woolner LB, Stillwell GK. Palpation thyroiditis (multifocal granulomatous folliculitis). Am J Clin Pathol 1975;64:639–47.

187. Helling CA. Colloidopathy of the human thyroid gland. Science 1985;60:836–43.

188. Lever EG, Refetoff S, Scherberg NH, Carr K. The influence of percutaneous fine needle aspiration on serum thyroglobulin. J Clin Endocrinol Metab 1983;56:26–9.

Alterations Following Fine Needle Aspiration Biopsy

189. Baloch ZW, LiVolsi VA. Post fine-needle aspiration histologic alterations of thyroid revisited [Review]. Am J Clin Pathol 1999;112:311–6.

190. Baloch ZW, Wu H, LiVolsi VA. Post fine-needle aspiration spindle cell nodules of the thyroid (PSCNT). Am J Clin Pathol 1999;111:70–4.

191. Layfield LJ, Lones MA. Necrosis in thyroid nodules after fine needle aspiration biopsy. Acta Cytol 1991;35:427–30.

192. LiVolsi VA, Merino MJ. Worrisome histologic alterations following fine-needle aspiration of the thyroid (WHAFFT). Pathol Ann 1994;29:99–120.

Hashimoto's Thyroiditis

193. Amino N, Hagen SR, Yamada N, Refetoff S. Measurement of circulating thyroid microsomal antibodies by the tanned red cell hemagglutination technique: its usefulness in the diagnosis of autoimmune thyroid diseases. Clin Endocrinol 1976;5:115–25.

194. Bagchi N, Brown TR, Parish RF. Thyroid dysfunction in adults over 55 years. A study in an urban U.S. community. Arch Intern Med 1990;150:785–7.

195. Baloch ZW, LiVolsi VA. Post-fine needle aspiration histologic alterations of thyroid revisited. Am J Clin Pathol 1999;112:311–6.

196. Burman P, Totterman TH, Oberg K, Karlsson FA. Thyroid autoimmunity in patients on long-term therapy with leukocyte-derived interferon. J Clin Endocrinol Metab 1986;63:1086–90.

197. Chopra JJ, Solomon DH, Chopra V, Yoshihara E, Terasaki PI, Smith F. Abnormalities in thyroid function in relatives of patients with Graves' disease and Hashimoto's thyroiditis: lack of correlation with inheritance of HLA-B8. J Clin Endocrinol Metab 1977;45:45–54.

198. Davies TF, Martin A, Concepcion ES, Graves P, Cohen L, Ben-Nun A. Evidence of limited variability of antigen receptors on intrathyroidal T cells in autoimmune thyroid disease. N Engl J Med 1991;325:238–44.

199. Dayan CM, Daniels GH. Chronic autoimmune thyroiditis. N Engl J Med 1996;335:99–107.

200. Dayan CM, Londei M, Corcoran AE, et al. Autoantigen recognition by thyroid-infiltrating T cells in Graves' disease. Proc Natl Acad Sci USA 1991;88:7415–9.

201. de Kerdanet M, Lucas J, Lemee F, Lecornu M. Turner's syndrome with X-isochromosome and Hashimoto's thyroiditis. Clin Endocrinol 1994;41:673–6.

202. Del Prete GF, Maggi E, Mariotti S, et al. Cytolytic T lymphocytes with natural killer activity in thyroid infiltrates of patients with Hashimoto's thyroiditis: analysis at the clonal level. J Clin Endocrinol Metab 1986;62:52–7.

203. Doniach D, Boltazzo GF, Russell RC. Goitrous autoimmune thyroiditis (Hashimoto's disease). Clin Endocrinol Metab 1979;8:63–80.

204. Eguchi K, Matsuoka N, Nagataki S. Cellular immunity in autoimmune thyroid disease. Balliere's Clin Endocrinol Metab 1995;9:71–94.

205. Ewins DL, Rossor MN, Butler J, Roques PK, Mullan MJ, McGregor AM. Association between autoimmune thyroid disease and familial Alzheimer's disease. Clin Endocrinol 1991;35:93–6.

206. Fatourechi V, McConahey WM, Woolner LB. Hyperthyroidism associated with histologic Hashimoto's thyroiditis. Mayo Clin Proc 1971;46:682–9.

207. Hanafusa T, Pujol-Borrell R, Chiovato L, Russell RC, Doniach D, Bottazzo GF. Aberrance expression of HLA-DR antigen on thyrocytes in Graves' disease: relevance for autoimmunity. Lancet 1983;2:1111–5.

208. Harach HR, Escalante DA, Onativia A, Lederer Outes J, Sarvia Duy E, Williams ED. Thyroid carcinoma and thyroiditis in endemic goiter region before and after iodine prophylaxis. Acta Endocrinol (Copenh) 1985;108:55–60.

209. Harris M. The cellular infiltrate in Hashimoto's disease and focal lymphocytic thyroiditis. J Clin Pathol 1969;22:326–33.

210. Hashimoto H. Zur Kenntnis der lymphomatöen Veränderung der Schilddrüse (Struma lymphomatosa). Arch F Klin Chir 1912;97:219–48.

211. Holm LE, Blomgren H, Lowhagen T. Cancer risks in patients with chronic lymphocytic thyroiditis. N Engl J Med 1985;312:601–4.

212. Honda K, Tamai H, Morita T, Kumar K, Nishimura Y, Sasazuki T. Hashimoto's thyroiditis and HLA in Japanese. J Clin Endocrinol Metab 1989;69:1268–73.

213. Isaccson PG, Androulakis-Papachristou A, Diss TC, Pan L, Wright DH. Follicular colonization in thyroid lymphoma. Am J Pathol 1992;141:43–52.

214. Kato I, Tajima K, Suchi T, et al. Chronic thyroiditis as a risk factor for B cell lymphoma in the thyroid gland. Jpn J Cancer Res 1985;76:1085–90.

215. Katz SM, Vickery AL Jr. The fibrous variant of Hashimoto's thyroiditis. Hum Pathol 1974;5:161–70.

216. Kennedy RL, Jones TH, Cuckle HS. Down's syndrome and the thyroid. Clin Endocrinol 1992;37:471–6.

217. Knecht H, Hedinger CE. Ultrastructural Hashimoto's thyroiditis and focal lymphocytic thyroiditis with reference to giant cell formation. Histopathology 1982;6:511–38.

218. Kurihara H, Susaki J, Takamatsu M. Twenty cases with Hashimoto's disease clinging to Graves' disease. In: Nagataki S, Mori T, Turizuka K, eds. 80 years of Hashimoto's disease. Amsterdam: Elsevier Science, 1993;249:53.

219. Larsen PR, Davies TF, Hay ID. The thyroid gland. In: Wilson JD, Foster DW, Kronenberg AM, Larsen PR, eds. Williams textbook of endocrinology, 9th ed. Philadelphia: WB Saunders, 1998:389–515.

220. Lazarus JH, John R, Bennie EH, Crockett RJ, Crockelt G. Lithium therapy and thyroid function: a long-term study. Psychol Med 1981;11:85–92.

221. LiVolsi VA. The pathology of autoimmune thyroid disease: a review. Thyroid 1994;4:333–9.

222. Lloyd RV, Johnson TL, Blaivas M, Sisson JC, Wilson BS. Detection of HLA-DR antigens in paraffin-embedded thyroid epithelial cells with a monoclonal antibody. Am J Pathol 1985;120:106–11.

223. Londei M, Bottazzo GF, Feldmann M. Human T-cell clones from autoimmune thyroid gland: specific recognition of autologous thyroid cells. Science 1985;228:85–9.

224. Louis DN, Vickery AL Jr, Rosai J, Wang CA. Multiple branchial cleft-like cysts in Hashimoto's thyroiditis. Am J Surg Pathol 1989;13:45–9.

225. Maran AG, Buchanan DR. Branchial cysts, sinuses, and fistulae. Clin Otol 1978;3:77–92.

226. Mariotti S, Caturegli P, Piccolo P, Barbesino G, Pinchera A. Antithyroid peroxidase autoantibodies in thyroid diseases. J Clin Endocrinol Metab 1990;71:661–9.

227. Matsuzuka F, Miyauchi A, Katayama S, et al. Clinical aspects of primary thyroid lymphoma: diagnosis and treatment based on our experience of 119 cases. Thyroid 1993;3:93–9.

228. Nordmeyer JP, Shafeh TA, Heckmann C. Thyroid sonography in autoimmune thyroiditis: a prospective study on 123 patients. Acta Endocrinol 1990;122:391–5.

229. Oertel JE, Hefferss CS. Lymphoma of the thyroid and related disorders. Semin Oncol 1987;14:333–42.

230. Okayasu I, Hara Y, Nakamura K, Rose NR. Racial- and age-related differences in incidence and severity of focal autoimmune thyroiditis. Am J Clin Pathol 1994;101:698–702.

231. Parle JV, Franklyn JA, Cross KW, Jones SC, Sheppard MC. Prevalence and follow-up of abnormal thyrotropin (TSH) concentration in the elderly in the United Kingdom. Clin Endocrinol 1991;34:77–83.

232. Rallison ML, Dobyns BM, Keating FR, Rall JE, Tyler FH. Occurrence and natural history of chronic lymphocytic thyroiditis in childhood. J Pediatr 1975;86:675–82.

233. Rallison ML, Dobyns BM, Meikle AW, Bishop M, Lyon JL, Stevens W. Natural history of thyroid abnormalities: prevalence, incidence, and regression of thyroid disease in adolescents and young adults. Am J Med 1991;91:363–70.

234. Ramtoola S, Maisey MN, Clarke SE, Fogelman I. The thyroid scan in Hashimoto's thyroiditis: the great mimic. Nucl Med Commun 1988;9:639–45.

235. Reidbord HE, Fisher ER. Ultrastructural features of subacute granulomatous thyroiditis and Hashimoto's disease. Am J Clin Pathol 1973;59:327–37.

236. Roitt IM, Doniach D. A reassessment of studies on the aggregation of thyroid autoimmunity in families of thyroiditis patients. Clin Exp Immunol 1967;2:727–36.

237. Sauter NP, Atkins MB, Mier JW, Lechan RM. Transient thyrotoxicosis and persistent hypothyroidism due to acute autoimmune thyroiditis after interleukin 2 and interferon alpha therapy for metastatic carcinoma: a case report. Am J Med 1992;92:441–4.

238. Sostre S, Reyes MM. Sonographic diagnosi and grading of Hashimoto's thyroiditis. J End rinol Invest 1991;14:115–21.

239. Stagnaro-Green A. Postpartum thyroiditis: prevalence, etiology, and clinical implications. Thyroid Today 1993;16:1–11.

240. Takasu N, Yamada T, Takasu M, et al. Disappearance of thyrotropin-blocking antibodies and spontaneous recovery from hypothyroidism in autoimmune thyroiditis. N Engl J Med 1992;326:513–8.

241. Tamai H, Kimura A, Dong RP, et al. Resistance to autoimmune thyroid disease is associated with HLA-DQ. J Clin Endocrinol Metab 1994;78:94–7.

242. Tomer Y, Davies TF. Infection, thyroid disease, and autoimmunity. Endocr Rev 1993;14:107–20.

243. Trip MD, Wiersinga W, Plomp TA. Incidence, predictability, and pathogenesis of amiodarone-induced thyrotoxicosis and hypothyroidism. Am J Med 1991;91:507–11.

244. Valtonen VV, Ruutu P, Varis K, Ranki N, Malkamaki M, Makela PH. Serological evidence for the role of bacterial infections in the pathogenesis of thyroid diseases. Acta Med Scand 1986;219:105–11.

245. Vanderpump MP, Tunbridge WM, French JM, et al. The incidence of thyroid disorders in the community: a twenty-year follow-up of the Wickham Survey. Clin Endocrinol 1995;43:55–68.

246. Weetman AP, McGregor AM. Autoimmune thyroid disease: further developments in our understanding. Endocr Rev 1994;15:788–830.

247. Williams ED, Doniach I. Post-mortem incidence of focal thyroiditis. J Pathol Bacteriol 1962;83:255–64.

248. Woolner LB. Thyroiditis classification and clinicopathologic correlation. In: Hazad JB, Smith DE, eds. The thyroid. Baltimore: Williams & Wilkins, 1964:123–42.

249. Woolner LB, McConahey WM, Beahrs OH. Struma lymphomatosa (Hashimoto's thyroiditis) and related thyroidal disorders. J Clin Endocrinol Metab 1959;19:53–83.

250. Zinzani PL, Magagnoli M, Galieni P, et al. Nongastrointestinal low-grade mucosa-associated lymphoid tissue lymphoma: analysis of 75 patients. J Clin Oncol 1999;17:1254–60.

Graves' Disease

251. Brown RS. Immunoglobulins affecting thyroid growth: a continuing controversy. J Clin Endocrinol Metab 1995;80:1506–8.

252. Carter JK, Smith RE. Rapid induction of hypothyroidism by an avian leukosis virus. Infect Immun 1983;40:795–805.

253. Chang DC, Wheeler MH, Woodcock JP, et al. The effect of preoperative Lugol's iodine on thyroid blood flow in patients with Graves' hyperthyroidism. Surgery 1987;102:1055–61.

254. Cooper DS, Ladenson PW, Nisula BC, Dunn JF, Chapman EM, Ridgway EC. Familial thyroid hormone resistance. Metabolism 1982;31:504–9.

255. Cooper DS, Wenig BM. Hyperthyroidism caused by an ectopic TSH-secreting pituitary tumor. Thyroid 1996;6:337–43.

256. Curran RC, Eckert H, Wilson GM. The thyroid gland after treatment of hyperthyroidism by partial thyroidectomy or I-131. J Pathol Bacteriol 1958;76:541–60.

257. Eguchi K, Matsuoka N, Nagataki S. Cellular immunity in autoimmune thyroid disease. Balliere's Clin Endocinol Metab 1995;9:71–94.

258. Feldberg NT, Sergott RC, Savino PJ, Blizzard JJ, Schatz NJ, Amsel J. Lymphocyte subpopulation in Graves' ophthalmology. Arch Ophthalmol 1985;103:656–9.

259. Fradkin JE, Wolff J. Iodide-induced thyrotoxicosis. Medicine 1983;62:1–20.

260. Grubeck-Boebenstein B, Trieb K, Holter W. Retrobulbar T cells from patients with Graves' ophthalmology are CD8+ and specifically autologous fibroblasts. J Clin Invest 1994;93:2738–43.

261. Hamburger JI. Solitary autonomously functioning thyroid lesions. Diagnosis, clinical features and pathogenic considerations. Am J Med 1975;58:740–8.

262. Hanson GA, Komorowski RA, Cerlety JM, Wilson SD. Thyroid gland morphology in young adults: normal subjects versus those with prior low-dose neck irradiation in childhood. Surgery 1983;94:984–8.

263. Hedberg CW, Fishbein DB, Janssen RS, et al. An outbreak of thyrotoxicosis caused by the consumption of bovine thyroid gland in ground beef. N Engl J Med 1987;316:993–8.

264. Johnson JR. Some aspects of relationship of microscopic appearance to hyperthyroidism. Adenomatous goiters with and without hyperthyroidism. Arch Surg 1949;59:1088–99.

265. Kabel PJ, Voorbij HA, Deltaan M, et al. Intrathyroidal dendritic cells. J Clin Endocrinal Metab 1988;65:199–207.

266. Larsen PR, Davies TF, Hay ID. The thyroid gland. In: Wilson JD, Foster DW, Kronenberg AM, Larsen PR, eds. William's textbook of endocrinology, 9th ed. Philadelphia: WB Saunders, 1998:389–515.

267. Leclere J, Weryha G. Stress and auto-immune endocrine diseases. Horm Res 1989;31:90–3.

268. Lee KS, Kim K, Hur KB, Kim CK. The role of propranolol in the preoperative preparation of patients with Graves' disease. Surg Gynecol Obstet 1986;162:365–9.

269. Lloyd RV, Johnson TL, Blairas M, Sisson JC, Wilson BS. Detection of HLA-DR antigens in paraffin-embedded thyroid epithelial cells with a monoclonal antibody. Am J Pathol 1985;120:106–11.

270. Madec AM, Allannic H, Genetet N, et al. T lymphocyte subsets at various stages of hyperthyroid Graves' disease: effect of carbimazole treatment and relationship with thyroid-stimulating antibody levels of HLA status. J Clin Endocrinol Metab 1986;62:117–21.

271. McKenzie JM. Hyperthyroidism caused by thyroid adenomata. J Clin Endocrinol Metab 1966;26:779–81.

272. Miyai K, Tanizawa O, Yamamoto T, Azukizawa M, Kawai Y. Pituitary-thyroid function in trophoblastic disease. J Clin Endocrinol Metab 1976;42:254–9.

273. Mori H, Amino N, Iwatani Y, et al. Decrease of immunoglobulin G-Fc receptor-bearing T lymphocytes in Graves' disease. J Clin Endocrinol Metab 1982;55:399–402.

274. Noppakun N, Bancheun K, Chandraprasert S. Unusual locations of localized myxedema in Graves' disease. Report of three cases. Arch Dermatol 1986;122:85–8.

275. Okita N, How J, Topliss D, Lewis M, Row VV, Volpe R. Suppressor T lymphocyte dysfunction in Graves' disease: role of the H-2 histamine receptor-bearing suppressor T lymphocytes. J Clin Endocrinol Metab 1981;53:1002–7.

276. Patchefsky AS, Hoch WS. Psammoma bodies in diffuse toxic goiter. Am J Clin Pathol 1972;57:551–6.

277. Ramtoola S, Maisey MN, Clarke SE, Fogelman I. The thyroid scan in Hashimoto's thyroiditis: the great mimic. Nucl Med Commun 1988;9: 639–45.

278. Reinwein D, Benker G, Konig MP, Pinchera A, Schatz H, Schleusener A. The different types of hyperthyroidism in Europe. Results of a prospective survey of 924 patients. J Endocrinol Invest 1988;11:193–200.

279. Ross DS. Syndromes of thyrotoxicosis with low radioactive iodine uptake. Endocrinol Metab Clin N Am 1998;27:169–85.

280. Salvi M, Fukazama H, Bernard N, Hiromatsu Y, How J, Wall JR. Role of autoantibodies in the pathogenesis and association of endocrine autoimmune disorders. Endocr Rev 1988;9:450–66.

281. Shapiro SJ, Friedman NB, Perzik SL, Catz B. Incidence of thyroid carcinoma in Graves' disease. Cancer 1970;26:1261–70.

282. Sridama V, Pacini F, DeGroot LJ. Decreased suppressor T lymphocytes in autoimmune thyroid diseases detected by monoclonal antibodies. J Clin Endocrinol Metab 1982;54:316–29.

283. Stout BD, Wiener L, Cox JW. Combined alpha and beta sympathetic blockade in hyperthyroidism. Clinical and metabolic effects. Ann Intern Med 1969;70:963–70.

284. Tachiwaki O, Wollman SH. Shedding of dense cell fragments into follicular lumen early in involution of the hyperplastic thyroid gland. Lab Invest 1982;47:91–8.

285. Tollefsen HR, Shah JP, Huvos AG. Follicular carcinoma of the thyroid. Am J Surg 1973;126:523–8.

286. Tomer Y, Davies TF. Infection, thyroid disease, and autoimmunity. Endocr Rev 1993;14:107–20.

287. Tunbridge WM, Evered DE, Hall R, et al. The spectrum of thyroid disease in a community: the Wickham Survey. Clin Endocrinol 1977; 7:481–493.

288. Valenta L, Lemarchand-Beraud T, Nemec J, Griessen M, Bednor J. Metastatic thyroid carcinoma provoking hyperthyroidism with elevated circulating thyrostimulators. Am J Med 1970;40:72–6.

289. Wall JR, Bernard N, Boucher A, et al. Pathogenesis of thyroid-associated ophthalmopathy: an autoimmune disorder of the eye muscle associated with Graves' hyperthyroidism and Hashimoto's thyroiditis. Clin Immuno Immunopathol 1993;68:1–8.

290. Wang PW, Hiromatsu Y, Laryea E, Wosu L, How J, Wall JR. Immunologically mediated cytotoxicity against human eye muscle cells in Graves' ophthalmology. J Clin Endocrinol Metab 1986;63:316–22.

291. Winsa B, Adami HO, Bergstrom R, et al. Stressful life events and Graves' disease. Lancet 1991;338:1478–9.

292. Zellmann HE. Iatrogenic and factitious thyroidal disease. Med Clin N Am 1979;63:329–35.

Postpartum Thyroiditis

293. Gorman CA, Duick DS, Woolner LB, et al. Transient hyperthyroidism in patients with lymphocytic thyroiditis. Mayo Clin Proc 1978;53:359–65.

294. Lucas A, Pizarro E, Granada ML, et al. Postpartum thyroiditis: epidemiology and clinical evolution in a nonselected population. Thyroid 2000;10:71–7.

295. Roti E, Emerson CH. Clinical review 29: postpartum thyroiditis. J Clin Endocrinol Metab 1992;74:3–5.

296. Taylor HC, Sheeler LR. Recurrence and heterogeneity in painless thyrotoxic lymphocytic thyroiditis. Report of five cases. JAMA 1982;248:1085–8.

Silent Thyroiditis

297. LiVolsi VA. The pathology of autoimmune thyroid disease: a review. Thyroid 1994;4:333–9.

298. Mizukami Y, Michigishi T, Hashimoto T, et al. Silent thyroiditis: a histologic and immunohistochemical study. Hum Pathol 1988;19:423–31.

299. Nikolai TF, Brosseau J, Kettnernick MA, Roberts R, Beltaos E. Lymphocyte thyroiditis with spontaneously resolving hyperthyroidism (silent thyroiditis). Arch Intern Med 1980;140:478–82.

Focal Lymphocytic Thyroiditis

300. Goudie RB, Anderson JR, Gray KG. Complement-fixing antithyroid antibodies in hospital patients with asymptomatic thyroid lesions. J Path Bact 1959;77:389–400.

301. Harach HR, Williams ED. Fibrous thyroiditis—an immunopathological study. Histopathology 1983;7:739–51.

302. Harland WA, Frantz VK. Clinicopathologic study of 261 surgical cases of so-called thyroiditis. J Clin Endocrinol Metab 1956;16:1433–7.

303. Williams ED, Doniach I. Post-mortem incidence of focal thyroiditis. J Pathol 1962;83:255–64.

Riedel's Thyroiditis

304. Heufelder AE, Goellner JR, Bahn RS, Gleich GJ, Hay ID. Tissue eosinophilia and eosinophil degranulation in Riedel's invasive fibrous thyroiditis. J Clin Endocrinol Metab 1996;81:977–84.

305. Kurashima C, Hirokawa K. Focal lymphocytic infiltration of thyroids in elderly people. Histopathological and immunohistochemcial studies. Survey Synth Pathol Res 1985;4:457–66.

306. Larsen PR, Davies TF, Hay ID. The thyroid gland. In: Wilson JP, Foster DW, Kronenberg HM, Larsen PR, eds. Williams textbook of endocrinology, 9th ed. Philadelphia: WB Saunders, 1998:389–515.

307. Munro JM, Van der Walt JD, Cox EL. A comparison of cytoplasmic immunoglobulins in retroperitoneal fibrosis and abdominal aortic aneurysms. Histopathology 1986;10:1163–9.

308. Schwaegerle SM, Bauer TW, Esselstyn CB Jr. Riedel's thyroiditis. Am J Clin Pathol 1988; 90:715–22.

309. Wold LE, Weiland LH. Tumefactive fibro-inflammatory lesions of the head and neck. Am J Surg Pathol 1983;7:477–82.

Simple Nontoxic or Multinodular Goiter

310. Aeschimann S, Kopp PA, Kimura ET, et al. Morphological and functional polymorphism within clonal thyroid nodules. J Clin Endocrinol Metab 1993;77:846–51.

311. Al-Moussa M, Beck JS. Histometry of thyroids containing few and multiple nodules. J Clin Pathol 1986;39:483–8.

312. Apel RL, Ezzat S, Bapat BV, Pan N, Livolsi VA, Asa SL. Clonality of thyroid nodules in sporadic goiter. Diagn Mol Pathol 1995;4:113–21.

313. Berghout A, Wiersinga WM, Drexhage HA, et al. The long-term outcome of thyroidectomy for sporadic non-toxic goitre. Clin Endocrinol 1989;31:193–9.

314. Borowski GD, Garofaro CD, Rose LI, et al. Effect of long-term amiodarone therapy on thyroid hormone levels and thyroid function. Am J Med 1985;78:443–50.

315. Bray GA. Increased sensitivity of the thyroid in iodine-depleted rats to the goitrogenic effects of thyrotropin. J Clin Invest 1968;47:1640–7.

316. Brown RS. Immunoglobulins affecting thyroid growth: a continuing controversy. J Clin Endocrinol Metab 1995;80:1506–8.

317. Burke G, Silverstein GE, Sorkin AI. Effect of long-term sulfonylurea therapy on thyroid function in man. Metabolism 1967;16:651–7.

318. Dige-Petersen H, Hummer L. Serum thyrotropin concentration under basal conditions and after stimulation with thyrotropin-releasing hormone in idiopathic nontoxic goiter. J Clin Endocrinol Metab 1977;44:1115–20.

319. Drexhage HA, Bottazzo GF, Doniach D, Bitensky L, Chayen J. Evidence for thyroid growth stimulating immunoglobulins in some goitrous thyroid diseases. Lancet 1980;2:287–92.

320. Fujita M, Enomoto T, Wada H, Inoue M, Okudaira Y, Shroyer KR. Application of clonal analysis. Differential diagnosis for synchronous primary ovarian and endometrial cancers and metastatic cancer. Am J Clin Pathol 1996;105: 350–9.

321. Ghossein RA, Rosai J, Heffess C. Dyshormonogenetic goiter: a clinicopathologic study of 56 cases. Endocr Pathol 1997;8:283–92.

322. Glinoer D. Radioiodine therapy of non-toxic multinodular goiter. Clin Endocrinol 1994; 41:713–4.

323. Glinoer D, Leone M. Goiter and pregnancy: a new insight into an old problem. Thyroid 1992; 2:65–70.

324. Greer MA, Astwood EB. Treatment of simple goiter with thyroid. J Clin Endocrinol 1953;13: 1312–31.

325. Greig WR, Boyle JA, Duncan A, et al. Genetic and non-genetic factors in simple goitre formation: evidence from a twin study. Q J Med 1967;36:175–88.

326. Hicks DG, LiVolsi VA, Neidich JA, Puck JM, Kant JA. Clonal analysis of solitary follicular nodules in the thyroid. Am J Pathol 1990;137:553–62.

327. Hull OH. Critical analysis of two hundred twenty-one thyroid glands—study of thyroid glands obtained at necropsy in Colorado. Arch Pathol 1955;59:291–311.

328. Izembart M, Heshmati HM, Dagousset F, de Cremoux P, Boutteville C, Vallee G. Serum thyroglobulin is elevated in patients with heterogeneous goiter during radioiodine scintography but normal in those with homogeneous goiter. Schweiz Med Wochenschr 1986;116:634–7.

329. Kopp P, Kimura ET, Aeschimann S, et al. Polyclonal and monoclonal thyroid nodules coexist within human multinodular goiters. J Clin Endocrinol Metab 1994;79:134–9.

330. Lyon MF. Clones and X-chromosomes. J Pathol 1988;155:97–9.

331. Lyon MF. X-chromosome inactivation and the location and expression of X-linked genes. Am J Hum Genet 1988;42:8–16.

332. Marine D. Etiology and prevention of simple goiter. Medicine 1924;3:453–79.

333. Mehbod H, Swartz CD, Brest AN. The effect of prolonged thiazide administration on thyroid function. Arch Intern Med 1967;119:283–6.

334. Murray IP, Thompson JA, McGirr EM, MacDonald EM, Kennedy JS, McLennan I. Unusual familial goiter associated with intrathyroidal calcification. J Clin Endocrinol Metab 1966;26:1039–49.

335. Nygaard B, Faber J, Hegedus I, Hansen JM. 131I treatment of nodular non-toxic goitre. Eur J Endocrinol 1996;134:15–20.

336. Papotti M, Fara E, Ardeleanu C, Bussolati G. Occurrence and significance of vascular invasion in multinodular adenomatous goiter. Endocr Pathol 1994;5:35–9.

337. Rieu M, Bekka S, Sambor B, Berrod JL, Fombeur JP. Prevalence of subclinical hyperthyroidism and relationship between thyroid hormonal status and thyroid ultrasonographic parameters in patients with non-toxic nodular goitre. Clin Endocrinol 1993;39:67–71.

338. Ross DS. Thyroid hormone suppressive therapy of sporadic nontoxic goiter. Thyroid 1992;2: 263–9.

339. Smyth PP, Neylan D, O'Donovan DK. The prevalence of thyroid-stimulating antibodies in goitrous disease assessed by cytochemical section bioassay. J Clin Endocrinol Metab 1982;54:357–61.

340. Studer H, Peter HJ, Gerber H. Natural heterogeneity of thyroid cells: the basis for understanding thyroid function and nodular goiter growth. Endocr Rev 1989;10:125–35.

341. Thomas GA, Williams D, Williams ED. The clonal origin of thyroid nodules and adenomas. Am J Pathol 1989;134:141–7.

342. Valente WA, Vitti P, Rotellar CM, et al. Antibodies that promote thyroid growth. A distinct population of thyroid-stimulating autoantibodies. N Engl J Med 1983;309:1028–34.

343. Vickery AL Jr. The diagnosis of malignancy in dyshormonogenic goiter. Clin Endocrinol Metab 1981;10:317–35.

Dyshormonogenetic Goiter

344. Barsano CP, De Groot LJ. Dyshormonogenic goitre. Clin Endocrinol Metab 1979;8:145–65.

345. Batsakis JG, Nishiyama RH, Schmidt RW. "Sporadic goiter syndrome": a clinicopathologic analysis. Am J Clin Pathol 1963;39:241–51.

346. Fisher DA, Klein AH. Thyroid development and disorders of thyroid function in the newborn. N Engl J Med 1981;304:702–12.

347. Ghossein RA, Rosai J, Heffess C. Dyshormonogenetic goiter: a clinicopathologic study of 56 cases. Endocr Pathol 1997;8:283–92.

348. Kennedy JS. The pathology of dyshormonogenic goitre. J Pathol 1969;99:251–64.

349. Lever EG, Medeñros-Neto GA, De Groot LJ. Inherited disorders of thyroid metabolism. Endocr Rev 1983;4:213–39.

350. Moore GH. The thyroid in sporadic goitrous cretinism. A report of three new cases, description of the pathologic anatomy of the thyroid glands, and a review of the literature. Arch Pathol 1962;74:35–46.

351. Ramalingaswani V. Iodine and thyroid cancer in man. In: Hedinger CE, ed. Thyroid cancer (VICC monography). New York: Springer-Verlag, 1969;12:113–23.

Toxic Multinodular Goiter

352. Grubeck-Loebenstein D, Derfler K, Kassal H, et al. Immunological features of nonimmunogenic hyperthyroidism. J Clin Endocrinol Metab 1985;60:150–5.

353. Huysmans DA, Hermus AR, Corstens FH, et al. Large compressive goiters treated with radioiodine. Ann Intern Med 1994;121:757–62.

354. Larsen PR, Davies TF, Hay ID. The thyroid gland. In: Wilson JD, Fasler DW, Kronenberg HM, Larsen PR, eds. Williams textbook of endocrinology, 9th ed. Philadelphia: W.B. Saunders, 1998:389–515.

355. Studer H, Peter HJ, Gerber H. Toxic nodular goitre. Clin Endocrinol Metab 1985;14:351–72.

356. Van Sande J, Parma J, Tonacchera M, Swillens S, Dumont J, Vassart G. Somatic germline mutations of the TSH receptor gene in thyroid disease. J Clin Endocrinol Metab 1995;80:2577–85.

Endemic Goiters

357. Correa P, Castro S. Survey of pathology of thyroid glands from Cali, Columbia—a goiter area. Lab Invest 1961;10:39–50.

358. Day TK, Powell-Jackson PR. Fluoride, water hardness, and endemic goitre. Lancet 1972;1:1135–8.

359. Hetzel BS. Iodine deficiency disorders (IDD) and their eradication. Lancet 1983;2:1126–9.

360. Maberly GF, Corcoran JM, Eastman CJ. The effect of iodized oil on goitre size, thyroid function, and the development of the Jod Basedow phenomenon. Clin Endocrinol (Oxf) 1982;17:253–9.

361. McCarrison R. Observations on endemic cretinism in the Chitral and Gilgit valleys. Lancet 1908;2:1275–80.

362. Scrimshaw NS. The geographic pathology of thyroid disease. In: Hazard JB, Smith DV, eds. The thyroid. Publication 5. International Academy of Pathology Monograph. Baltimore: Williams & Wilkins, 1964:100–22.

363. Versmiglio F, Benvenga S, Melluso R, et al. Increased serum thyroglobulin concentrations and impaired thyrotropin response to thyrotropin-releasing hormone in euthyroid subjects with endemic goiter in Sicily: their relation to goiter size and nodularity. J Endocrinol Invest 1986;9:389–96.

364. Weetman AP. Is endemic goiter an autoimmune disease? J Clin Endocrinol Metab 1994;78:1017–9.

Amyloid Goiter

365. Amado JA, Ondiviela R, Palacios S, Casanova D, Manzanos J, Freijanls J. Fast growing goitre as the first clinical manifestation of systemic amyloidosis. Postgrad Med J 1982;58:171–2.

366. Arean VM, Klein RE. Amyloid goiter. Review of literature and report of a case. Am J Clin Pathol 1961;36:341–55.

367. Hirota S, Miyamoto M, Kasugai T, Kitamura Y, Morimura Y. Crystalline light chain deposition of amyloidosis in the thyroid gland and kidneys of a patient with myeloma. Arch Pathol Lab Med 1990;114:429–31.

368. Kanoh T, Shimada H, Uchino H, Matsumura K. Amyloid goiter with hypothyroidism. Arch Pathol Lab Med 1989;113:542–4.

C-Cell Hyperplasia

369. Albores-Saavedra J. C-cell hyperplasia [Letter]. Am J Surg Pathol 1989;13:987–9.

370. Albores-Saavedra J, Monforte H, Nadji M, Morales AR. C-cell hyperplasia in thyroid tissue adjacent to follicular cell tumors. Hum Pathol 1988;19:795–9.

371. Asaadi AA. Ultrastructure in C-cell hyperplasia in asymptomatic patients with hypercalcitonemia and a family history of medullary thyroid carcinoma. Hum Pathol 1981;12:617–22.

372. Biddinger PW, Brennan MF, Rosen PP. Symptomatic C-cell hyperplasia associated with chronic lymphocytic thyroiditis. Am J Surg Pathol 1991;15:599–604.

373. Carney JA, Moore SB, Northcutt RC, Woolner LB, Stillwell GK. Palpation thyroiditis (multifocal granulomatous folliculitis). Am J Clin Pathol 1975;64:639–47.

374. DeLellis RA, Nunnemacher G, Wolfe HJ. C-cell hyperplasia: an ultrastructural analysis. Lab Invest 1977;36:237–48.

375. DeLellis RA, Wolfe HJ. The pathobiology of the human calcitonin (C) cell: a review. Pathol Annu 1981;16:25–52.

376. Dralle H, Gimm O, Simon D, et al. Prophylactic thyroidectomy in 75 children and adolescents with hereditary medullary thyroid carcinoma: German and Austrian experience. World J Surg 1998;22:744–50.

377. Eng C. The RET proto-oncogene in multiple endocrine neoplasia type 2 and Hirschsprung's disease. N Engl J Med 1996;335:943–51.

378. Eng C, Thomas GA, Neuberg DS, et al. Mutation of the RET proto-oncogene is correlated with RET immunostaining in subpopulations of cells in sporadic medullary thyroid carcinoma. J Clin Endocrinol Metab 1998;83:4310–13.

379. Gagel RF, Tashjian AH Jr, Cummings T, et al. The clinical outcome of prospective screening for multiple endocrine neoplasia type 2a. An 18-year experience. N Engl J Med 1988;318:478–84.

380. Gibson WC, Peng TC, Croker BP. C-cell nodules in adult human thyroid. A common autopsy finding. Am J Clin Pathol 1981;75:347–50.

381. Guyetant S, Rousselet MC, Durigon M, et al. Sex-related C-cell hyperplasia in the normal human thyroid: a quantitative autopsy study. J Clin Endocrinol Metab 1997;82:42–7.

382. Kaserer K, Scheuba C, Neuhold N, et al. C-cell hyperplasia and medullary thyroid carcinoma in patients routinely screened for serum calcitonin. Am J Surg Pathol 1998;22:722–8.

383. Komminoth P, Kunz EK, Matias-Guiu X, et al. Analysis of RET proto-oncogene point mutations distinguishes heritable from nonheritable medullary thyroid carcinomas. Cancer 1995;76:479–89.

384. Lallier M, St-Vil D, Giroux M, et al. Prophylactic thyroidectomy for medullary thyroid carcinoma in gene carriers of MEN 2 syndrome. J Pediatr Surg 1998;33:846–8.

385. Libbey NP, Nowakowski KJ, Tucci JR. C-cell hyperplasia of the thyroid in a patient with goitrous hypothyroidism and Hashimoto's thyroiditis. Am J Surg Pathol 1989;13:71–7.

386. Lips CJ, Leo JR, Berends MJ, et al. Thyroid C-cell hyperplasia and micronodules in close relatives of MEN-2A patients: pitfalls in early diagnosis and re-evaluation of criteria for surgery. Henry Ford Hosp Med J 1987;35:133–8.

387. LiVolsi VA, Feind CR, Lo Gerfo P, Tashjian AH Jr. Demonstration by immunoperoxidase staining of hyperplasia of parafollicular cells in the thyroid gland in hyperparathyroidism. J Clin Endocrinol Metab 1973;37:550–9.

388. Lloyd RV. RET proto-oncogene mutations and rearrangements in endocrine diseases. Am J Pathol 1995; 147:1539–44.

389. McGregor LM, McCune BK, Graff JR, et al. Roles of the trk family neurotropin receptors in medullary thyroid carcinoma development and progression. Proc Natl Acad Sci USA 1999;96:4540–5.

390. Melvin KE, Miller HH, Tashjian AH Jr. Early diagnosis of medullary carcinoma of the thyroid gland by means of calcitonin assay. N Engl J Med 1971;285:1115–20.

391. O'Toole K, Fenoglio-Preiser C, Pushparaj N. Endocrine changes associated with the human aging process: III. Effect of age on the number of calcitonin immunoreactive cells in the thyroid gland. Hum Pathol 1985;16:991–1000.

392. Perry A, Molberg K, Albones-Saavedra J. Physiologic versus neoplastic C-cell hyperplasia of the thyroid: separation of distinct histologic and biologic entities. Cancer 1996;77:750–6.

393. Rosai J, Carcangiu ML, DeLellis RA. Tumors of the thyroid gland. Atlas of Tumor Pathology, 3rd Series, Fascicle 5. Washington, DC: Armed Forces Institute of Pathology, 1992.

394. Saad MF, Ordonez NG, Rashid RK, et al. Medullary carcinoma of the thyroid. A study of the clinical features and prognostic factors of 161 patients. Medicine 1984;63:319–42.

395. Schroder S, Bocker W, Baisch H, et al. Prognostic factors in medullary thyroid carcinomas. Survival in relation to age, sex, stage, histology, immunocyto-chemistry, and DNA content. Cancer 1988;61:806–16.

396. Schürch W, Babäi F, Boivin Y, Verdy M. Light-electron microscopic and cytochemical studies on the morphogenesis of familial medullary thyroid carcinoma. Virchows Arch [A] 1977;376:29–46.

397. Scopsi L, DiPalma S, Ferrari C, Holst JJ, Rehfeld JF, Rilke F. C-cell hyperplasia accompanying thyroid diseases other than medullary thyroid carcinoma: an immunocytochemical study by means of antibodies to calcitonin and somatostatin. Mod Pathol 1991;4:297–304.

398. Vollenweider I, Hedinger C. Solid cell nests (SCN) in Hashimoto's thyroiditis. Virchows Arch [A] 1988;412: 357–63.

399. Wells SA Jr, Ontjes DA, Cooper CW, et al. The early diagnosis of medullary carcinoma of the thyroid in patients with multiple endocrine neoplasia type II. Ann Surg 1975;182:362–70.

400. Wolfe HJ, DeLellis RA, Scott RT, Tashjian AH Jr. C-cell hyperplasia in chronic hypercalcemia in man [Abstract]. Am J Pathol 1975;78:20A.

401. Wolfe HL, Melvin KE, Cervi-Skinner SJ, et al. C-cell hyperplasia preceding medullary thyroid carcinoma. N Engl J Med 1973;289:437–41.

402. Yamaoka Y. Solid cell nest (SCN) of the human thyroid gland. Acta Pathol Jpn 1973;23:493–506.

4
ADRENAL GLAND

NORMAL ADRENAL GLAND

Embryology

The adrenal cortex develops from the mesoderm, with the steroidogenic cells arising from the coelomic mesothelium. The studies of Crowder (1), based on the Carnegie Embryological Collection (2), showed that around the 25th day of gestation (5 to 6 mm embryo), the coelomic epithelium medial to the mesonephros and urogenital ridge proliferates, resulting in cords of large polyhedral cells which extend to the overlying mesenchyme to form the adrenal primordium bilaterally. Around the 30th day of gestation (9 mm embryo), cells from the mesonephric glomerulus migrate toward the adrenal primordium, and by the 35th day (10 mm embryo), the coelomic epithelial cells adjacent to the adrenal primordium penetrate into the primordium. Between days 35 and 45 of gestation, the adrenal glands enlarge significantly and the primitive sympathetic cells, along with nerve tracts, migrate to form the medulla. By the 45th day of gestation, the gland is elliptical in shape and weighs about 1 mg.

At 8 weeks of gestation the adrenal glands weigh 4 to 6 mg each and there is marked proliferation of the outer cortical zone. The definitive cortex can be distinguished from the inner or fetal cortex (3). At 4 months, the adrenal glands are slightly larger than the kidneys and are mostly composed of fetal cortex. Recent studies have shown that cortical cells from the zona glomerulosa migrate inward, suggesting that these are capable of producing all three classes of adrenal cortical steroids (6).

During the third trimester, the glands continue to increase in weight and at birth each gland weighs about 4 g. There is no difference in the weight of the adrenal gland by sex during embryonic development.

The medulla becomes visible, and by 37 days of development (11 mm embryo), bundles of nerve fibers and sympathicoblasts in primitive small cells enter the glands. Immediate paraganglia or pheochromoblasts are dispersed along the course of the nerve fibers (1). Around 56 days (27 to 31 mm embryo), the paraganglionic cells replicate and develop into chromaffin cells. The primitive sympathicoblasts may persist until birth or early infancy, forming neuroblastic nodules (4,5). These nodules increase with age, and peak at 17 to 20 weeks of gestation, and then may regress in older fetuses. Nodules range in diameter from 60 µm to 400 µm, and they may be confused with small neuroblastomas (1,4).

Anatomy

Gross Anatomy. The adrenal glands are located anterior to the upper poles of the kidneys (fig. 4-1). The weight of the normal adrenal gland varies significantly from childhood to puberty. Data from sudden death cases have shown that the mean unfixed weight does not exceed 2 g per gland up to 5 years of age and then increases to just over 2 g during early puberty (14,15,27). There is a substantial increase during the pubertal period of rapid growth. With chronic illness and elevated corticotropin (ACTH) levels, the weight can increase by 0.5 to 1.0 g per gland.

The fetal zone of the adrenal gland involutes markedly starting at about 2 weeks after birth, and by the end of the first month of life, about 50 percent of the weight of this zone has been lost (7,13,26). By the end of the first year of life, only the stroma of the degenerated fetal cortex remains. Recent studies have shown a role for apoptosis in this involution, especially during the first 2 to 4 weeks of life (9,24).

The adrenal glands of neonates have a smooth external surface. Cut sections show a dark red-brown color caused by regression of the fetal cortex and congestion. Medullary tissue is not visible in the neonatal gland, since it is less than 1 percent of the total gland volume at this time. In adults, the right gland is pyramidal and the left crescentic in shape (figs. 4-2, 4-3). The adrenal cortex is bright yellow due to

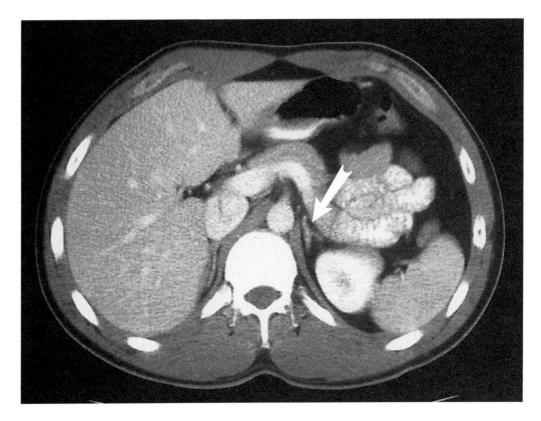

Figure 4-1

NORMAL ADULT ADRENAL GLAND

Contrast-enhanced CT of the upper abdomen demonstrates the normal left adrenal gland (arrow) as an inverted, Y-shaped structure anterior to the upper pole of the left kidney.

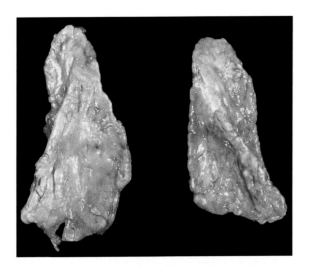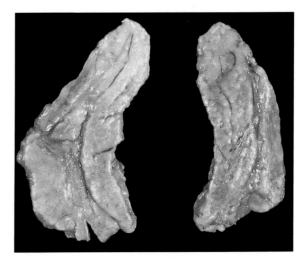

Figure 4-2

NORMAL ADULT ADRENAL GLAND

The gross appearance of the adult adrenal glands from their anterior (left) and posterior (right) aspects. The right adrenal (left in the photo) is more triangular while the left adrenal is crescentic.

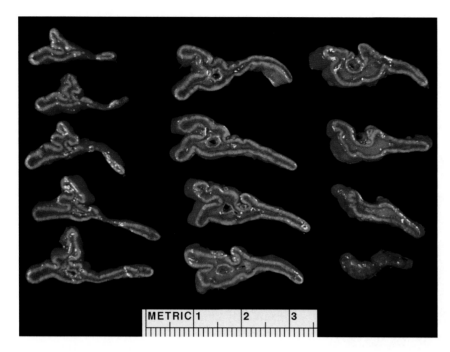

Figure 4-3

NORMAL ADULT
ADRENAL GLAND

This transverse section through the left adrenal gland shows the bright yellow center and gray medulla which occupies about 10 percent of the volume of the gland.

lipid accumulation. The zona reticularis or inner zone is thinner and darker.

The medulla has an ellipsoid shape near the head of the gland and a pickle shape at the body. The medulla is gray-tan and is best seen in the head and body of the gland (fig. 4-3). Qualitative measurement has shown that the cortical/medullary ratio is 10 to 1 overall (12). If the cortex becomes atrophic, the medulla appears more prominent. In some areas of the adrenal gland the medulla is absent, and if parts of the cortex abut on other parts of the cortex, a raphé is visible (18). The adrenal gland can be divided grossly into the head, which contains most of the medulla; the body, which has some medullary tissue; and the tail, which consists only of cortical tissue (10,21,25). The wings or alae are 2- to 3-mm–thick structures adjacent to the long axis of the body; they do not contain medulla, except when medullary hyperplasia develops.

The weight of the adrenal gland in adults who die suddenly without prior illness is 4.0 to 4.2 g ± 15 percent (95 percent confidence limit of 2.8 to 5.5 g) (21). Ninety percent of the gland weight is contributed by the cortex (23). The mean weight of adrenal glands of black individuals dying suddenly is 3.8 ± 0.8 g, suggesting racial differences in weight (21). There is no correlation between absolute body weight and adrenal weight, and no difference between the weight of the left and right gland. Although historically it has been reported that the adrenal gland is heavier in males than in females (17), these observations are not supported by more recent studies (21). Pregnancy- and sex-related changes in adrenal weights are seen in some mammals (11), but not humans (21). When death is preceded by a chronic illness, there is a significant increase in the mean adrenal weight (mean, 5.8 to 6.2 g ± 25 percent).

To obtain accurate adrenal gland weights, the glands should be carefully dissected and all excess fat removed. The results should be correlated with endocrinologic and other clinical data to make a precise diagnosis.

Blood Supply. The adrenal gland is supplied by three principal arteries, which divide into many (50 to 60) smaller branches, some of which partially supply the adrenal capsule. There is a single central main adrenal vein which is enveloped by cortical tissue as it exits the glands. The right adrenal vein is shorter than the left vein. It has been proposed that the shortness and decreased compliance of the right adrenal vein may be responsible for the higher incidence of perinatal adrenal hemorrhage in the right compared to the left gland (18).

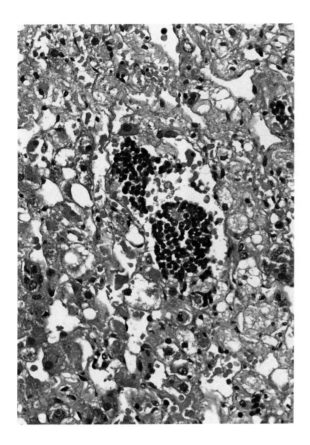

Figure 4-4

DEVELOPING FETAL ADRENAL GLAND

Provisional or fetal adrenal cortex at 3 months of development shows eosinophilic adrenal cortical cells and small nodules of primitive neuroblastic cells admixed with the fetal cortex.

There is collateral drainage of the adrenal gland which may be important in unusual circumstances (16). Emissary veins run centrifugally from the central veins and branch through the cortex to join the pericapsular veins, which collect into the venial comitantes. These veins follow the superior and inferior groups of adrenal arteries and drain into a variety of contiguous veins including the inferior phrenic and inferior adrenal veins (21).

Because there is no direct arterial supply to the deeper cortical layers, these cells rely on the blood that has passed through the center zones and which contains secreted steroids. This relationship is preserved even in large mammals such as elephants and whales (21). Most of the cortical tissue is perfused by blood that enters the parenchyma from the capsular arterial plexus. Thus, the blood supply to the cortex is derived from capillary sinusoids which are lined by endothelial cells with fenestrae or pores closed by a single membrane. Most of the blood entering the cortex in the head of the gland eventually reaches the medulla, where there is a corticomedullary portal system. The zona glomerulosa always lies nearest the source of arterial blood. The medulla is also supplied by the arterial medullae which pass directly to it from the capsular arterial plexus (21).

The major effluent vessels have eccentrically arrayed bundles of longitudinal smooth muscle. These muscles are absent in neonates and are not well developed in young children. They may have important functions during hemorrhage (8).

Lymphatic Supply. Lymphatic vessels are present only in the capsule of the gland. Cortical and medullary parenchymal tissues are devoid of lymphatics, which are present only in the adventitia of the central vein and its major tributaries (25). Abnormalities of the adrenal lymphatic vessels may contribute to adrenal cysts.

Innervation. The adrenal gland receives an abundant supply of nerves through a capsular nerve plexus that traverses the cortex with the arterial medullae. Most of the nerves terminate in the medulla or in the smooth muscle of the major vessels. These include preganglionic sympathetic fibers innervating the pheochromocytes and postganglionic fibers (20).

Microscopic Anatomy. In the neonate, between 70 and 85 percent of the adrenal cortex is made up of the provisional cells of the fetal zone (fig. 4-4). This zone regresses during the first few weeks to months of life. Anencephalic fetuses have a normal-appearing cortex up to 20 weeks' gestation, but at birth the cortex is much thinner than that of the normal neonate (19).

Microscopic cystic changes have been reported in the adrenal glands of some neonates as well as premature and stillborn infants. These microcystic changes have been attributed to in utero stress (22). Other degenerative changes including vacuolization of the cortical cells have been reported in infants with erythroblastosis fetalis and thalassemia major, and these conditions may also be related to intrauterine stress caused by hypoxia (17).

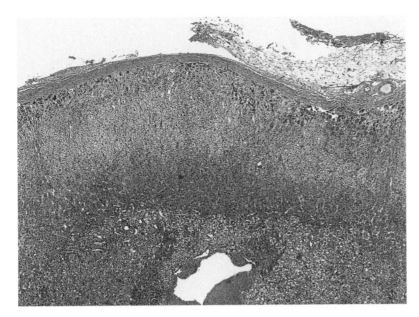

Figure 4-5

NORMAL ADULT ADRENAL
GLAND

Normal adrenal cortex and medulla
in an adult shows lipid-rich cortical cells
of the zona fasciculata and medullary
cells with basophilic cytoplasm adjacent
to the central vein.

The neonatal adrenal definitive cortex is 0.1 to 0.2 mm in thickness; by 9 days after birth it is 0.5 mm thick and by the 12th year of life, it is 1.0 cm thick. The normal adrenal cortex is 2 cm thick in healthy adults (figs. 4-5–4-8). The thickness varies in different parts of the gland. The zona glomerulosa, which is the outer zone, comprises 5 to 10 percent of the cortex. The cells here are smaller with less cytoplasm than the other cortical cells. The middle zone or fasciculata makes up about 70 percent of the cortex. It is formed by radial cords of cells with abundant lipid-filled cytoplasm which are pale staining with the hematoxylin and eosin (H&E) stain. The inner portion of the zona fasciculata merges with the inner cortical zone or zona reticularis. This zone is composed of cells with compact, finely granular, eosinophilic cytoplasm. These cells have variable amounts of lipochrome pigment which contribute to its brown color and are designated as compact cells. Adrenal cortical cells are also found around the central vein and its branches, and are termed the "cortical cuff." All three zones may be present in the cuff.

The adrenal medulla is made up of chromaffin cells that are organized in nests and anastomosing cords (figs. 4-9–4-11). The cells have basophilic to amphophilic granular cytoplasm and indistinct cytoplasmic cell borders. There is moderate variation in cell size and mitotic figures are extremely uncommon. Intracytoplasmic

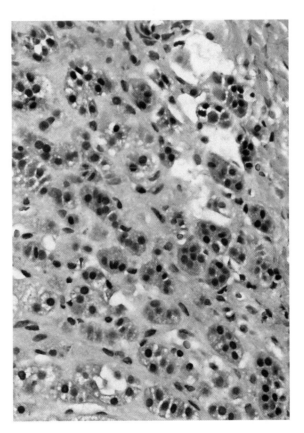

Figure 4-6

NORMAL ADULT ADRENAL GLAND

Higher magnification of the zona glomerulosa shows small cells with a high nuclear /cytoplasmic ratio and lipid in the clear cytoplasm.

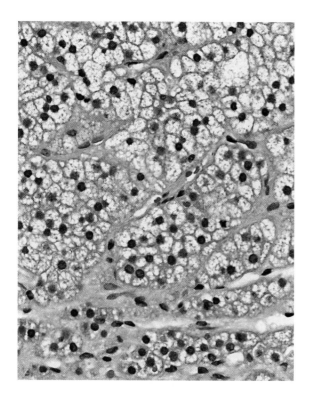

Figure 4-7

NORMAL ADULT ADRENAL GLAND

The zona fasciculata consists of larger cells with predominantly clear cytoplasm organized in columns.

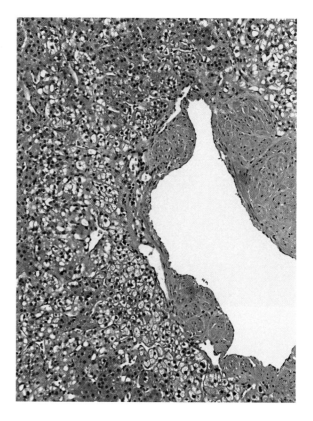

Figure 4-9

NORMAL ADRENAL MEDULLA

The central adrenal vein in the medulla has a thick wall of smooth muscle.

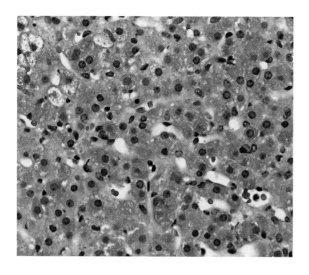

Figure 4-8

NORMAL ADULT ADRENAL GLAND

The zona reticularis consists of cells with less cytoplasmic lipid than the fasciculata. The cytoplasm is composed of eosinophilic compact cells organized in cords and containing brown lipofuscin pigment.

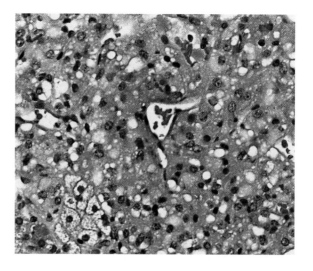

Figure 4-10

NORMAL ADRENAL MEDULLA

The adrenal medulla consists of rounds cells with basophilic cytoplasm arranged in nests and anastomosing cords.

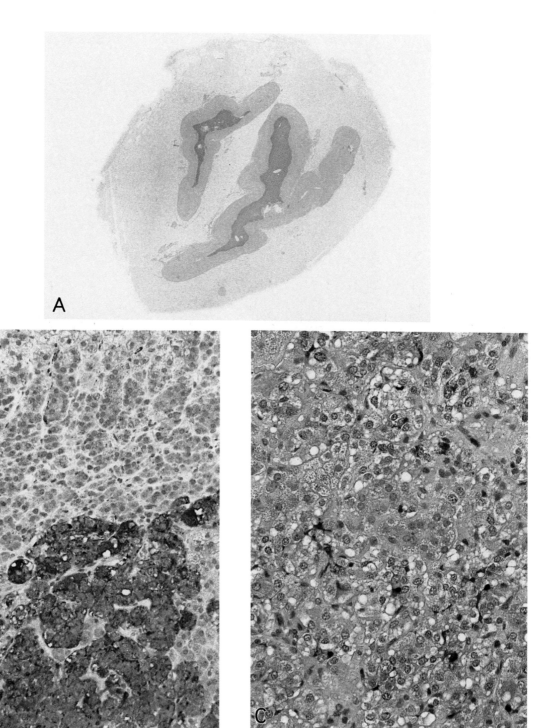

Figure 4-11

NORMAL ADRENAL MEDULLA

A: Immunostain for chromogranin outlines the adrenal medulla in brown. The tail and wing of the normal gland are usually devoid of medullary tissue. The adrenal cortex is negative for chromogranin A (diaminobenzidine chromogen).

B: Synaptophysin strongly stains the adrenal medulla. The adrenal cortex is weakly positive.

C: S100 protein immunostain highlights the sustentacular cells which are intimately associated with the pheochromocytes (diaminobenzidine chromogen).

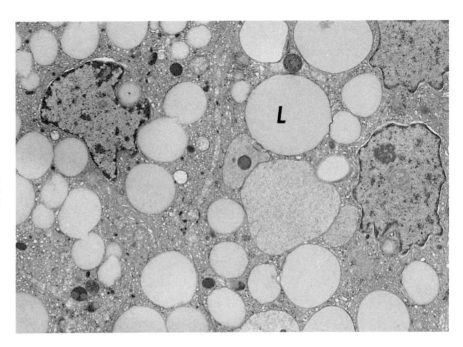

Figure 4-12

ULTRASTRUCTURE OF
NORMAL ZONA
FASCICULATA

Cells of the zona fasciculata have abundant large lipid droplets (L) (X3,810).

hyaline globules are present in some normal chromaffin cells and are thought to represent dense core secretory granules. They may be present in up to 80 percent of adrenal medullae and are more common in patients with chronic neurological disorders such as Parkinson's disease (19).

Two other cell types present in the medulla are ganglion cells and sustentacular cells. Ganglion cells are found singly or in association with myelinated nerve bundles. Sustentacular cells, also known as supporting or satellite cells, are present at the periphery of the medullary cords and are readily recognized by their spindle shape and staining for S100 acidic protein (fig. 4-11C).

Ultrastructure

The ultrastructural features of each adrenal cortical zone are quite distinct, which allows for easy recognition and separation of optimally fixed, surgically excised tissue (30,32). Cells of the zona glomerulosa have sparse amounts of intracellular lipid and mitochondria that are elliptical with lamellar or plate-like cristae. Microvillus projections may be present on the cell surface. Lysosomes and lipofuscin granules are uncommon in this zone. Very little smooth endoplasmic reticulum is present in the zona glomerulosa.

Cells of the zona fasciculata have distinct mitochondria that are round to oval, with short and long tubular cristae (figs. 4-12, 4-13). Variably sized lipid droplets are present in the cytoplasm of these cells. Smooth endoplasmic reticulum is prominent, especially in the inner fasciculata. Rough endoplasmic reticulum is present in moderate amounts. Microvillus cytoplasmic projections are more prominent in the inner fasciculata, and lysosomes are increased in number compared to those in the glomerulosa.

Cells of the zona reticularis have spherical to ovoid mitochondria with short and long tubular invaginations of the inner membrane (figs. 4-14, 4-15) (30,32). The cells have abundant lipofuscin granules, lysosomes, and microvilli, while lipid droplets are sparse in these compact cells.

The fetal adrenal cortex contains spherical to ovoid mitochondria with tubular cristae. The cells have abundant smooth endoplasmic reticulum and short cytoplasmic microvilli (31).

The chromaffin cells of the adrenal medulla have unique ultrastructural features including dense core secretory granules that are quite pleomorphic and range in size from 150 to 300 nm in diameter (figs. 4-16, 4-17) (28). Moderate amounts of rough endoplasmic reticulum are present. The cells have interdigitating

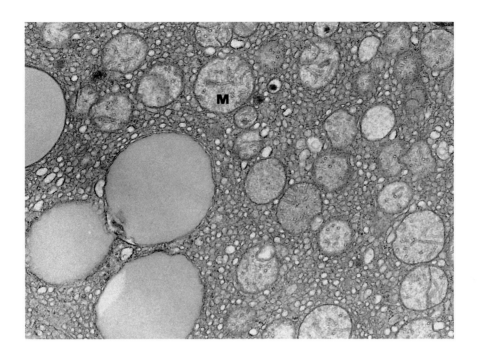

Figure 4-13

ULTRASTRUCTURE OF NORMAL ZONA FASCICULATA

The mitochondria (M) have tubular or vesicular cristae. Abundant smooth endoplasmic reticulum, which is one of the sites of steroid synthesis, is present in the cytoplasm (X10,000).

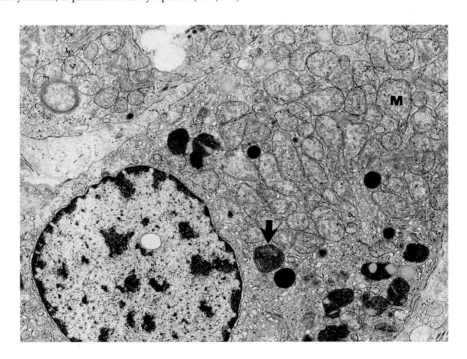

Figure 4-14

ULTRASTRUCTURE OF NORMAL ZONA RETICULARIS

The cytoplasm of the cells of the zona reticularis has abundant tubulovesicular mitochondria (M) and lipofuscin bodies (arrow) (X6,300).

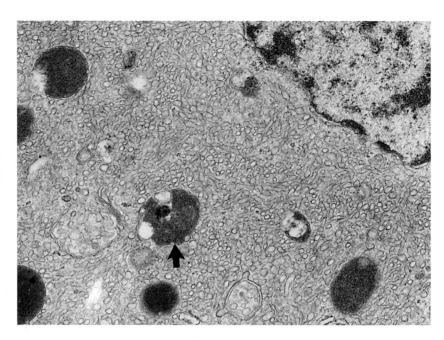

Figure 4-15

ULTRASTRUCTURE OF NORMAL ZONA RETICULARIS

A higher magnification of figure 4-14 shows the smooth endoplasmic reticulum and lipofuscin bodies (arrow) (X13,000).

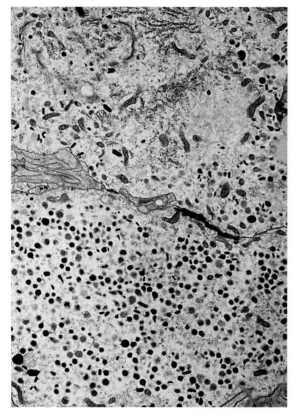

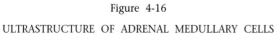

Figure 4-16

ULTRASTRUCTURE OF ADRENAL MEDULLARY CELLS

Numerous cytoplasmic, dense core secretory granules containing catecholamines, chromogranin, and dopamine beta-hydroxylase are present (X3,810).

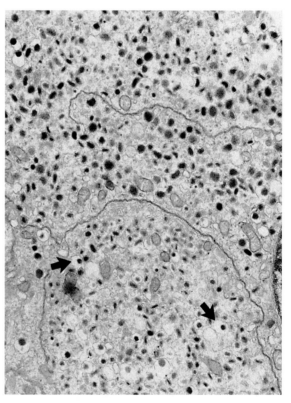

Figure 4-17

ULTRASTRUCTURE OF ADRENAL MEDULLARY CELLS

There are a few norepinephrine-type secretory granules with a clear halo between the granule core and membrane (arrows) and many epinephrine-type granules in the cytoplasm (X3,500).

180

blunt cytoplasmic processes with poorly developed cell junctions. Historically, "light" and "dark" cells were recognized, which probably relate to the density of the cytoplasmic organelles. The morphology of the secretory granule correlates with the type of catecholamine stored. The norepinephrine-type granules have a prominent halo between the granule membrane and the dense core, while the epinephrine-type granules have a very small space between the dense core and the granule membrane.

The stellate cells are in close proximity to the chromaffin cells. They have oval indented nuclei and thin elongated cytoplasmic processes (29). These cells partially surround the chromaffin cells without the interposition of a basal lamina. They have moderate amounts of rough endoplasmic reticulum and occasional lipid droplets, but no secretory granules.

Immunohistochemistry

The adrenal cortex is immunoreactive for intermediate filaments, including cytokeratins (34,36,46). Vimentin immunostaining is variably positive. Various lectin-binding sites, including those for wheat germ agglutinin and concanavilin A, have been reported in the adrenal cortex (52). Alpha-inhibin protein is also expressed in adrenal cortical cells. This dimeric 32 kd peptide is composed of an alpha and beta subunit; higher concentrations of the alpha subunit are present in the adrenal cortex. Inhibin is not specific for adrenal cortical cells, because other tissues such as placenta, pituitary gland, and gonad also produce this peptide (45,49). Other peptides detected in the adrenal cortex are the antiapoptotic protein, bcl2 (35); growth factors such as transforming growth factor alpha, epidermal growth factor (57), and insulin-like growth factor II; and class II major histocompatibility complexes including human leukocyte antigen, D-related (HLA-DR) (40). The anti-melanoma monoclonal antibody, melan A (A103), has been useful in differentiating adrenal cortical cells and neoplasms because of its selective immunoreactivity with steroid-producing cells (39). The Dax-1 protein acts as a transcriptional repressor in the adrenal cortex. Mutations of the gene lead to adrenal hypoplasia (47,48). These proteins are present in both the nucleus and cytoplasm of the cortical cells.

Recent studies have shown that the immune mediatory protein, interleukin 6, which is involved in communication between the immune and endocrine systems, is also produced by cells in the inner zone (reticularis) of the adrenal cortex (37). The presence of HLA-DR and interleukin 6 (37) in these cells suggests an important immunologic function for some adrenal cortical cells.

Antibodies against adrenal cortical steroidogenic enzymes and cytochrome P450 have provided a great deal of useful information about the functional activity of the adrenal cortex (50, 51,53,54,56). Immunohistochemical analyses support the functional classification of the three zones based on historical biochemical studies and provide a direct method to study corticosteroidogenesis in situ.

Immunohistochemical studies of the adrenal medulla show that the cells are diffusely positive for chromogranin (fig. 4-11A) and synaptophysin (fig. 4-11B). The adrenal cortex is also positive for synatophysin, but is negative for chromogranin. Immunostaining for synaptophysin is stronger in the medulla than in the cortex (fig. 4-11B). Adrenal medullary cells and the tumors derived from these cells are usually negative for keratin and vimentin, but often express neurofilament protein (41). A wide spectrum of peptides has been identified in the adrenal medulla including methionine enkephalin and corticotropin. In addition, antibodies against catecholamine-synthesizing enzymes as well as catecholamines can be detected by immunohistochemistry (figs. 4-18, 4-19) (42–44). The stellate cells in the medulla stain strongly for S100 protein (fig. 4-11C) (33,42).

Molecular Biology and Physiology

The homeostasis of adrenal cortical function is regulated by a feedback mechanism between the hypothalamus, pituitary gland, and adrenal cortex. Glucocorticoids exert a negative feedback influence on the hypothalamus and pituitary gland to maintain normal homeostasis (fig. 4-19).

Adrenal Cortex. Steroid hormones are derived from cholesterol which can be synthesized de novo from acetate (60). The cytochrome P450s (CYP) are the enzymes involved in adrenal steroid biosynthesis, while the transcription

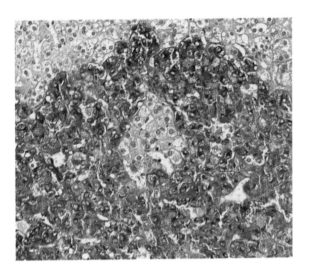

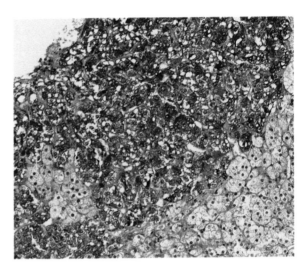

Figure 4-18

CATECHOLAMINE-SYNTHESIZING ENZYMES IN THE ADRENAL MEDULLA

Left: Tyrosine hydroxylase is present diffusely in all of the cells of the adrenal medulla (diaminobenzidine chromogen).
Right: Detection of epinephrine with a specific antiepinephrine antibody in the adrenal medulla. The adrenal cortical cells are negative for epinephrine (diaminobenzidine chromogen).

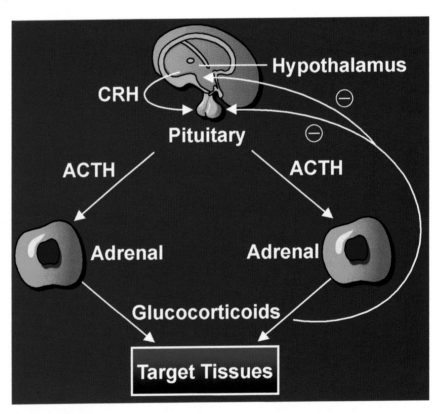

Figure 4-19

HYPOTHALAMIC-PITUITARY-
ADRENAL AXIS

Schematic diagram show-
ing the hypothalamic-pituitary-
adrenal axis and the effects of
glucocorticoids on the regulation of the synthesis and release
of corticotropin-releasing hormone (CRH) from the hypo-
thalamus and ACTH from the
anterior pituitary.

factor AdBP/SF-1 regulates the expression of the CYP genes (60). The principal glucocorticoids are deoxycorticosteroid, 11-deoxycortisol, corti-costeroid, and cortisol (fig. 4-20). Aldosterone is the principal mineralocorticoid and is derived from corticosteroid.

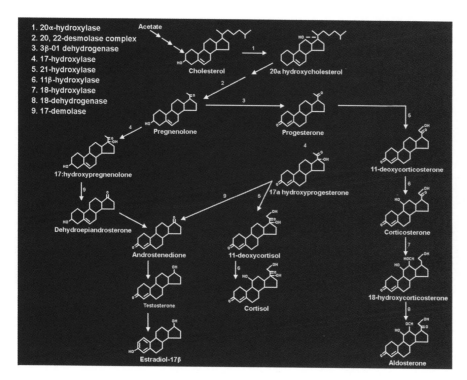

1. 20α-hydroxylase
2. 20, 22-desmolase complex
3. 3β-01 dehydrogenase
4. 17-hydroxylase
5. 21-hydroxylase
6. 11β-hydroxylase
7. 18-hydroxylase
8. 18-dehydrogenase
9. 17-demolase

Figure 4-20

ADRENAL CORTICAL STEROIDOGENESIS

Biosynthesis of adrenal steroid hormone from acetate and cholesterol is shown diagrammatically. The principal enzymes involved in these biosynthetic pathways are also indicated.

The fetal adrenal gland is deficient in 3 beta-hydroxysteroid dehydrogenase (3β-HSD), and produces abundant dihydroepiandrosterone sulfate, but little cortisol. The definitive zone of the fetal gland produces cortisol, which is the principal glucocorticoid in humans. In the adult, different zones produce different glucocorticoids. The zona glomerulosa and outer fasciculata produce aldosterone, while the fasciculata produces mainly cortisol. Dihydroepiandrosterone and other adrenal androgens, as well as estrogens, are produced by the zona fasciculata and zona reticularis (60).

Specific drugs can inhibit adrenal steroidogenesis. Mitotane (2, 2-bis [2-chlorophenyl-4-chlorophenyl]-1, 1-dichloroethane or o,p'DDD) is cytotoxic to human adrenal glands and can be used to produce a "medical adrenalectomy" (60). Other drugs that can inhibit adrenal steroidogenesis include aminoglutethimide which inhibits CYPIIAI (cholesterol side chain cleavage enzyme) and results in a decrease in cortisol levels, and metyrapone which inhibits CYPII BI (11 beta-hydroxylase), which in turn inhibits cortisol and aldosterone synthesis.

Secretion of corticotropin-releasing hormone (CRH) from the hypothalamus, ACTH from the pituitary, and glucocorticoids from the adrenal cortex is regulated by the endocrine feedback system. The hypothalamic-pituitary-adrenal axis is critical in maintaining normal adrenal cortical function. Various factors, including physical and psychological stress, can affect this axis and lead to an increase in ACTH and cortisol levels. Physical stress factors include major surgery, burns, severe trauma, fever, exercise, cold exposure, and cigarette smoking (60,61); psychological stress includes endogenous depression and chronic anxiety.

Aldosterone secretion is regulated mainly by the renin-angiotensin system. Specific serum electrolytes including potassium and sodium are important in regulating aldosterone secretion.

Glucocorticoids exert their effects by regulating carbohydrate metabolism throughout the body. These steroids interact with soluble intracellular receptors. The glucocorticoid receptor is a 94 kd protein that is associated with heat shock protein 90 as well as several others. These proteins assist in the folding and assembly of the glucocorticoid receptor protein complex (58).

Glucocorticoids regulate the transcriptional activity of many genes including those for pro-opiomelanocortin (POMC), prolactin, and the glycoprotein hormones.

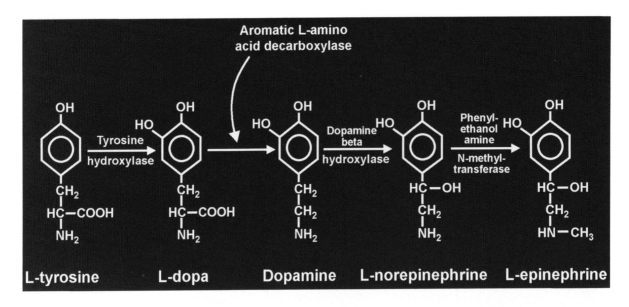

Figure 4-21

ADRENAL MEDULLARY HORMONE BIOSYNTHESIS

Synthesis of norepinephrine and epinephrine in the adrenal medulla. The enzymes that participate in catecholamine biosynthesis are indicated.

Adrenal Medulla. Catecholamines are synthesized from tyrosine which is derived from phenylalanine (fig. 4-21). The enzymes that regulate catecholamine synthesis are in turn regulated by some of the catechols such as norepinephrine. The phenylethanolamine N-methyltransferase enzyme, which converts norepinephrine to epinephrine, is in turn regulated by glucocorticoids. Recent evidence from experimental animal studies indicates that the POMC pituitary gene is needed for the development of the adrenal medulla as well as the adrenal cortex (62).

The chromaffin granules contain catecholamines and various peptides. Chromogranins are the major soluble proteins within the chromaffin granule. These proteins are part of a large family of acid proteins that are present in all neuroendocrine cells that have secretory granules (59). Other proteins in the secretory granule are dopamine beta-hydroxylase and cytochrome b-561. The latter is involved in transmembrane electron transport linking the ascorbic acid cycle with dopamine beta-hydroxylase and other mono-oxygenases (63). Other peptides present in the chromaffin granules include neuropeptide Y, a 36-amino acid peptide stored

in the adrenal medulla that acts to decrease norepinephrine release, and galanin, a 29-amino acid peptide of the adrenal medulla and nerve tissue that has various functions including contraction of smooth muscle, inhibition of ion transport, and participation with neuropeptide Y in the regulation of feeding behavior.

REACTIVE, HEREDITARY, AND DEVELOPMENTAL DISORDERS

Adrenal Cytomegaly

Definition. Adrenal cytomegaly is an enlargement of the adrenocortical cells of the fetal cortex.

General Remarks. Adrenal cytomegaly may be seen in neonates but is more common in premature infants (3 to 7 percent) (68). It is also common in infants with Rh incompatibility (66) and is probably associated with fetal stress. Cytomegaly is not usually found in other tissues in these cases. However, fetal stress often occurs without the development of adrenal cytomegaly. Adrenal cytomegaly is usually only present up to a few months of age, but may persist in older children or adults (69,74,82).

There is no good evidence to support the suggestion that the presence of cytomegalic cells is a precursor of childhood adrenal tumors; these cells do not represent carcinoma in situ (72,74).

Microscopic Findings. The cytomegalic cells are present in the adrenal cortex. They may be as large as 150 μm in diameter and have enlarged pleomorphic and hyperchromatic nuclei (fig. 4-22). They contain up to 25 times the normal amount of DNA (69). Nuclear pseudoinclusions or cytoplasmic invaginations into the nucleus are present, but mitotic figures are rare.

Differential Diagnosis. Cytomegalic inclusion disease may be confused with adrenal cytomegaly. Cytomegalic inclusion disease is seen most commonly in infants. The virally infected cells have basophilic rather than eosinophilic cytoplasm, and the large intranuclear inclusion is surrounded by a clear halo. Cytomegalovirus infection does not occur with neonatal adrenal cytomegaly, and the pseudoinclusions represent cytoplasmic invaginations into the nucleus. Patients with Beckwith-Wiedemann syndrome often have cytomegalic cells in the adrenal glands. However, the adrenal glands are hyperplastic and many other clinical findings are associated with this syndrome.

Focal Adrenalitis

Focal adrenalitis is a focal accumulation of benign lymphocytes and plasma cells in the adrenal cortex. It is fairly common and may be present in up to half of autopsied patients (75). The focal infiltrates of lymphocytes and plasma cells are commonly associated with chronic inflammatory disorders in the retroperitoneum such as chronic pyelonephritis, but should be distinguished from autoimmune adrenalitis (70).

Ovarian Thecal Metaplasia

Ovarian thecal metaplasia is the mesenchymal proliferation of spindle cells in the adrenal capsule, which extends between or surrounds small nests of cortical cells. Other terms for this disorder include *nodular hyperplasia of adrenocortical blastema* or *thecal metaplasia* (fig. 4-23).

This lesion is present in a significant percentage of women (about 4 percent) and is usually detected postmenopausally. On rare occasion, it may also occur in men. The lesion ranges from

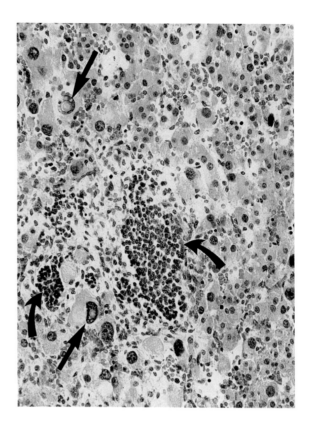

Figure 4-22

ADRENAL CYTOMEGALY IN A STILLBORN INFANT

Enlarged cells with pleomorphic nuclei, some of which have "pseudoinclusions" (straight arrows), and small nests of neuroblastic cells (curved arrows) are present. (Fig. 1-40 from Fascicle 19, 3rd Series.)

0.1 to 2.0 cm (70); half the nodules are multifocal and some may be bilateral (78). These metaplastic foci should be distinguished from the spindle cell proliferation in the adrenal glands described by Carney (67) which usually involves a large part of the adrenal cortex.

Adrenal Hypoplasia

This is the presence of hypoplastic or atrophic adrenal glands. It may be present at birth or may develop later in life. The most common cause of hypoplastic adrenal glands is anencephaly.

Complete absence of the adrenal gland is very rare and in some cases may be familial (64,77). A recently described familial condition is associated with mutations in the POMC gene leading to adrenal insufficiency, obesity, ACTH deficiency, and alteration in pigmentation (71).

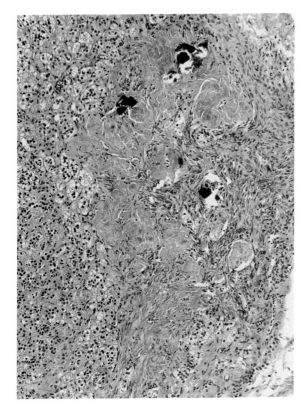

Figure 4-23

OVARIAN THECAL METAPLASIA

A focus of ovarian thecal metaplasia with dystrophic calcification is attached to the adrenal capsule. There are small nests of cortical cells between some of the hyalinized connective tissue bands. (Fig. 1-42 from Fascicle 19, 3rd Series.)

The mutation in one patient was present in exon 3 of the POMC gene, while in another, in exon 2. Unilateral absence of the adrenal gland occurs in 1/10,000 live births (81). Bilateral hypoplasia results in adrenal insufficiency.

Anencephaly can occur in up to 1 in 450 live births, with a female to male ratio of 4 to 1 (79). In anencephalics the neurohypophysis is usually absent or very small while the anterior pituitary gland is present but may lack some cell types. With the absence of an intact hypothalamic-pituitary-adrenal axis, the sella turcica is frequently flat and filled with spongy vascular tissue. The pituitary has decreased numbers of ACTH cells while the other cells of the anterior pituitary gland are usually normal in number (76, 80). Other central nervous system defects such as microcephalia, occipital cephalomeningocele, and hydrocephalus may be associated with adrenal hypoplasia. Rare cases of congenital absence or hypoplasia of the pituitary gland and neurohypophyseal aplasia may be associated with adrenal hypoplasia, resulting in perinatal adrenal failure (64,73).

A common cause of adrenal atrophy is chronic treatment with exogenous glucocorticoids (figs. 4-24, 4-25). The adrenal glands can become quite atrophic and patients usually have to be weaned slowly from the exogenous therapy to allow their adrenal gland to return to normal function.

Figure 4-24

ADRENAL ATROPHY

An atrophic adrenal gland secondary to chronic glucocorticoid therapy is shown on the top. The gland on the bottom is normal.

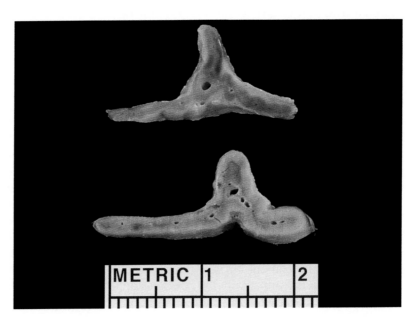

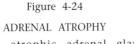

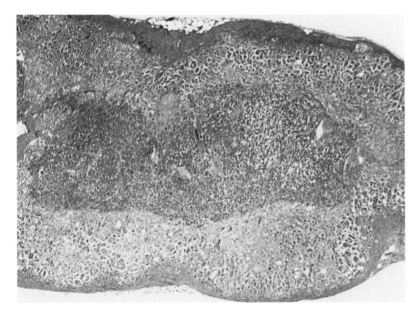

Figure 4-25

ADRENAL ATROPHY

Microscopic view shows a prominent adrenal medulla with decreased thickness of the cortex.

Adrenal Malformations and Heterotopias

Adrenal midline fusion or union is a developmental abnormality that leads to a single butterfly- or horseshoe-shaped adrenal gland above the aorta. Union occurs in embryos and neonates with central nervous system defects such as spina bifida, meningomyelocele, indeterminate visceral situs, and the Cornelia de Lange syndrome (associated with mental and growth retardation, low-set ears, antiverted nostrils, and spade-like hands with short tapering fingers). The histologic appearance of the glands is usually normal (83).

In adrenal adhesion, two tissues adhere to each other, but there is an intervening connective tissue capsule separating them. In contrast, with adrenal union there is an intermingling of different parenchymal cells (fig. 4-26). Adrenorenal and adrenohepatic unions occur in 0.4 to 3.0 percent of unselected autopsy cases (84). In these cases, the organs share a common capsule, but there is no intermingling of the parenchymal elements. The embryologic defect in adhesion and fusion or union is most likely related to failure of the periadrenal capsular mesenchyme to separate completely early in development.

Adrenal Rests and Accessory Adrenal Tissues

Adrenocortical tissue can be found outside the adrenal gland proper. Adrenal rests and

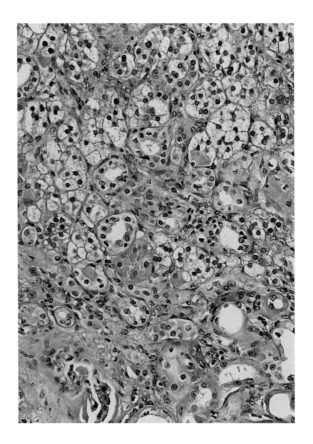

Figure 4-26

ADRENAL-RENAL UNION

Adrenal and renal parenchyma are united without an intervening capsule. (Fig. 2-1 from Fascicle 19, 3rd Series.)

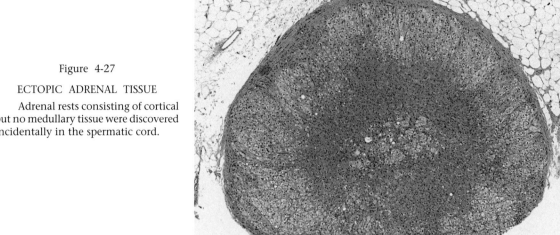

Figure 4-27

ECTOPIC ADRENAL TISSUE

Adrenal rests consisting of cortical but no medullary tissue were discovered incidentally in the spermatic cord.

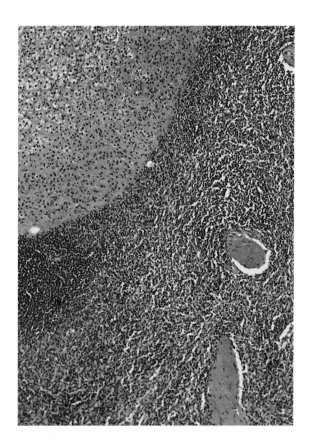

Figure 4-28

ECTOPIC ADRENAL TISSUE

Ectopic adrenal cortex in the spleen. These adrenal rest tissues can become hyperplastic in disorders associated with excessive ACTH production.

accessory adrenal glands are usually accompanied by orthotopic adrenal glands, so they do not represent true heterotopias (85–91). The presence of nests of accessory adrenocortical tissue outside of the gland proper is fairly common (figs. 4-27, 4-28) (86). Although these nests are not in themselves pathological, they can be associated with adrenocortical hyperplasia or neoplastic development (95). The aberrant adrenal tissue may originate at the time the adrenal primordium is disrupted by the nerve tracts as the neural crest cells migrate to form the medulla; this occurs prior to encapsulation of the glands. Most rests have been found close to the adrenal gland; however, other sites include the celiac plexus, broad ligament, kidney, uterus, spermatic and ovarian vessels, scrotum, and hernia sacs. Rarer sites of accessory tissue are the pancreas, spleen, liver, mesentery, lung, brain, and spinal nerves (93). The more distal sites usually contain only cortical tissue, but the larger rests close to the orthotopic gland may contain both cortex and medulla.

Adrenal rests within the spermatic cord are common in children (fig. 4-27). In one study they were present in almost 4 percent of children at the time of inguinoscrotal surgery (93). They have also been found in 9 percent of children operated on for an undescended testis (94). In contrast to the spermatic cord and paraovarian vessels, accessory adrenal tissue within the testis or ovary is rare (90).

Ectopic adrenal tissue in the pancreas may be confused with metastatic renal cell tumors or with clear cell neuroendocrine pancreatic tumors. Similarly, rare adrenal cortical tumors have been reported in the liver (93) and scrotum (92).

Adrenal rests should be distinguished from the heterotopias of the adrenal glands such as adrenal-hepatic and adrenal-renal heterotopias. In true heterotopias, the adrenal gland is located within the renal capsule or within Glisson's capsule of the liver.

Congenital Adrenal Hypoplasia

In congenital adrenal hypoplasia the small adrenal glands may be sporadic or inherited. Various causes of adrenal hypoplasia have been recognized: 1) an autosomal recessive pattern of inheritance, 2) a sporadic condition, 3) an X-linked pattern associated with cytomegaly, or 4) deficiency of the enzyme glycerol kinase (97–99). The X-linked congenital type of hypoplasia is associated with hypogonadotropic hypogonadism in young men (99). Congenital adrenal hypoplasia is most likely due to a developmental problem during embryogenesis. Infants with this disorder usually present with weight loss, vomiting, and dehydration with severe electrolyte disturbances. The adrenal glands are small for age with a decreased fetal zone. Scattered cytomegalic cells and cells with decreased cytoplasmic lipid are usually present.

Hereditary Adrenal Cortical Unresponsiveness to Adrenocorticotropic Hormone

This rare condition is associated with glucocorticoid deficiency related to abnormalities of the ACTH receptor. The condition has only recently been described (100–102). The causal defect is thought to be impaired ACTH signaling to the receptor on adrenocortical cells. Symptoms begin during childhood and include seizures, hypoglycemia, muscle weakness, and a cutaneous hyperpigmentation that is similar to that of Addison's disease. The clinical work-up shows low plasma cortisol levels and because of the negative feedback system, increased serum ACTH.

Histologic secretions show a normal zona glomerulosa, which is the ACTH-independent zone, while the zone fasciculata and reticularis are atrophic (102).

EXOGENOUS INJURY

Drugs

Some pharmacologic agents inhibit adrenal steroidogenesis and have been used therapeutically to control excessive production of glucocorticoids. In dogs, mitotane or 2,2-bis (2-chlorophenyl-4-chlorophenyl)-1, 1-dichloroethane or o,p'-DDD causes necrosis and hemorrhage of the two inner zones of the adrenal cortex while sparing the zona glomerulosa (110). Normal and neoplastic human adrenal glands are sensitive to this cytotoxic drug which can produce a medical adrenalectomy (fig. 4-29) (103,110). Mitotane alters cortisol metabolism by leading to formation of 6-hydroxycortisol rather than the 17-hydroxycorticosteroids.

Aminoglutethimide is used to control hypercortisolism in patients with Cushing's syndrome by inhibiting CYPIIAI, the enzyme that converts cholesterol to pregnenolone (105). This leads to decreased cortisol and mineralocorticoid biosynthesis.

Metyrapone inhibits the enzyme that catalyzes the final step in cortisol biosynthesis, CYPIIBI, and it also inhibits aldosterone synthesis (107). It is used mainly for the diagnostic testing of the hypothalamic-pituitary-adrenal axis and for treating patients with Cushing's syndrome.

Radiation

Radiation to the adrenal glands can lead to fibrosis although the cortex is relatively radioresistant compared to other endocrine tissues (108). High-dose X irradiation (more than 5,000 roentgens) to the abdominal, pelvic, and lumbar regions can lead to hyaline fibrosis (108). The fibrosis is usually present in the inner cortex (reticularis) and there is a reduction of the zona fasciculata, but in one reported study there was no apparent change in cortical function (108).

Miscellaneous Drugs and Chemicals

Other drugs may have a direct or indirect effect on the adrenal cortex. 12-methylbenzanthracene and hexadimethane can cause selective necrosis of the cortex. The chemotherapeutic drug, 5-fluorouracil, has been reported to cause toxicity in vitro (106). Ketoconazole, etomidate, cyanoketone, and trilostane have inhibitory effects on adrenal steroidogenesis (106).

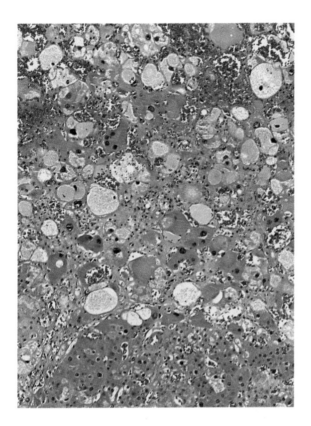 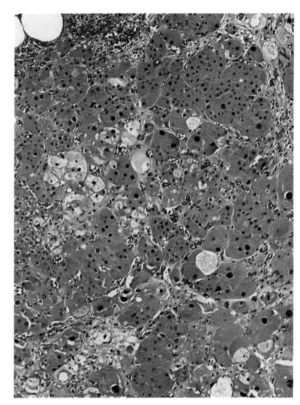

Figure 4-29

MITOTANE TREATMENT

Left: This patient with Cushing's syndrome had been treated with mitotane before resection of the adrenal glands. The cells of the atrophic adrenal cortex are of variable size. Many clear cells with swollen cytoplasm are present.
Right: There are clusters of more compact eosinophilic cells with fatty metaplasia (lower left).

Rifampin and dilantin can lead to increased breakdown of glucocorticoids (106).

Iron overload can lead to excess deposition of iron in the adrenal cortex, especially in the zona glomerulosa. This may be seen in patients with hemochromatosis and in those who receive multiple transfusions. Patients with hemolytic anemia may have the adrenal glands affected indirectly via iron deposition in the pituitary, which leads to destruction of anterior pituitary cells and decreased ACTH production (104).

INFECTIOUS DISEASES AND MISCELLANEOUS CONDITIONS

Infectious agents, especially *Mycobacterium tuberculosis,* used to be a common cause of hypocorticalism associated with Addison's disease (Table 4-1). Cases of tuberculous adrenalitis are still prevalent, but other infectious agents such as cytomegalovirus and the virus that causes acquired immunodeficiency disease (AIDS) as well as fungi and bacteria may be encountered in the adrenal gland.

Tuberculous Adrenalitis

Definition. Tuberculous adrenalitis is a primary or secondary infection of the adrenal glands caused by the *Mycobacterium* species.

General Remarks. Historically, tuberculosis of the adrenal gland was a common cause of chronic, acquired hypoadrenocorticalism, but it is now an uncommon cause. To induce Addison's disease, tuberculosis must involve both glands, with complete or near complete destruction of the adrenal cortex. Some cases may be secondary to pulmonary involvement, but in other cases, active extra-adrenal tuberculosis may be absent.

Table 4-1

CAUSES OF ADRENAL INSUFFICIENCY
(ADDISON'S DISEASE)

Idiopathic
    Autoimmune adrenalitis - primary, secondary,
      and tertiary

Inflammatory
    Bacterial/Fungal
      Tuberculosis
      Histoplasmosis
      Blastomycosis
      Coccidiomycosis
      Candidiasis
      Cryptococcosis
      Sarcoidosis
    Viral
      Human immunodeficiency virus
      Cytomegalovirus
      Herpes simplex virus

Metabolic
    Amyloidosis

Neoplastic
    Metastatic malignancies

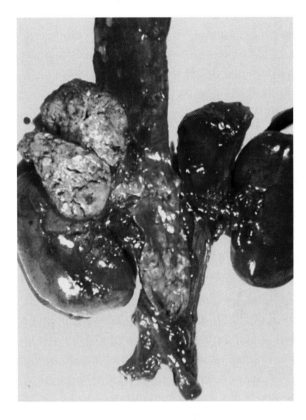

Figure 4-30

TUBERCULOUS ADRENALITIS

A tumefactive lesion is present in both adrenal glands.
The right gland is opened and shows caseous necrosis.

Early studies have shown that once tuberculous adrenalitis begins it progresses to destruction of the glands (112,115,123). Immunopathologic studies of patients with tuberculous adrenalitis do not show antibodies involved in the pathogenesis or progression of this disease. However, steroid cell antibodies have been detected in patients with tuberculous adrenalitis (116).

Macroscopic Findings. The adrenal glands are variably enlarged, with a mean combined weight of 25 g, although weights of up to 50 g have been reported (115). The glands are yellow-gray, with gray-red nodules depending on the stage of the lesion (fig. 4-30). The cut surface shows a diffuse firm mass with a thin rim of normal residual cortex and fibrovascular tissue. Focal areas of calcification may be seen, but extensive calcification is not usually present.

Microscopic Findings. Large areas of caseous necrosis with a variable thin rim of peripheral fibrovascular tissue and variable amounts of residual cortex, usually as a thin rim, may be present (figs. 4-31, 4-32). Inflammatory cells consisting of lymphocytes and Langerhans'-type giant cells are present. The tubercle bacilli can be detected in about half the cases with special stains such as Ziehl-Neelsen (fig. 4-32), and in even more cases with fluorescent stains. Fibrosis is usually minimal which may be related to the inhibitory effects of the glucocorticoids produced in the adrenal glands.

Medullary tissue is usually obliterated as well. It is thought that the destruction starts in the medulla and extends to the cortex, with sparing of a thin rim of outer cortex which may contain a few clusters of viable clear cells (112,115).

Differential Diagnosis. The differential diagnosis of tuberculous adrenalitis includes other granulomatous diseases such as fungal infections. Special stains with methenamine silver and Ziehl-Neelsen can usually detect diagnostic organisms. Immunosuppressed patients may have multiple

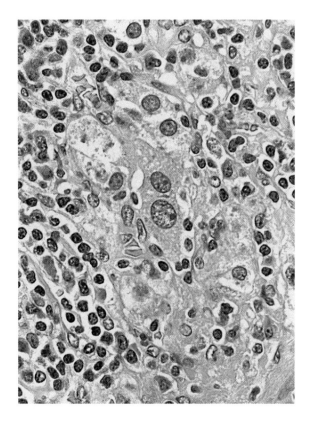

Figure 4-31

TUBERCULOUS ADRENALITIS

The histologic view shows reactive epithelial histiocytes and lymphocytes in the areas of infection.

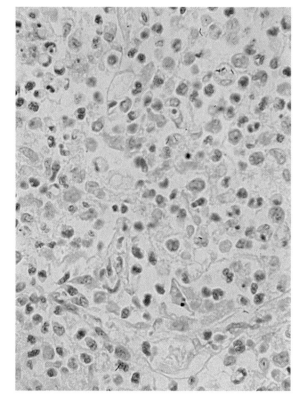

Figure 4-32

TUBERCULOUS ADRENALITIS

Ziehl-Neelsen stain shows a positive (red) reaction for acid-fast organisms.

infections, so special stains should be used in these cases.

Prognosis and Treatment. Historically, patients usually developed adrenal insufficiency with tuberculous adrenalitis. Patients are treated with antituberculosis drugs today, but necrosis of adrenal function can occur after antituberculous treatment in rare cases (119).

Fungal Infections

General Remarks. Fungal infections may involve the adrenal glands and lead to Addison's disease (111,113,114,117,118,120,122,124). Some investigators have suggested that the high level of glucocorticoids in the gland may predispose to fungal and other opportunistic infections (115). Adrenal insufficiency may be caused by *Histoplasma* and *Cryptococcus*, which are the most common etiologic fungi in nontropical regions; in tropical areas *Paracoccidioides* is the most common fungus associated with adrenal insufficiency.

Macroscopic Findings. The adrenal glands are enlarged, and variable degrees of necrosis and fibrosis may be present. Calcification may be detected radiologically or on sectioning.

Microscopic Findings. Histologic examination shows granulomatous inflammation with lymphocytes, histiocytes, and multinucleated giant cells. Special stains for fungal organisms can help to establish the diagnosis (fig. 4-33).

Differential Diagnosis. Tuberculous adrenalitis often has a similar histologic picture, so the use of special stains, cell cultures, and even polymerase chain reaction analysis is important.

Prognosis and Treatment. Patients with extensive fungal infections involving both adrenal glands can develop adrenal insufficiency. Recovery of adrenal function after antifungal

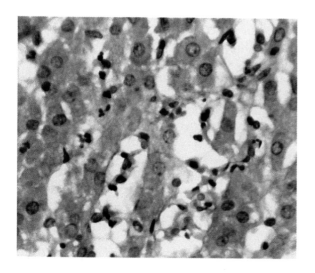 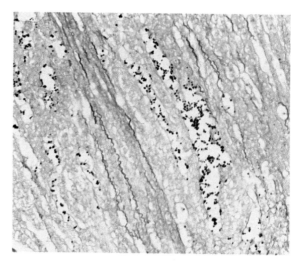

Figure 4-33

CRYPTOCCOCAL ADRENALITIS

Left: Periodic acid–Schiff (PAS) stain is positive for cryptococcal organisms in an immunosuppressed patient.
Right: Grocott's methenamine silver (GMS) stain is positive for fungal organisms.

treatment has been reported (111,118). Ketoconazole has been used to treat patients with paracoccidioidomycosis or South American blastomycosis. Ketoconazole treatment is a double-edged sword in the treatment of this disease, since it has an inhibitory effect on adrenal steroidogenesis (121).

Acquired Immunodeficiency Syndrome Adrenalitis

Definition. This adrenal inflammation is associated with infectious agents in patients with human immunodeficiency virus (HIV).

General Remarks. Acquired immunodeficiency syndrome (AIDS)-related adrenal dysfunction may be present in patients that are HIV positive as well as those with frank AIDS (125–131). The changes in the adrenal gland may be secondary to effects of opportunistic infections (127,131) or neoplasms such as Kaposi's sarcoma (127). Some patients develop adrenal insufficiency (128). Most AIDS patients have decreased adrenal reserves; a defect in the production of 17-deoxycorticosteroid by the zona fasiculata has been reported (126,129). Peripheral resistance to glucocorticoids has been noted in some patients with AIDS, which may be related to a decreased affinity of type II glucocorticoid receptors in spite of increased receptor density (130).

Macroscopic Findings. The gross appearance of the glands is variable depending on the etiologic agent. With *Mycobacterium avium-intracellulare* or fungal infections, caseous necrosis is often present in the enlarged adrenal gland. Cytomegalovirus infection is not associated with marked gland enlargement (127,131).

Microscopic Findings. The histologic features also depend on the etiologic agents. With mycobacterial or fungal infections, there is caseous necrosis with lymphocytes, histiocytes, and multinucleated giant cells. Infections with cytomegalovirus and herpes simplex adenovirus are associated with intranuclear inclusions in the adrenocortical cells and necrotic adrenal cells while toxoplasma infections are associated with cytoplasmic inclusions of the organisms.

Differential Diagnosis. A plethora of organisms may be present in the adrenal glands of patients with AIDS, such as opportunistic viruses and fungi. Careful examination of the H&E-stained sections may detect the intranuclear organism associated with cytomegalic inclusion disease and adenovirus. Special stains for fungal and acid-fast organisms are useful in the presence of caseous necrosis with multinucleated giant cells.

Miscellaneous Causes of Adrenalitis

Viral infections with cytomegalovirus and herpes simplex virus can lead to adrenal necrosis (134,135). These cases are only rarely associated with adrenal insufficiency. Bacterial infections such as secondary syphilis can lead to adrenal insufficiency in rare cases. A sclerotic adrenal gland with a lymphoplasmocytic infiltrate and the delineation of the spirochete with special stains such as Warthin-Starry, clarify the diagnosis (132). Other diseases such as African trypanosomiasis can lead to adrenal insufficiency (133). This insufficiency has been shown to be unrelated to treatment with suramin, although this drug can impair adrenocortical function (133).

ADRENAL CORTICAL HYPOFUNCTION

Decreased function of the adrenal cortex (which sometimes involves the adrenal medulla) may be due to multiple causes. Primary adrenal insufficiency or Addison's disease (Table 4-1), secondary adrenocortical insufficiency related to pituitary failure with decreased or absent ACTH production, and tertiary adrenal insufficiency related to hypothalamic failure in which corticotropin-releasing hormone (CRH) or other factors regulating pituitary ACTH production are reduced or absent, are all uncommon. The incidence of adrenal insufficiency is six cases per one million adults per year and the prevalence is 40 to 110 cases per million adults (159). Once diagnosed, adrenal cortical insufficiency can be easily treated medically. However, the general signs and symptoms of fatigue, weight loss, weakness, and gastrointestinal problems are not specific, so the diagnosis may be difficult to make initially.

Primary Adrenal Insufficiency

Autoimmune Adrenalitis. In autoimmune adrenalitis, also known as *idiopathic primary adrenal sufficiency,* there is decreased function or loss of function of the adrenal cortex due to destruction by an autoimmune process. Clinical signs and symptoms do not become apparent until 90 percent of the adrenal cortex is destroyed.

A wide range of diseases can lead to primary adrenal insufficiency including autoimmune adrenalitis; infectious disease caused by mycobacterial, fungal, or bacterial infection such as meningococcemia; polyglandular autoimmune syndromes; metastatic disease to the adrenal gland; or uncommon hereditary disorders (141,143,144,148, 151,160,166,172). Historically, tuberculosis was the most common cause of primary adrenal insufficiency; however, autoimmune destruction of the adrenal gland is the most common cause today (70 to 90 percent of cases). This is followed by tuberculosis (about 10 percent of cases) (140, 171). The decreased secretion of glucocorticoids and mineralocorticoids leads to adrenocorticoid insufficiency. The development of insufficiency is usually gradual.

In primary adrenal insufficiency due to autoimmune adrenalitis, there is evidence of immunologic involvement including cellular and humoral immunity, multiple and familial clustering, prevalence of specific HLA types, and involvement of other endocrine glands. Immunologic studies show evidence of cell-mediated immunity with decreased suppressor T-cell function and increased circulating Ia-positive T lymphocytes (142, 163,174). The histopathologic findings of infiltrating lymphocytes and fibrosis are similar to findings in other T cell-mediated diseases such as tuberculosis.

Evidence of a humoral-mediated immunity, including the presence of antibodies that react to the three zones of the adrenal cortex, is seen in up to three fourths of patients with autoimmune adrenalitis (136,138,144,156,162, 167,173). These antibodies are not found in normal subjects or in patients with other diseases. The detection of antibodies is more common in women than men. With longstanding disease, the antibody titers may decrease or even disappear (159). In general, autoantibodies directed at all three zones of the adrenal cortex appear months to years before the onset of adrenocortical insufficiency (136,138). The zona glomerulosa is probably affected first (138) and may precede failure of the fasciculata by months to years (136). Antigens against specific steroidogenic enzymes have been identified in patients with primary insufficiency and in those with associated endocrine autoimmunity (162,167,173).

Many patients with autoimmune adrenal disease have antibodies against other endocrine glands; in contrast, these antibodies are uncommon in normal populations without adrenal or other endocrine diseases (137,152). About 60 percent of patients with autoimmune adrenal disease also have thyroid antimicrosomal antibodies (177). The presence of antibodies to gastric parietal cells and intrinsic factor usually correlates with atrophic gastritis and pernicious anemia (159). The detection of antigonadal antibodies is associated with gonadal failure; there is a higher incidence of ovarian failure than testicular failure. At the opposite end of the spectrum, patients who have other autoimmune endocrine diseases, but do not have autoimmune adrenalitis, usually do not have antiadrenal antibodies in their serum, except for patients with hypoparathyroidism (137).

The genetics of autoimmune adrenal insufficiency have been studied extensively (145, 150,155,161). This condition may be familial or sporadic. If adrenal insufficiency occurs as part of the polyglandular autoimmune syndrome, it is more likely to be familial. Genetic susceptibility to autoimmune adrenal insufficiency is linked to HLA-B8, DR3, and HLA-DR4. Sporadic autoimmune adrenal insufficiency is associated with the various HLA types, as is polyglandular autoimmune syndrome II (145, 161). However, some cases associated with polyglandular autoimmune syndrome II, such as Hashimoto's thyroiditis, pernicious anemia, and premature primary gonadal failure, do not have a strong HLA linkage. Normal adrenocortical cells express HLA-DR type II antigens, so inappropriate expression of these antigens is probably not linked directly to the pathogenesis of autoimmune adrenal insufficiency (145,159).

Polyglandular Autoimmune Syndrome. Adrenal insufficiency is associated with the polyglandular autoimmune syndrome (PGA) type II in 100 percent of cases and with PGA type I in 60 percent of cases (150,157). In general, about 50 percent of patients with autoimmune adrenal insufficiency have one or more autoimmune endocrine disorders (159). In contrast, patients with the more common autoimmune endocrine disorders such as Hashimoto's thyroiditis or insulin-dependent diabetes mellitus rarely develop adrenal insufficiency (159).

PGA type I is primarily associated with hypoparathyroidism, chronic mucocutaneous candidiasis, and adrenal insufficiency (150,157). The adrenal insufficiency develops at 12 to 13 years of age, usually after the other two principal disorders. PGA I is associated with the long arm of chromosome 21 and is inherited in an autosomal recessive pattern, with an approximately 1.5 greater frequency in females.

PGA type II is more common; half the cases are familial with onset between 20 and 40 years of age. It is not associated with a specific HLA linkage, but is slightly more common in women. About half of the patients present with adrenal insufficiency that may be associated with autoimmune thyroid disease (Graves' disease, Hashimoto's thyroiditis) and diabetes mellitus. Hypoparathyroidism does not occur with the type II syndrome. This disorder is inherited as a polygenic, autosomal dominant or autosomal recessive condition (139,145,150,161). These syndromes are discussed further in chapter 5.

Clinical and Radiologic Findings. Patients with autoimmune adrenal insufficiency and with PGA are predominantly female (about 70 percent) while patients with isolated autoimmune adrenal insufficiency are predominantly males in the first two decades of life (71 percent) and predominantly females after the third decade (82 percent) (159). Adrenal insufficiency is often insidious in onset and may go undetected until increased stress precipitates a crisis. A major pathophysiologic factor precipitating an adrenal crisis is mineralocorticoid deficiency, even when synthetic glucocorticoids are being administered (159). The most common clinical manifestation of acute insufficiency is shock, either in a patient without a previous diagnosis of primary adrenal insufficiency after a major physiological stress or in a patient who is being treated for adrenal insufficiency but requires more glucocorticoids because of bacterial infection or some other major illness. Nonspecific symptoms include nausea, vomiting, abdominal pain, weakness, fatigue, confusion, and even coma. Hypoglycemia may sometimes be the presenting problem. The adrenal insufficiency may be due to adrenal infarction, hemorrhage, sepsis, or thromboembolism.

Adrenal shock can progress to coma and death without appropriate diagnosis and therapy (159). Adrenal hemorrhage and death may be associated with the Waterhouse-Friderichsen syndrome which is secondary to sepsis from *Meningococcus* or *Pseudomonas aeruginosa* (136,159).

Chronic adrenal insufficiency is associated with signs and symptoms of glucocorticoid, mineralocorticoid, and androgen deficiencies. The most common findings in these patients, seen in 100 percent, are weakness, fatigue, weight loss, and anorexia while most patients have gastrointestinal symptoms, hyperpigmentation, and hypotension. The hyperpigmentation is due to the increased content of melanin in the skin resulting from the increased stimulation of melanocytes by high ACTH levels. Cardiovascular manifestations include postural dizziness and syncope. Joint pain, calcification of articular cartilage, splenomegaly, and lymphadenopathy may develop. Psychiatric manifestations include organic brain syndrome, depression, and psychosis (159).

Radiologic findings vary with the etiology of the disease. With tuberculous or fungal adrenalitis, metastatic malignancies or hemorrhage may be associated with adrenal enlargement, but this is not seen in patients with autoimmune adrenal disease (146,164). While tuberculous adrenalitis is usually associated with enlarged glands initially, atrophic, calcified glands may be present with chronic tuberculosis (146). In chronic primary adrenal insufficiency, the sella turcica may be enlarged on skull radiograph secondary to ACTH cell hyperplasia; this enlargement may be reduced by steroid treatment (149,155).

Laboratory Findings. Patients with primary adrenal insufficiency have decreased cortisol secretion that does not increase with acute or chronic ACTH administration. Serum ACTH levels are elevated, while serum testosterone levels in men are normal, but low in women (because the adrenal cortex is the source for approximately 50 percent of androgen in women). Serum thyroxine levels are normal or low, while TSH levels are often increased. Serum prolactin (PRL) may also be slightly elevated. Both thyroid-stimulating hormone (TSH) and PRL levels return to normal after treatment with glucocorticoids.

Electrolyte abnormalities, including hyponatremia and hypercalcemia, are present in most patients. The hyponatremia is related to aldosterone deficiency from the zona glomerulosa. Liver aspartate transaminase levels may be abnormal but usually return to normal after glucocorticoid therapy.

Macroscopic Findings. Patients with primary autoimmune adrenalitis have small adrenal glands which are largely replaced by hyalinized fibrous tissue in chronic cases. Gland weights vary from 1.9 to 4.6 g, but smaller glands of 0.2 g have been reported (163).

Microscopic Findings. The adrenal glands show loss of the normal cortical cells or islands of residual cortical cells. The capsule of the gland is thickened, and is more prominent in smaller glands (fig. 4-34) (169). The residual cells are compact, with eosinophilic cytoplasm, and show lipid depletion. Hypertrophy of these residual cells may be secondary to stimulation by the increased concentrations of serum ACTH. The medulla is usually spared and may extend to the inner aspect of the capsule because of the destruction of the overlying cortex. Chronic inflammatory cell infiltrates include lymphocytes, plasma cells, and histiocytes. In some cases, there are lymphoid nodules with germinal centers. When accessory adrenal cortical tissue is present outside the cortex, similar histologic changes are usually present.

Differential Diagnosis. Other conditions leading to atrophic adrenal glands include chronic glucocorticoid therapy, treatment with o,p'DDD or mitotane, end-stage tuberculosis, and fungal infections. Inflammatory infiltrates can also be seen in other conditions such as lymphocytic adrenalitis, myelolipomatous changes in the adrenal cortex, and Carney's complex with bilateral pigmented adrenocortical disease.

Chronic glucocorticoid treatment leads to diffuse atrophy of the glands, but there is no destruction of the adrenocortical cells. Lipid-laden cells are seen histologically. Treatment with mitotane can lead to atrophic adrenal glands with areas of fibrosis and residual islands of cortical cells. In atrophic adrenal glands due to chronic tuberculosis, multinucleated giant cells in a background of necrosis and fibrosis are seen (140). Myelolipomatous changes are often associated with hypercortisolism. The presence of fat cells, lymphocytes, and bone marrow elements including myeloid and erythroid precursors can help make the distinction. In bilateral pigmented adrenocortical disease (Carney's complex), the glands may be of normal or slightly increased size. The presence of lymphocytes is usually associated with enlarged

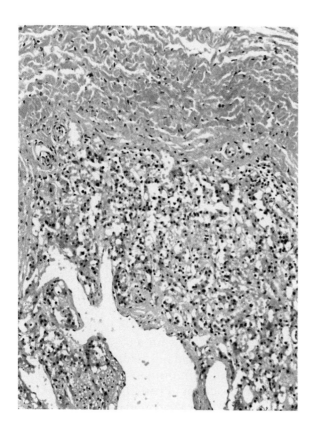 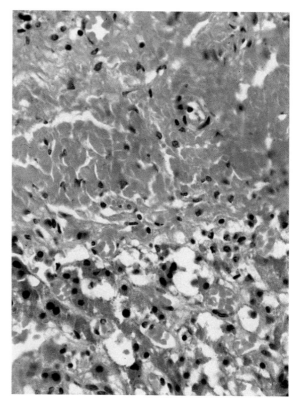

Figure 4-34

PRIMARY ADRENAL INSUFFICIENCY

Left: The adrenal glands are small and composed mainly of cortex with few residual cortical cells.
Right: Higher magnification shows that the cortex is composed mainly of hyalinized fibrous tissue. The medullary cells have prominent basophilic cytoplasm.

zona reticularis–type cells which form nodules, mainly at the corticomedullary junction.

Treatment and Prognosis. Treatment of the adrenal crisis by intravenous fluids and glucocorticoids may be life-saving in an emergency. Lifelong glucocorticoid and mineralocorticoid treatment is needed for primary adrenal insufficiency. Patients undergoing surgery usually require high-dose glucocorticoid prophylaxis to combat the stress of surgery (159). During pregnancy the usually required maintenance dose of glucocorticoids is increased in the third trimester and/or during labor and delivery (159).

Historically, the prognosis of patients with chronic adrenal insufficiency was grim, and more than 80 percent died during the first 2 years after diagnosis (167). Today most patients live a normal life span with full physical activity (136). The prognosis depends largely on the underlying disease. Heart failure, essential hypertension, and osteopenia are some complications in patients with chronic adrenal insufficiency treated with replacement therapy (159).

Secondary and Tertiary Adrenal Insufficiency

Definition. These adrenal insufficiencies are related to the failure of the pituitary gland to secrete adequate amounts of ACTH (secondary) or of the hypothalamus to secrete corticotropin-releasing hormone (CRH) (tertiary).

General Remarks. Patients with isolated ACTH deficiency may present with hypoglycemia (168,175). With chronic secondary or tertiary adrenal insufficiency, a mineralocorticoid deficiency develops, but this condition usually responds to glucocorticoid therapy.

The etiology of secondary adrenal insufficiency includes pituitary macroadenomas, craniopharyngioma, infections such as tuberculosis or fungal diseases, sarcoidosis, lymphocytic hypophysitis, head trauma, and large intracranial artery aneurysms that destroy the normal anterior pituitary gland. Postpartum pituitary necrosis secondary to infarction (Sheehan's syndrome), pituitary apoplexy, and metastasis to the pituitary can also disrupt ACTH secretion and lead to secondary adrenal insufficiency.

Isolated ACTH deficiency has been reported in some patients (147,176), including cases due to mutation of the pro-opiomelanocortin gene (175). Isolated ACTH deficiency may be associated with other autoimmune endocrine disorders including lymphocytic hypophysitis; some patients have antipituitary antibodies in the serum limiting these cases to an autoimmune process. Congenital deficiency of a post-translational cleavage enzyme for ACTH has also been reported (158).

Tertiary adrenal insufficiency may be caused by suppression of hypothalamic-pituitary-adrenal function after chronic administration of high dosages of glucocorticoids (159). This leads to a decrease in the number of corticotrophic cells and atrophy of the zona fasciculata and reticularis cells. Prolonged ACTH administration can restore cortisol production.

Clinical and Radiologic Findings. The clinical features of secondary and tertiary adrenal insufficiency are similar to those of the primary disease, but patients do not develop hyperpigmentation and they are less susceptible to hypotension or dehydration. However, the other generalized signs and symptoms including weakness, myalgias, arthralgias, and psychological manifestations that are related to glucocorticoid deficiency are present. Hypoglycemia is more common in secondary than primary adrenal insufficiency. Patients usually present with evidence of chronic glucocorticoid deficiency rather than acute insufficiency.

Evidence of metastatic or primary lesions involving the pituitary or hypothalamic region may be detected by computed tomography (CT) or magnetic resonance imaging (MRI). However, adrenal atrophy is often difficult to detect even with sensitive radiologic techniques.

Laboratory Findings. In secondary and tertiary insufficiency, some laboratory findings are similar to findings in primary adrenal insufficiency. The differences, however, include a low level of plasma ACTH, absence of elevated potassium because of relatively normal mineralocorticoid production, and a higher incidence of hypoglycemia (159).

Cortisol production is usually decreased in secondary insufficiency because of low or absent ACTH production. In tertiary insufficiency, there is decreased or absent CRH secretion (153, 154). Because the pituitary gland is normal in tertiary insufficiency, stimulation with exogenous CRH leads to increased ACTH secretion (153). Men with secondary or tertiary adrenal insufficiency present with glucocorticoid deficiency while women have both glucocorticoid and androgen deficiency. In both secondary and tertiary insufficiency, mineralocorticoid secretion is usually normal, so adrenal crisis is less common than with primary adrenal failure.

Macroscopic Findings. The adrenal glands are variably decreased in size depending on the etiology and duration of the disease. Cut sections show a prominent medulla and a normal zona glomerulosa while the fasciculata and reticularis are thinner than normal.

Microscopic Findings. Histologic examination shows atrophy of the zona fasciculata and reticularis while the zona glomerulosa, which is largely ACTH-independent, and the medulla are relatively normal. If the patient has been treated with glucocorticoids before the adrenal glands are examined, the atrophic zone may respond to therapy with enlargement of individual cells. Patients with longstanding secondary or tertiary adrenal insufficiency may develop atrophy of the zona glomerulosa, but these cells respond to substitution therapy with glucocorticoids.

Differential Diagnosis. Distinguishing primary from secondary or tertiary adrenal insufficiency can usually be made by clinical and pathologic correlation. Since most cases of primary adrenal insufficiency are autoimmune in origin, the presence of lymphocytes and plasma cells along with fibrosis and involvement of all three cortical zones can help to distinguish it from secondary or tertiary insufficiency in which only the two inner zones are affected.

Treatment and Prognosis. Treatment is similar to that of primary chronic insufficiency, with the exception that mineralocorticoid replacement is usually not required (159). For secondary adrenal insufficiency, replacement of other pituitary hormones may be needed depending on their status.

The prognosis depends on the underlying cause of the insufficiency. Metastatic tumors to the pituitary gland are associated with a poor prognosis while craniopharyngiomas can often be treated successfully by surgery. For isolated ACTH deficiency, target hormone replacement therapy (hydrocortisone) is usually effective.

Isolated Mineralocorticoid Deficiency

A deficiency of aldosterone production by the zona glomerulosa of the adrenal gland is called isolated mineralocorticoid deficiency. There are various causes for this hypoaldosteronism. The most common is impaired release of renin from the kidney due to diabetes mellitus, autoimmune diseases, amyloidosis, sickle cell anemia, and other causes (159,165). Primary hypoaldosteronism may be caused by a congenital condition in which an autosomal recessive inherited disorder is associated with a deficiency of the terminal enzyme in aldosterone biosynthesis (CYP11B2), which converts the 18-hydroxyl group to an aldehyde (170). Infants with this condition usually have recurrent dehydration, salt wasting, and failure to thrive.

Acquired hypoaldosteronism may be caused by certain drugs. Heparin-suppressed aldosterone synthesis can lead to primary hypoaldosteronism in the presence of an impaired renin-angiotensin system. In rare cases, metastatic carcinoma to the adrenal gland may lead to primary hypoaldosteronism (160).

Adrenal Hemorrhage and Necrosis

Definition. Hemorrhage and necrosis of the adrenal gland are usually associated with bacterial infection.

General Remarks. This is an uncommon condition which may occur in neonates, children, and adults. When the condition occurs in children, it is known as the *Waterhouse-Friderichsen syndrome*. Unilateral hemorrhage, which is usually more common in the right adrenal gland, is seen in newborn infants (178). The Waterhouse-Friderichsen syndrome is most common during the first 2 years of life (181,183).

The incidence of adrenal hemorrhage at autopsy has been reported to be between 0.14 and 0.60 percent (182), although others have reported bilateral adrenal hemorrhage in up to 1.1 percent of 2,000 consecutive autopsies in adults (184). In contrast, 0.5 to 1.0 percent of neonatal autopsies showed adrenal hemorrhage (179). Many infants survive small adrenal hemorrhages (178).

The pathogenesis of acute adrenal hemorrhage is mainly related to sepsis, but burns, myocardial infarction, cardiac failure, hypertensive cardiac disease, hypothermia, and hemorrhage into other organs may cause it (180,184). Anticoagulants may also precipitate adrenal hemorrhage.

In children, acute adrenal insufficiency (Waterhouse-Friderichsen syndrome) may be associated with severe bacterial infection with *Meningococcus* or *Pseudomonas*. Vascular collapse and adrenal hemorrhage develop after infection with these organisms. Children have petechial hemorrhages as part of the process of disseminated intravascular coagulation. Other bacteria including *Streptococcus pneumonia* and *Haemophilus influenzae* may also lead to the Waterhouse-Friderichsen syndrome.

Clinical and Radiologic Findings. Patients develop adrenal hemorrhage and necrosis which leads to acute adrenal insufficiency or adrenal crisis. There is associated hypotension, shock, nausea, vomiting, anorexia, fever, and abdominal pain.

Mineralocorticoid levels are usually normal early on, but later, dehydration and hypotension develop as levels decrease. Bilateral adrenal hemorrhage may be seen in neonates from birth trauma. Hemorrhage also occurs during pregnancy, following idiopathic adrenal vein thrombosis, or as a complication of venography such as with infarction of an adenoma.

Radiologically, the hemorrhage of acute adrenal crisis is seen as enlargement of one or both adrenal glands. Before the development of CT, the diagnosis of adrenal hemorrhage was usually made at autopsy (184).

Laboratory Findings. Evidence of occult or acute hemorrhage by a sudden fall in the hemoglobin and hematocrit as well as progressive hyperkalemia and hyponatremia, and evidence

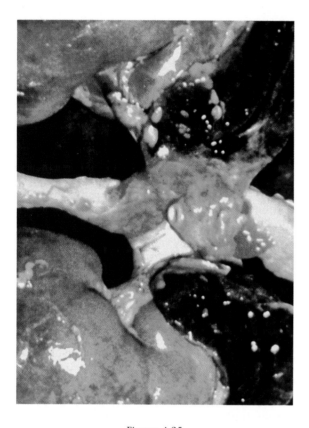

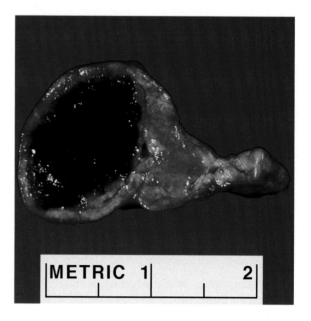

Figure 4-36

WATERHOUSE-FRIDERICHSEN SYNDROME

Cut section of the adrenal gland shows that the hemorrhage affects the medulla and inner cortex, with some sparring of the outer cortex during the earlier stages.

Figure 4-35

WATERHOUSE-FRIDERICHSEN SYNDROME

Both adrenal glands are quite hemorrhagic secondary to meningococcemia while the kidneys are not grossly affected.

of volume contraction are usually diagnostic, along with the clinical and radiologic findings.

Macroscopic Findings. The gross findings depend on the etiology of the hemorrhage. This may vary from massive hemorrhage, involving all of both adrenal glands, to small petechial hemorrhages in the adrenal cortex. In some cases a localized hematoma may be present. The adrenal glands are usually swollen but often retain their original shape. With acute hemorrhage, the changes are most striking in the zona reticularis and extend to the outer cortical layers. Necrosis, with sparing of the subcapsular cells, is often seen in the Waterhouse-Friderichsen syndrome (figs. 4-35, 4-36). Neonatal hemorrhage and necrosis usually involve predominantly the fetal cortex, with extension to the adult cortex.

Hemorrhage and necrosis are usually seen when the capsular and emissary veins are oc-cluded by adrenal vein thrombosis. In contrast to central vein thrombosis, the capsular and emissary veins may remain patent without the development of hemorrhage and necrosis (180).

Microscopic Findings. Histologic findings support the gross evidence of hemorrhage and necrosis (fig. 4-37), with fibrin deposition and acute infiltration by neutrophils. In the Waterhouse-Friderichsen syndrome, cells in the outer zona glomerulosa may be spared, while the medullary cells are also involved with hemorrhage and necrosis.

Differential Diagnosis. The gross and microscopic findings can be used to distinguish different patterns of hemorrhage. With central adrenal vein thrombosis, most of the cortex may be spared early in the disorder. In the Waterhouse-Friderichsen syndrome, the outer cortex is spared while the rest of the adrenal gland shows central hemorrhagic necrosis.

Treatment and Prognosis. Treatment consists of replacement of circulating glucocorticoid, sodium, and water deficits. Vasoconstrictive agents such as dopamine are used in extreme

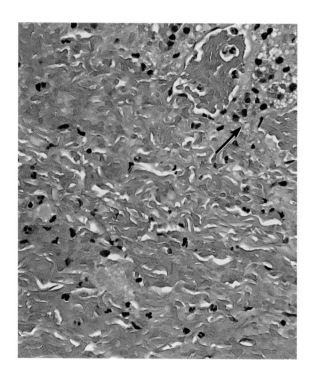

Figure 4-37

WATERHOUSE-FRIDERICHSEN SYNDROME

Microscopic examination shows extensive hemorrhagic necrosis of the adrenal glands with a few viable cortical cells (arrow).

cases to assist with volume replacement. The prognosis is much improved today compared to a few decades ago because of the availability of glucocorticoids for replacement therapy. Rapid diagnosis and initiation of treatment are critical for the successful treatment of acute adrenal hemorrhage and necrosis.

Metastatic Tumors Causing Adrenal Insufficiency

Definition. The massive replacement of adrenal cortical cells by metastatic tumors, leading to adrenal insufficiency.

General Remarks. The adrenal metastases have to be quite massive for patients to develop adrenal insufficiency. It is estimated that 80 to 90 percent of the adrenal gland must be lost before adrenal insufficiency develops (188–192,194). Recent studies have estimated that between 19 and 33 percent of patients with documented metastatic tumors and CT evi-

dence of bilateral adrenal enlargement develop adrenal insufficiency. The most common metastases to the adrenal gland are from lung and breast carcinomas; others include renal cell, gastric and colon carcinomas, as well as melanomas. Adrenal cortical carcinoma with metastasis to the contralateral gland has also been implicated in adrenal cortical insufficiency (195). Massive involvement of the adrenal gland by malignant lymphoma may sometimes lead to insufficiency (190).

Clinical and Radiologic Findings. The clinical findings of adrenal insufficiency secondary to massive bilateral metastases are similar to those of other causes of adrenal insufficiency: nausea, anorexia, dehydration, weight loss, and electrolyte imbalances which may be complicated by the underlying malignancy.

The use of MRI and CT scans have increased the sensitivity of detecting adrenal metastases in general. In one autopsy series, bilateral metastases were present in 23 percent of 91 patients who were studied by CT (185). Massive bilateral involvement of the adrenal glands on radiologic studies usually indicates metastatic disease. The glands are round to oval with soft tissue density unless there is extensive hemorrhage and necrosis. With hemorrhage, the MRI usually has a high signal intensity on T1- and T2-weighted images.

Macroscopic Findings. There is bilateral involvement with variable degrees of hemorrhage and necrosis. The tumors are usually tan-brown to black, which is different than the yellow of adrenal cortical tumors (fig. 4-38). Some metastases such as from renal cell carcinomas which have abundant lipid, may simulate an adrenal cortical neoplasm. Renal cell carcinomas metastatic to the adrenal gland have been reported in 19 percent of autopsy cases (186), but the involvement is usually unilateral, since bilateral involvement from renal cell carcinoma is uncommon (193).

Microscopic Findings. The histologic diagnosis is usually uncomplicated, especially when the primary tumor is known and the histologic slides are available for comparison (fig. 4-39). Immunohistochemical stains can be very useful in separating different types of poorly differentiated malignant tumors. This is especially true with malignant melanoma in which a

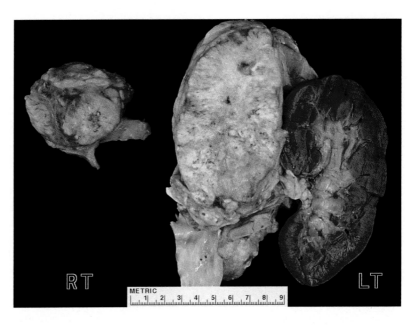

Figure 4-38

ADRENAL INSUFFICIENCY
SECONDARY TO
METASTATIC CARCINOMA

Lung adenocarcinoma metastatic to
the adrenal gland extensively replaces most
of the normal adrenal tissue.

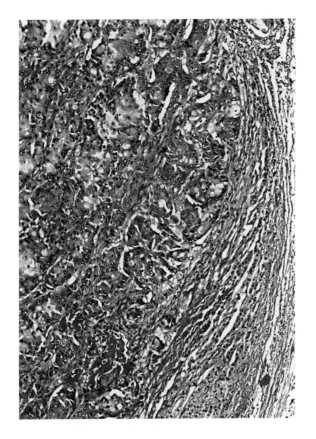

Figure 4-39

ADRENAL INSUFFICIENCY SECONDARY
TO METASTATIC CARCINOMA

Histologic examination shows a thin rim of residual
adrenal cortical tissue.

primary may not be known. Immunohistochemical stains for S100 protein, HMB45, vimentin, and keratin can be diagnostic in these cases, since all of these markers, except keratins, are positive in malignant melanoma. Massive involvement of the adrenal glands by lymphoma can be diagnosed readily by immunohistochemical characterization with CD45, along with specific B- and T-cell markers.

Differential Diagnosis. The differential diagnosis may be difficult when it is necessary to separate bilateral metastatic clear cell renal carcinoma from adrenal metastasis to the contralateral gland. Immunostaining for vimentin, keratin, inhibin, and synaptophysin can help distinguish these lesions since the latter is usually positive for inhibin, synaptophysin, and vimentin and weakly positive for keratin, whereas renal cell carcinomas are positive for keratin and vimentin.

Treatment and Prognosis. In most cases of bilateral metastases, clinical recognition of adrenal insufficiency is uncommon since most of the adrenal cortex (more than 90 percent) has to be destroyed before hypofunction is manifested (187). Recent studies suggest that one-fifth to one-third of patients with bilateral adrenal metastases have partial adrenal insufficiency and benefit from glucocorticoid therapy (191,192). The prognosis is usually poor because of the extensive primary disease in these patients.

OTHER CONDITIONS ASSOCIATED WITH HYPOFUNCTION

Adrenal Amyloidosis

Definition. Deposition of amyloid in the adrenal glands may lead to adrenal insufficiency.

General Remarks. Historically, amyloid deposits in the adrenal glands were a frequent finding at autopsy, but today are uncommon. Amyloidosis is a rare cause of adrenal insufficiency (199). The glands have to be bilaterally and extensively involved to cause adrenal insufficiency. Amyloid deposits in the adrenal gland may be the result of aging (198,201,202). In a recent study of 108 consecutive autopsies, interstitial amyloid was present in 73 (68 percent) adrenal glands (201). Multinodular amyloid deposits have been seen older patients (202). Biochemical analysis shows a serum amyloid P component and serum amyloid A protein.

In a study of the functional significance of amyloid deposits in the adrenal gland, Arik et al. (196) found that of 15 patients with renal amyloidosis without clinical evidence of adrenal insufficiency, 7 had abnormal cortisol responses, suggesting amyloid involvement of the adrenal cortex. In another study of 10 patients with renal amyloidosis, 2 had adrenal cortical dysfunction (197).

Macroscopic Findings. The adrenal glands may be normal in size or slightly enlarged. The cut surface is gray-yellow. Enlarged glands weighing up to 30 to 34 g together have been reported (200).

Microscopic Findings. Amyloid deposits are usually present in the zona fasciculata and reticularis. The deposits are present between the adrenal cells and the capillary endothelium. With increasing deposition of amyloid, the inner zone becomes a hyaline acellular mass with obliteration of most adrenocortical cells resulting in adrenal cortical insufficiency (fig. 4-40).

With senile and other secondary forms of amyloid deposition in the adrenal glands, the degree of involvement can be quite variable but is often focal.

Differential Diagnosis. Amyloid deposits should be distinguished from the hyaline sclerosis that may be seen in organizing infarction. Special stains for amyloid and ultrastructural studies can readily distinguish these conditions.

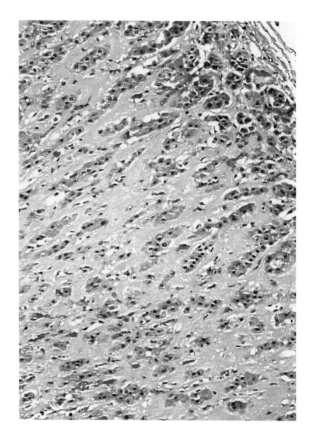

Figure 4-40

ADRENAL AMYLOIDOSIS

There is diffuse replacement of most of the adrenal cortical cells by amyloid, which has a characteristic acellular hyaline appearance.

Adrenoleukodystrophy

Definition. Primary adrenal insufficiency associated with progressive neurologic dysfunction, also known as *Addison-Schilder's disease*.

General Remarks. Adrenoleukodystrophy is inherited as a X-linked recessive disorder. It affects 1 in 120,000 males, begins in childhood, and progresses rapidly to dementia, blindness, and quadriplegia.

Adrenomyeloneuropathy is an adult form of the disease which starts in adolescence and early adulthood. Affected individuals have weakness, spasticity, and distal polyneuropathy. It is usually a slowly progressive disorder (203,206,212).

These disorders are caused by defective fatty acid beta-oxidation in peroxisomes which is associated with elevated plasma concentrations of very long chain saturated fatty acids.

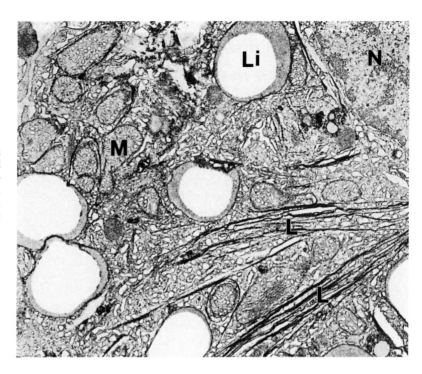

Figure 4-41

ADRENOLEUKODYSTROPHY

Ultrastructural examination shows a striated cell with lamellar-lipid (L) profiles (Li-lipid droplet, M-mitochondria, N-nucleus) (X16,900). (Fig. 18-5 from Neville AM, O'Hare MJ. The human adrenal cortex. New York: Springer-Verlag, 1982:260.)

Cholesterol esters and gangliosides accumulate in the membranes of the adrenal cortex, brain, and other organs (206). The defective gene is on chromosome Xq28, and it encodes a peroxisomal membrane protein (207). Various point mutations with single amino acid substitutions are associated with adrenoleukodystrophy (213).

Macroscopic Findings. The adrenal glands are smaller than usual, although the normal shape is retained. Each gland weighs less than 2 g and may be less than 1 g.

Microscopic Findings. Cortical cells are variably enlarged with abundant cytoplasmic material that causes a waxy appearance in the cytoplasm. Swollen ballooned cells have strictures and clefts, the result of lipid extraction during processing by xylene and alcohol. Ballooned cells are pathognomonic for adrenoleukodystrophy (209). Groups of ballooned cells are multifocal and tend to form small nodules. They may undergo lysis to form macrovacuoles.

Ultrastructural studies usually show that the ballooning and striations result from proliferation of smooth endoplasmic reticulum and accumulation of lamellar-lipid profiles (fig. 4-41) (210). The adrenal medulla is usually not affected, so in extreme cases in which most of the cortical cells are destroyed, only medullary tissues remain.

Lymphocytic infiltrates are uncommon and found only in the most atrophic glands. Other tissues affected include the cerebral white matter in which demyelinating changes and inflammation occur along with gliosis and macrophage infiltrates (212). The Schwann cells of the peripheral nerves and the Leydig cells of the testis are also abnormal. Spermatogenic arrests may be present in the testis in cases that develop in adulthood (211).

Differential Diagnosis. Distinction from autoimmune idiopathic Addison's disease may be difficult in the end stage of adrenoleukodystrophy since both disorders may be associated with cortical cells replaced by hyalinized connective tissue. However, the presence of ballooned cells, characteristic of adrenoleukodystrophy, is diagnostic. In addition, a lymphocytic infiltrate is characteristic of autoimmune Addison's disease but is rare in adrenoleukodystrophy.

Treatment and Prognosis. Dietary therapy such as Lorenzo's oil may prevent or delay the neurological manifestations of adrenoleukodystrophy, but does not improve the neurological symptoms after their inception (204,205). The effects of dietary therapy on adrenal function are not known (208).

Wolman's Disease

This rare autosomal recessive disorder is fatal in early infancy (213–215). It is associated with a deficiency of lysosome acid lipase. There is an accumulation of cholesterol esters and triglycerides in various tissues. Hepatosplenomegaly and bilateral enlargement of the adrenal glands with dystrophic calcification are frequently seen. The zonas fasciculata and reticularis have cells with vacuolated cytoplasm that were once filled with cholesterol esters but now show clefts from the losses during processing. There is usually necrosis, calcification, and fibrosis of the inner cortex. Affected individuals are usually dead by 6 months of age.

Adrenal Cysts

Definition. Adrenal cysts are tumefactive cystic lesions of the adrenal gland that involve primarily the cortex.

General Remarks. These are uncommon lesions usually involving one adrenal gland (216,218,221), but in a small percentage of cases, they may be bilateral (216). The frequency of adrenal cysts at autopsy has been reported as 0.06 percent (218). Adrenal cysts are rare in neonates and children (217,228,232).

Adrenal cysts have been subtyped into various groups by different investigators (216–218). *Endothelial cysts* are the most common type and constituted 45 percent of the cases in a review of the literature (216,217). They are usually made up of lymphatic channels, but true vascular channels may also be present. *Adrenal pseudocyst* is the second most common type, comprising up to 39 percent of cases in the above literature review. This is the most common clinically or surgically recognized type. Some primary adrenal pseudocysts have been shown to have a true vascular lining; immunohistochemistry (219,221,223, 230,231) shows components suggesting a vascular origin including elastic tissue and adrenal vein smooth muscle (225). Although the origin of adrenal pseudocyst is unclear, some authors have suggested a mesothelial origin (231). *Epithelial cysts* represent less than 10 percent of adrenal gland cysts (216,218,226). The possible eti-

ology of the epithelial cell in such cysts is uncertain. *Parasitic cysts* also represent less than 10 percent of adrenal cysts. They are often discovered incidentally at autopsy. Ecchinococcal organisms are usually involved. A review of 40 adrenal cysts operated on at the Mayo Clinic over the past 40 years found that most were pseudocysts (80 percent), followed by endothelial cysts (17.5 percent), and one epithelial cyst (2.5 percent).

Adrenal cysts may occasionally simulate metastatic disease (219,228) or may represent cystic degeneration of cortical or medullary neoplasms. The frequency with which adrenal pseudocysts are reported is increasing, which may reflect improved radiologic imaging methods. The possible etiology of these cysts includes cystic degeneration of an adrenal cortical or medullary neoplasm, a vascular neoplasm or malformation, and hemorrhagic degeneration in the adrenal gland parenchyma (224,225,234).

Clinical and Radiologic Findings. Women have a 2- to 4-fold greater incidence of adrenal cysts than men. Patients may present with nonspecific signs and symptoms including flank pain, epigastric discomfort, and a palpable abdominal mass with larger cysts. Rare patients may have fever and leukocytosis. Chronic hemorrhage into large cysts can lead to anemia. Most adrenal cysts are not associated with endocrine symptoms. A few patients may have hypertension which is cured by surgical removal of the cyst. The hypertension may be related to compression of the renal vein (229,233). In a series of eight adrenal pseudocysts reported by Medeiros et al. (230), four patients had symptoms of abdominal and/or flank pain attributable to their adrenal lesion, and three had hypertension which resolved in one patient after surgery. There was a remote history of trauma in two of the eight patients.

Radiologic findings of adrenal pseudocysts include a well-defined cystic mass with areas of calcification in some cysts. CT scans show a density close to that of water. MRI usually shows a low signal intensity on T1-weighted images and a high signal intensity on T2-weighted images with enhancement (fig. 4-42) (227).

Macroscopic Findings. The cysts vary greatly in size from microcysts that are 0.1 to 1.0 mm in diameter and are seen in the adrenal cortex of older fetuses and infants (232,233) to

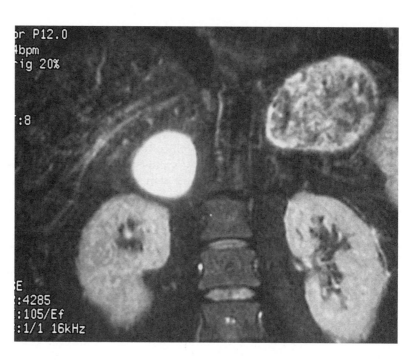

Figure 4-42

ADRENAL CYST

Right adrenal pseudocyst presenting as a round, uniformly high-signal mass superior to the right kidney on T2-weighted MRI in the coronal place. Ultrasound confirms the presence of an anechoic adrenal cyst.

pseudocysts that are usually 4 to 10 cm in diameter but may be as large as 33 cm. Pseudocysts may contain dark brown fluid from hemorrhage (figs. 4-43–4-46) (218). Most cysts are unilocular with a thickened fibrous wall. The lining is usually irregular. Areas of calcification are often present within the wall. The focal yellowish areas present in the cyst wall usually represent residual adrenal cortical cells (fig. 4-46).

Microscopic Findings. The histologic features reflect the type of adrenal cyst present. Pseudocysts are among the most common and do not contain any endothelial or epithelial cell lining (figs. 4-47–4-49). They may originate from hemorrhage and expand into a previously normal adrenal gland. Liquefaction and organization of the necrotic material follows, with subsequent enlargement due to further hemorrhage and fluid accumulation. Parasitic cysts usually contain echinococcal or other organisms and the wall has many eosinophils. Epithelial-lined cysts have been described but are rare (fig. 4-50). They may represent a lymphangiomatous or angiomatous origin from the maldevelopment of lymphatics associated with blood vessels in the adrenal capsule and the capillary sinusoids. Alternatively, the endothelial lining may represent recanalization in a hemorrhagic pseudocyst.

Immunohistochemical Findings. Analyses of pseudocysts have found factor VIII immunoreactivity in the inner wall, but no vimentin and keratin (230). In one case report of an epithelial-lined cyst of the adrenal gland, the lining cells were positive for keratin but were negative for factor VIII, vimentin, and epithelial membrane antigen, and a mesothelial origin of the epithelial lining was proposed (231). Another study of a primary adrenal pseudocyst showed staining for laminin and type IV collagen, suggesting a vascular origin.

Differential Diagnosis. The major differential diagnosis is a cystic neoplasm. Cystic adrenal cortical or medullary neoplasms as well as cystic metastatic carcinomas (219) can simulate adrenal cysts. Histologic identification of neoplastic adrenal cortical cells, pheochromocytoma cells, or metastatic carcinoma cells on H&E-stained sections usually provides the diagnosis. Occasionally, immunohistochemical stains may be needed to distinguish between cystic adrenal neoplasms and metastatic tumors.

Treatment and Prognosis. Surgical excision of the cyst is the treatment of choice. Laparoscopic surgery, which is used for benign adrenal disease, may be an option for smaller cysts (235–237). The prognosis for patients with benign adrenal cysts is excellent (216,230).

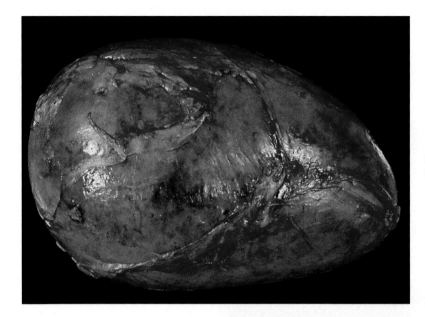

Figure 4-43

ADRENAL CYST

Right adrenal pseudocyst with a tan-gray wall and portions of yellow residual adrenal cortex on the surface.

Figure 4-44

ADRENAL CYST

Adrenal pseudocyst with a thickened fibrous wall. Focal calcification may be present in the wall.

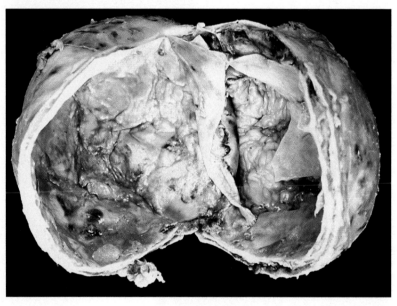

ADRENAL CORTICAL NODULES AND HYPERPLASIA

A wide spectrum of conditions can lead to adrenal cortical hyperplasia, ranging from congenital hyperplasia due to inborn errors of metabolism to Cushing's syndrome and even rarer conditions such as primary pigmented adrenocortical disease. These conditions are usually associated with a hyperfunctioning adrenal cortex that produces excessive amounts of steroid hormones.

Many adrenal cortical nodules, especially small nodules, discovered incidentally at autopsy or during surgical removal of the adrenal glands for other reasons, are nonfunctional. These nodules occur in asymptomatic patients and are often associated with age-related changes in the adrenal vasculature.

Adrenal cortical hyperplasia associated with hypercorticalism can be pathophysiologically classified into ACTH-dependent and ACTH-independent conditions (Table 4-2). Alternatively, a

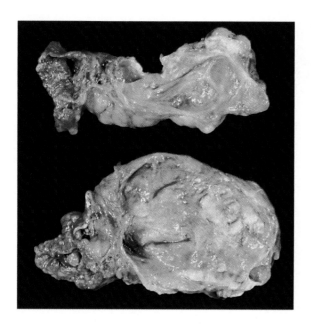

Figure 4-45

ADRENAL CYST

This adrenal pseudocyst has an irregular wall and adjacent adrenal cortical tissues on the left.

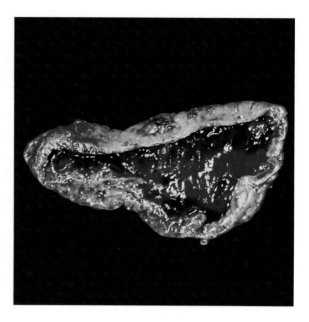

Figure 4-46

ADRENAL CYST

Hemorrhagic adrenal pseudocyst with central cavitation surrounded by adrenal cortex.

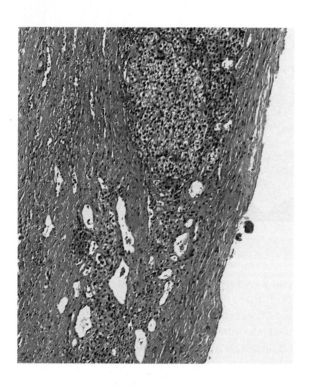

Figure 4-47

ADRENAL CYST

There are residual adrenal cortical cells in the wall of this adrenal pseudocyst.

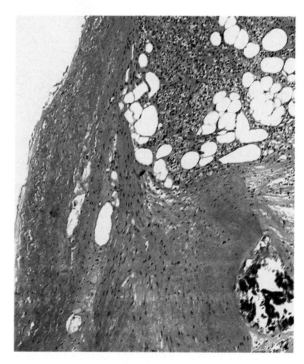

Figure 4-48

ADRENAL CYST

Fibrosis and dystrophic calcification in the wall of this adrenal pseudocyst.

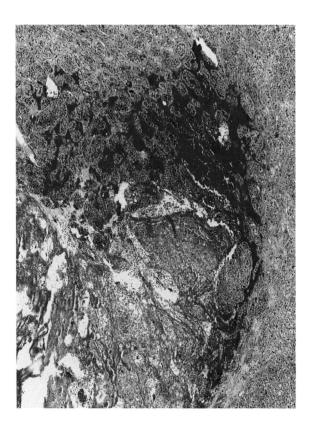

Figure 4-49

ADRENAL CYST

Adrenal pseudocyst with recent and old hemorrhage in the wall.

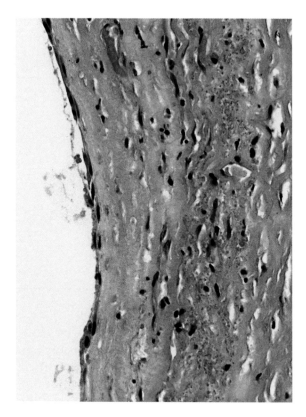

Figure 4-50

ADRENAL CYST

Adrenal cyst with an endothelial lining above the fibrotic cyst wall.

morphologic classification, which is probably more useful for pathologists, takes into account the nodule size, pattern of distribution, color, and other features that may be used to classify adrenal cortical hyperplasia.

Other conditions associated with adrenal cortical hyperplasia include congenital adrenal hyperplasia and the adrenogenital syndrome secondary to deficiencies of the enzymes needed for steroid biosynthesis.

Incidental Nonfunctional Adrenal Cortical Nodules

Definition. One or more nodules are present in the adrenal cortex in an asymptomatic patient.

General Remarks. A great deal of confusion exists regarding the classification of nonfunctional adrenal cortical nodules. Many of these nodules are discovered incidentally at autopsy,

while others may be diagnosed incidentally during radiologic studies (248–250,252–254). The designation of these nodules as neoplasms rather than hyperplastic nodules has often been done arbitrarily, without documentation of the monoclonal nature of the lesion as would be expected with true neoplasms. If the historical definition of an adenoma as a solitary nodule in the adrenal gland measuring at least 3 to 5 mm in diameter is used, then 1 to 3 percent of autopsied adrenal glands would contain adenomas (239,247, 249,252). These nodules are more common in older patients and in patients with hypertension. In one study a solitary nodule was found in 29 percent of 100 consecutive autopsies in women of an average age of 81 years (241). Solitary nodules were found in up to 20 percent of autopsied patients with a history of hypertension (253). Patients with diabetes mellitus also have an increased incidence of solitary adrenal nodule at autopsy (245).

Table 4-2

ACTH-DEPENDENT AND -INDEPENDENT CUSHING'S SYNDROME

ACTH-Dependent Cushing's Syndrome
1. Cushing's disease - pituitary tumor
2. Ectopic ACTH syndrome
3. Ectopic corticotropin-releasing hormone syndrome

ACTH-Independent Cushing's Syndrome
1. Hyperplasia
   Macronodular hyperplasia
   Primary pigmented adrenocortical disease
2. Tumors
   Adrenocortical adenomas
   Adrenocortical carcinomas
3. Iatrogenic

Most small adrenal nodules probably represent localized overgrowth of adrenocortical cells, which may be related to aging and/or response to adrenal vascular changes (241,248). Dobbie (241) has elegantly outlined the various types and stages of nodule development. The earliest lesions are entirely within the cortex, while further enlargement leads to compression of the surrounding tissues. Nodules continue to grow and come to form a mushroom-like mass that protrudes through the capsule or expands within the gland, attaining a size of up to 2 to 3 cm. The term cortical extrusion refers to the extension of cortical nodules into the periadrenal tissue. The cortex may show an "hour-glass" pattern of extrusion or a mushroom pattern, or the cortical cells may stream into the adjacent periadrenal adipose tissue (241). These extrusions should not be mistaken for carcinomas. The capsular arteries of adrenal glands containing nodules often show hyalinization and intimal proliferation which are sometimes associated with obliteration of the lumen (241). These changes may result from ischemia, leading to focal cortical atrophy.

Recent molecular biological studies using the Lyon hypothesis have shown that many benign as well as malignant tumors are monoclonal (257). Similar studies have been done in the adrenal cortex (242,243). Although most adrenocortical carcinomas are monoclonal, adrenocortical adenomas may be monoclonal (43 percent) or polyclonal (28.5 percent) with various intermediate phases (28.5 percent) (243). The significance of polyclonal adenomas is that either they are not true adenomas or that some adenomas are truly polyclonal. Because some hyperplastic nodules, as in bilateral pigmented adrenocortical hyperplasias, have been shown to be monoclonal (256), clonality studies may not provide a direct answer when distinguishing hyperplastic nodules from adenomas.

In general, most small adrenocortical nodules are nonfunctional or at the very most minimally functional (fig. 4-51). Suzuki et al. (255) examined 15 small adrenocortical nodules that showed no clinical evidence of biological activity for steroid production. They found immunohistochemical evidence of various steroidogenic enzymes including 3-beta-hydroxysteroid dehydrogenase, C21-hydroxylase, 17-alpha-hydroxylase, and 11-beta-hydroxylase, indicating that these nodules were capable of producing cortisol. However, since the enzymatic activity of these proteins was not investigated, the possibility that the immunoreactivity was different than the enzymatic activity could not be excluded.

Some adrenal cortical nodules are pigmented when seen at autopsy or after surgical resection. In one series, there were focally pigmented nodules in 37 percent of autopsied adrenal glands (240). Multiple pigmented nodules, some of which are bilateral, have also been incidental findings. Neuromelanin has been detected in some of these pigmented nodules.

Some incidental nonfunctional nodules are discovered in patients undergoing radiologic studies of the upper abdomen; they have been reported in 0.6 to 1.3 percent of patients undergoing CT scans (238,244,250). In a Mayo Clinic series, the average age was 62 years, with females constituting more than half of the patients (246). The most common diagnosis of these nodules is a benign nonfunctioning adrenal cortical nodule and less commonly metastatic tumors from lung, breast, and other sites (257). The size of the nodule is important in determining whether a tumor is benign or malignant. In the Mayo Clinic series, 55 patients of a total of 342 who had incidentally discovered nodules underwent adrenal exploration. Malignant adrenal cortical nodules or carcinomas measured from 5.5 to 17.0 cm in diameter, indicating that smaller nodules or small tumors are usually benign.

Clinical and Radiologic Findings. Small nodules usually do not cause symptoms unless they are functional. Radiologic findings, including CT and MRI, often show one or more nodules in the adrenal gland. High resolution CT scans can detect nodules smaller than 1 cm in diameter.

Macroscopic Findings. Nonfunctional, benign nodules of the adrenal gland are usually multiple. The studies of Dobbie (241) and Neville (248) showed that nodularity of the adrenal gland is common, seen in 65 percent of more than 100 consecutive autopsies. Nodules are frequently bilateral and may extrude into the adrenal capsule. In some areas the cortical cells may be unencapsulated and stream into the adjacent periadrenal fat. Nodules may also completely detach from the capsule. Larger nodules may be greater than 2 cm in diameter.

Microscopic Findings. Various architectural patterns may be present in the nodules, including trabecular, pseudoglandular, solid, alveolar, and myxoid (fig. 4-52). Metaplastic changes include myelolipomatous and osseous metaplasia. The presence of cortical atrophy away from a dominant nodule may suggest that the nodule is functional, but this is uncommon in incidental nodules. Degenerative or retrogressive changes such as hyalinization, hemorrhage, or calcification may be present in larger nodules.

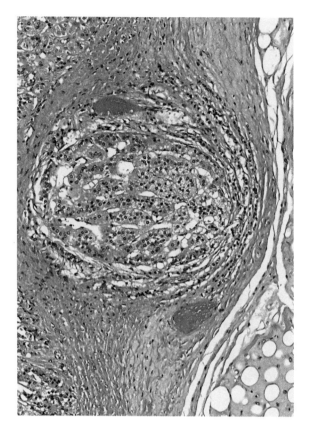

Figure 4-51

INCIDENTAL ADRENAL CORTICAL NODULE

An incidental nonfunctioning adrenal cortical nodule from a patient without evidence of cortical hyperfunction. The micronodule was present in the capsule and was composed of fasciculata-type cells.

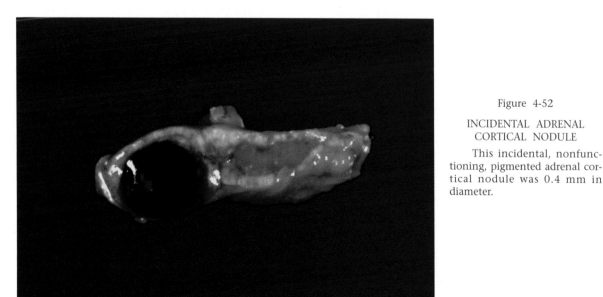

Figure 4-52

INCIDENTAL ADRENAL CORTICAL NODULE

This incidental, nonfunctioning, pigmented adrenal cortical nodule was 0.4 mm in diameter.

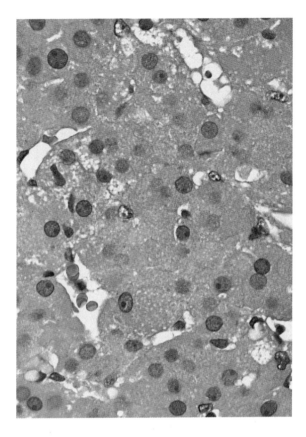

Figure 4-53

INCIDENTAL ADRENAL CORTICAL NODULE
Histologic examination shows zona reticularis-type cells with prominent cytoplasmic lipofuscin pigment.

Pigmented cortical nodules usually contain neuromelanin (figs. 4-52, 4-53) (240). These nodules are frequently located in the zona reticularis. They are unencapsulated and composed of eosinophilic cells with varying degrees of lipid depletion and lipofuscin pigment (fig. 4-53).

Differential Diagnosis. Incidental cortical nodules should be distinguished from adrenal cortical adenomas and carcinomas. The cytologic features of carcinomas, including increased mitotic activity with atypical mitoses and confluent necrosis in nodules that are larger than 5 cm, usually are diagnostic. Distinction of incidental nodules from adenomas or benign neoplasms may be more problematic. The presence of a solitary nodule that is often circumscribed usually indicates an adenoma. Nodular hyperplasia often consists of multiple nodules of varying sizes which may be bilateral.

Table 4-3

MORPHOLOGIC CLASSIFICATION OF ADRENAL CORTICAL HYPERPLASIA

I. Bilateral Disease
  a. Diffuse hyperplasia
  b. Nodular hyperplasia
    micronodular (less than 0.5 cm in diameter)
    macronodular (greater than 0.5 cm in diameter)
  c. Combined diffuse and nodular hyperplasia
  d. Marked macronodular hyperplasia
  e. Primary pigmented nodular adrenocortical disease (Carney's complex)
  f. Incidental pigmented nodule

II. Unilateral Disease
  a. Diffuse and/or nodular hyperplasia
  b. Incidental pigmented nodules

Treatment and Prognosis. Nonfunctioning incidental nodules may be followed clinically if they are small (less than 4 cm) and nonfunctional. Nodules greater than 4 cm are often treated surgically. Small nonfunctional nodules that are surgically excised and shown to be benign are associated with an excellent prognosis.

Adrenal Cortical Hyperplasia

Definition. This is a non-neoplastic condition in which there is an increase in the number of adrenal cortical cells.

General Remarks. Adrenocortical hyperplasia may be diffuse or nodular (Table 4-3). In adults, simple or diffuse hyperplasia is most common (62 percent), while nodular hyperplasia and hyperplasia with ectopic ACTH syndrome constitute 20 percent and 18 percent of cases, respectively (261,263). In children, simple hyperplasia is most common (62 percent), with nodular hyperplasia and hyperplasia with ectopic ACTH syndrome constituting 23 percent and 15 percent, respectively (263). An ACTH secretory pituitary adenoma is the most frequent cause of diffuse hyperplasia (263).

Nodular hyperplasia involving both adrenal glands can be seen in adults and children. These glands are characterized by the presence of one or more prominent yellow nodules greater than 0.5 cm in diameter in glands in which the cortex is clearly hyperplastic (261). The nodules can be as large as 2.0 to 2.5 cm. In children, bilateral nodular hyperplasia is seen most frequently in the first year of life. In adults, some investigators have suggested that the hyperplasia may develop secondary to the vascular damage to capsular arteries with continued increase in size of micronodules (274–276). In most cases of nodular hyperplasia, the adjacent adrenal cortex shows diffuse or simple hyperplasia and the clinical evidence of Cushing's syndrome is cured only by bilateral adrenalectomy, suggesting that diffuse and nodular hyperplasia are part of the same morphologic spectrum, probably representing one disease process (261–263). Some authors have observed unilateral nodular hyperplasia with low plasma ACTH levels (261,268). However, this may represent true adenomas rather than nodular hyperplasia (261). The existence of unilateral adrenal cortical hyperplasia associated with Cushing's syndrome has been reported (259,266). These patients are usually cured by unilateral adrenalectomy with no recurrent disease up to several years after surgery.

Hyperplasia due to ectopic ACTH or CRH production may occur in adults or children. In children, ectopic production of ACTH by pheochromocytoma, neuroblastoma, and thymic and islet cell tumors may lead to hyperplasia; in adults, ectopic ACTH and/or CRH production is usually associated with small cell lung carcinoma and bronchial carcinoid tumors, but other tumors such as islet cell tumors, pheochromocytomas, and thymic carcinoid tumor may also be involved (260,264,265).

In adults, Cushing's syndrome due to ectopic production of ACTH or CRH has been reported in about 15 percent of cases (265,272, 278,281,282). Although the etiology is normally a tumor such as small cell carcinoma of lung or carcinoid tumor, other non-neoplastic conditions may be associated with this syndrome (262, 263). CRH is commonly produced by bronchial carcinoid tumors although other tumors also produce this peptide ectopically (283,289). Unusual causes of ectopic Cushing's syndrome, such as a pituitary adenoma arising in a benign cystic teratoma of the ovary, have been reported (260).

Clinical and Radiologic Findings. Patients with Cushing's syndrome usually have progressive obesity in a centripetal distribution, involving the face, neck, trunk, and abdomen,

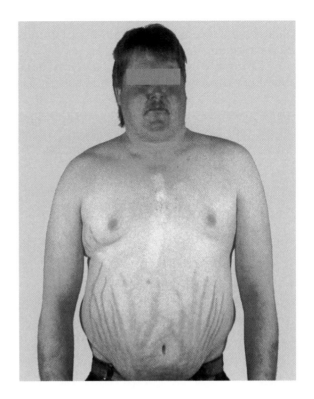

Figure 4-54

ADRENAL CORTICAL HYPERPLASIA

A 30-year-old man with pituitary-dependent Cushing's syndrome presented with hypertension, central obesity, facial plethora, purple-red abdominal and axillary striae, and proximal muscle weakness.

with sparing of the extremities (figs. 4-54–4-56). Proximal muscle wasting and weakness are common. Other signs and symptoms include cardiovascular complications, skin atrophy, glucose intolerance, easy bruisability, hirsutism, and psychiatric complications (271,277).

Radiologic findings depend on the etiology of Cushing's syndrome. In patients with Cushing's disease, a small pituitary ACTH adenoma can be detected by MRI in 50 percent of patients. Bilateral inferior petrosal sinus sampling for ACTH is required in most patients with ACTH-dependent Cushing's syndrome. Scintigraphy with ^{131}I-labeled cholesterol and adrenal arteriograms are occasionally performed (277). In patients with ectopic sources of ACTH or CRH, a tumor may be detected by CT or MRI. The adrenal glands appear normal in size or show bilateral diffuse or macronodular enlargement. Nodules smaller than 1 cm may be occasionally detected (261).

Laboratory Findings. Patients with Cushing's disease have elevated serum ACTH

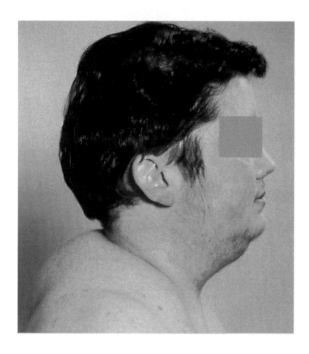

Figure 4-55

ADRENAL CORTICAL HYPERPLASIA

A 27-year-old woman with pituitary-dependent Cushing's syndrome. Hirsutism and dorsocervical fat pad are demonstrated.

levels. Some of the other pro-opiomelanocortin (POMC) peptides may also be elevated. Plasma concentration and urinary excretion of cortisol, 17-ketosteroids, and 17-ketogenic steroids are usually increased (277).

Patients with ectopic Cushing's syndrome have elevated serum ACTH levels as well as other POMC peptides. Plasma cortisol and precursors are also elevated (277).

Macroscopic Findings. Both adrenal glands are enlarged with diffuse hyperplasia. Each gland weighs between 6 and 12 g (figs. 4-57, 4-58). In children, depending on their age, the glands are heavier than normal, although the increased weight may be less than in adults (271). The glands are yellow to brown and have rounded edges. Cut sections show a thickened cortex with an inner brown layer and an outer yellow layer. Small nodules of less than 0.25 cm may be seen in diffuse hyperplasia. This may be most prominent in peripubertal children.

Glands with bilateral nodular hyperplasia are somewhat heavier than those with diffuse hyperplasia. A difference of 2 g or more between the two glands is seen with nodular hyperplasia, but less commonly with diffuse hyperplasia. Nodules are present in both glands and are greater than 0.5 cm in diameter, and many are 2.0 to 2.5 cm. The nodules are multiple and project from one pole of the gland or compress the adjacent cortex (fig. 4-59).

Figure 4-56

ADRENAL CORTICAL HYPERPLASIA

A 37-year-old woman presented with 9 kg weight gain over 2 years, new hypertension, secondary amenorrhea, hirsutism, emotional lability, and central redistribution of body fat. ACTH-dependent hypercortisolism was confirmed biochemically. Pituitary MRI showed an intra-sellar microadenoma. Left photograph taken at baseline. Right photograph taken 6 months after curative transsphenoidal surgery.

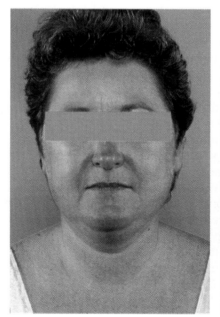
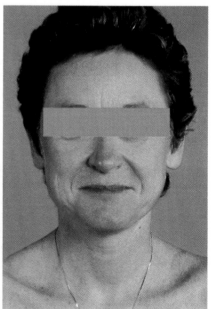

Microscopic Findings. Histologic examination of the adrenal glands in diffuse hyperplasia shows that the inner brown zone is associated with a thickened zona reticularis, and the yellow outer area shows a thickened zona fasciculata (figs. 4-60–4-62). The outer zona reticularis is usually not affected by the hyperplastic process, although in children with diffuse hyperplasia it may be more prominent than usual. In adrenal glands in which the weights are normal or near normal, the thickening of the zona reticularis is a distinct sign of hyperplasia. The individual cells are typically normal in size and appearance, although a slight hypertrophy may be present. The ultrastructural features are similar to those of the normal adrenal cortex (270,273).

At autopsy, the adrenal glands from patients with Cushing's syndrome contain all compact or zona reticularis–type cells, which extend out to the capsule or to the zona glomerulosa. These additional changes are probably related to the stresses associated with dying, in this case from Cushing's syndrome.

Another histologic change associated with Cushing's syndrome is the presence of small micronodules, usually around the central vein, consisting of lipid-laden clear cells similar to those of the zona fasciculata. Aggregates of fat cells may be present in the zona reticularis. Hypertrophy of the cells in the zona fasciculata and

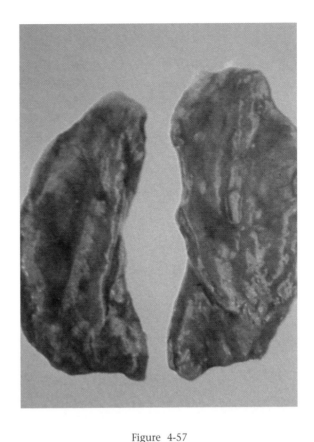

Figure 4-57

DIFFUSE ADRENOCORTICAL HYPERPLASIA

There is diffuse enlargement of both adrenal glands from a patient with an ACTH-producing pituitary adenoma. The gland weights were 10.2 g and 8.9 g for the right and left gland, respectively.

Figure 4-58

DIFFUSE ADRENOCORTICAL HYPERPLASIA

Cut section of the adrenal glands shows diffuse enlargement of the adrenal cortex.

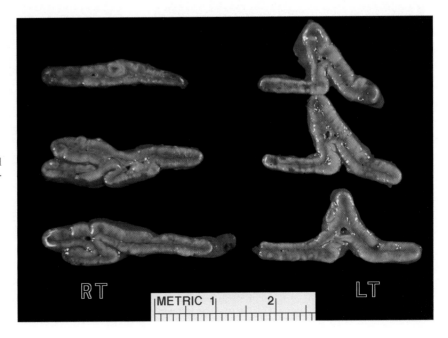

Figure 4-59

DIFFUSE ADRENOCORTICAL
HYPERPLASIA

There is diffuse expansion of the
adrenal cortex in a patient with an
ACTH-producing pituitary adenoma.

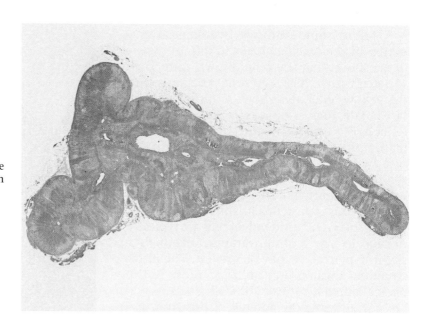

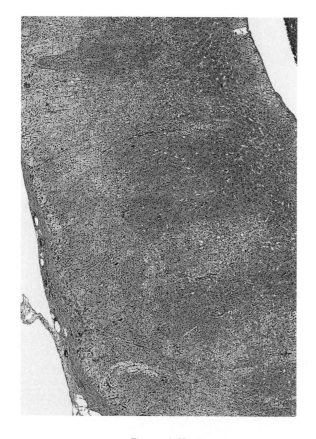

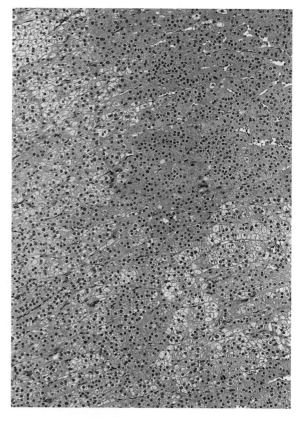

Figure 4-60

DIFFUSE ADRENOCORTICAL HYPERPLASIA

Higher magnification of figure 4-59 shows that the
zona fasciculata is the predominant region that is expanded.

Figure 4-61

DIFFUSE ADRENOCORTICAL HYPERPLASIA

A slight nodularity of lipid-rich and compact cells is
noted in this diffusely enlarged adrenal gland.

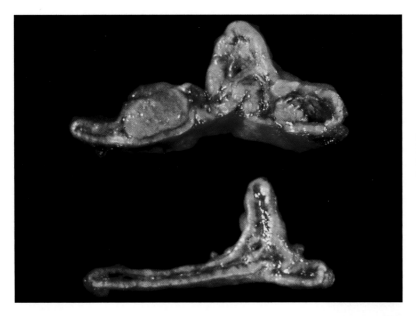

Figure 4-62

NODULAR HYPERPLASIA

Nodular hyperplasia secondary to an ACTH-producing adenoma. Multiple nodules are seen in the left adrenal gland, one of which is larger than 0.5 cm.

zona reticularis, along with nuclear pleomorphism, is probably secondary to the ACTH stimulation.

Occasional cases of spontaneous remission of Cushing's syndrome with bilateral adrenocortical hyperplasia have been reported (279, 286). Some of these have occurred after adrenal venography and administration of ACTH, which may be related to hemorrhage and necrosis of the glands (280).

The histologic features of adrenal glands with nodular hyperplasia include nodules of clear cells and compression of the adjacent cortex (fig. 4-63). Clusters of compact cells, corresponding to the brown color of some nodules, may be present. The capsular arteries usually show hyalinization and sclerosis. Cellular hypertrophy and nuclear pleomorphism may be seen in some nodules. Although some authors have equated cellular pleomorphism with tumor development in these nodules (258,267), this is probably not accurate, since in the adrenal glands and in other endocrine organs, pleomorphism is not related to anaplasia. Examination of the adjacent cortex in nodular hyperplasia shows evidence of hyperplasia, while in nonfunctioning nodules it is normal and in functioning adenomas it is atrophic. Ultrastructural examination shows normal-appearing adrenal cortical cells. In the areas adjacent to the nodules there is increased perivascular collagen and basement membrane material. The cells in the

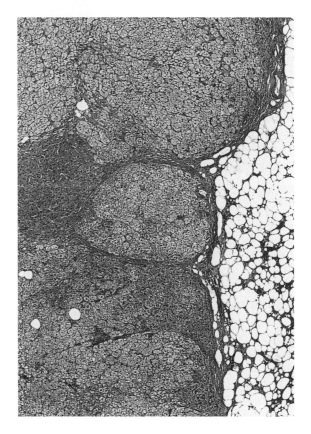

Figure 4-63

NODULAR HYPERPLASIA

Histologic view shows the multiple nodules of predominantly lipid-rich cells in a gland with nodular hyperplasia.

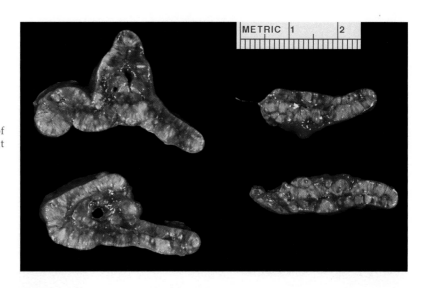

Figure 4-64

ECTOPIC ACTH SYNDROME

There is diffuse enlargement of both adrenal glands, with the right weighing 19 g and the left, 13 g.

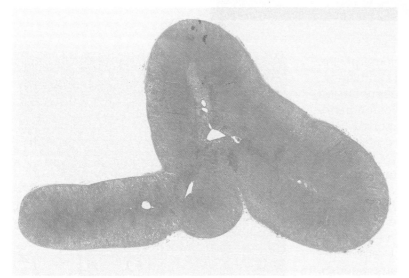

Figure 4-65

ECTOPIC ACTH SYNDROME

Diffuse hyperplasia secondary to ectopic ACTH syndrome caused by a small cell neuroendocrine carcinoma of the pancreas.

nodules may contain more prominent smooth endoplasmic reticulum (287).

The adrenal glands in ectopic ACTH or CRH syndrome weigh between 14 and 16 g each and may reach up to 20 g. Cut sections show a thickened cortex with a diffuse brown color (figs. 4-64, 4-65). Histologic examination shows more prominent compact or zona reticularis–type cells which extend from the medulla up to or almost to the zona glomerulosa or capsule (figs. 4-66, 4-67). Foci of clear cells are also present. The compact and clear cells are hypertrophic and show variable degrees of nuclear pleomorphism. Occasionally, metastatic tumor may be detected in the hyperplastic adrenal cortex (fig. 4-67).

Differential Diagnosis. The principal differential diagnosis is between nodular hyperplasia and benign neoplasms, usually adenomas of the adrenal cortex. Nodular hyperplasia usually consists of multiple nodules, while adenomas consist of a single nodule. To distinguish functional from nonfunctional nodules, it is necessary to examine the uninvolved cortex. In nodular hyperplasia, the other areas of the adrenal cortex away from the nodules are also hyperplastic, while in functional nodules, there is atrophy of the uninvolved cortex.

Treatment and Prognosis. Treatment of Cushing's disease includes surgical resection of the pituitary tumor. If the first surgical treatment

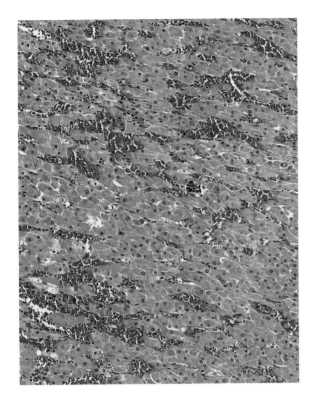

Figure 4-66

ECTOPIC ACTH SYNDROME

Histologic section of an adrenal gland from a patient with ectopic ACTH syndrome. There is diffuse hyperplasia with prominent compact or zona reticularis-type cells.

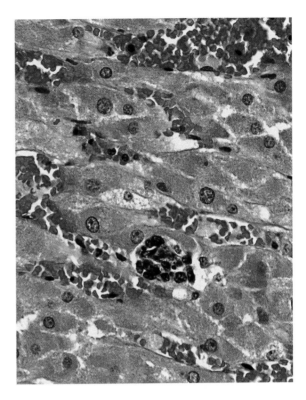

Figure 4-67

ECTOPIC ACTH SYNDROME

Diffuse hyperplasia showing cells with lipid depletion and a nest of metastatic pancreatic neuroendocrine carcinoma in the adrenal, which lead to a paracrine stimulation of the cortical cells.

is not curative, the options include reoperation, radiation of the pituitary, or performing a medical or surgical adrenalectomy (278,285). Mitotane has been used for medical adrenalectomy during or after pituitary radiation (269,274).

Open adrenalectomy by the anterior or posterior approach is associated with significant morbidity. Laparoscopic adrenalectomy is safe, effective, and curative; shortens hospitalization and convalescence; and produces less long-term morbidity than open adrenalectomy (264,288).

Ectopic ACTH or CRH syndrome is treated by removal of the tumor if possible. In most patients the tumor is not resectable at the time of diagnosis because of metastatic disease. Chemotherapy, radiation therapy, or both may be helpful. Hypercortisolism should be controlled as quickly as possible. Adrenal enzyme inhibition with drugs such as aminoglutethimide, ketoconazole, and metyrapone can be used. However,

in most cases bilateral adrenalectomy is the best treatment option for the hypercortisolism.

Previously, the prognosis of patients with Cushing's syndrome was often fatal due to cardiovascular, thromboembolic, or hypertensive complications and increased susceptibility to bacterial infection. Today, Cushing's syndrome is almost always curable. Untreated Cushing's syndrome in pregnancy is associated with spontaneous abortion, premature delivery, and rarely, neonatal adrenal insufficiency. Maternal deaths occur in 4 percent of patients (288).

The prognosis for patients with ectopic ACTH and CRH syndromes depends on the nature of the tumor, but it is usually very poor. Many patients succumb to the malignant disease within 1 year, while patients with indolent tumors may survive for more than a decade.

Adrenocortical Macronodular Hyperplasia

Definition. This primary adrenal cause of Cushing's syndrome is due to marked bilateral enlargement of the adrenal glands. Synonyms include *massive macronodular hyperplasia* and *macronodular adrenal dysplasia*.

General Remarks. This rare cause of Cushing's syndrome is associated with tumefactive enlargement of both adrenal glands (see fig. 4-3) (290,292). Pituitary studies, including petrosal sampling for ACTH, are normal (293, 295). Endocrinologic studies reveal elevated plasma cortisol levels with low levels of plasma ACTH. Dexamethasone testing does not suppress adrenal cortisol secretion (290,292,294). An activating mutation of G_s was associated with the syndrome in an infant (292). Abnormal adrenal expression and receptor function for various hormones including gastric inhibitory polypeptide (297), beta-adrenergic antagonists (298), and interleukin 1 (303) have been implicated in the etiology of macronodular hyperplasia with marked adrenal enlargement. A recent study (301) required the following features to be classified as macronodular hyperplasia with marked adrenal enlargement: bilateral adrenocortical nodules, an association with ACTH-independent hypercortisolism, and a histologically atrophic internodular cortex. Approximately 40 cases of this condition have been reported (302). Rare cases of familial clustering have also been noted (302).

Immunohistochemical and in situ hybridization studies by Sasano et al. (291,299,300) showed immunoreactivity for steroidogenic enzymes in the nodular cortical cells but not in the atrophied adrenal cortex. Immunoreactivity for P450 cholesterol side chain cleavage and P450 21-alpha-hydroxylase was observed in both clear and compact cells, while 3-beta-hydroxysteroid dehydrogenase was present only in clear cortical cells (299,300). These authors concluded that ineffective corticosteroidogenesis may contribute to the relatively low production of cortisol (299).

Clinical and Radiologic Findings. Clinical features include those of Cushing's syndrome with elevated plasma cortisol levels and low to undetectable ACTH levels (296,301,302). The mean age at diagnosis is 45 to 55 years. The sex distribution is quite variable from one series to the next but is probably equal. The time to diagnosis is usually between 1 to 2 years. CT studies often show bilateral adrenal nodules or massively enlarged glands (fig. 4-68). CT and MRI of the pituitary gland are within normal limits. Adrenal cortisol secretion is not suppressed by low and high dexamethasone treatment.

Macroscopic Findings. The glands are markedly enlarged and weigh up to 200 g combined. The nodules are multiple and may vary from 0.2 to over 4.0 cm in diameter (figs. 4-69, 4-70). The glands are coarsely nodular, with discrete nodules admixed with closely aggregated nodules. Cut sections show the nodule to be golden yellow with tan areas (fig. 4-70). The nodules are unencapsulated, and there may be compression of the adjacent cortex as well as the medulla.

Microscopic Findings. The cortical nodules consist of predominantly clear cells and some compact cells with variable amounts of lipid (figs. 4-71–4-73). Some cells may appear vacuolated; mitotic figures and cellular pleomorphism are uncommon. Myelolipomatous change may be present, which is probably a marker of cortical hyperactivity. Osseous metaplasia may also be present. Atrophy of the non-nodular cortex has been reported in some cases, but appears to be a variable finding (290,299,300).

The immunohistochemical and in situ hybridization studies of Sasano et al. (299) showed that ineffective steroidogenesis may contribute to the relatively low production of cortisol.

Differential Diagnosis. The differential diagnosis includes macronodular hyperplasia, without massive enlargement of the adrenal glands, secondary to pituitary-dependent Cushing's syndrome. Clinicopathologic correlations can assist in a morphologic diagnosis in difficult cases. Nodules are present in both cases, but the glands are much smaller in ACTH-dependent nodular hyperplasia. However, in a few cases of macronodular hyperplasia with marked adrenal enlargement one adrenal gland may weigh only 15 g or less (290). The serum ACTH is low in all cases, in spite of elevated serum cortisol. In ACTH-dependent nodular Cushing's syndrome, the adrenal glands are seldom more than 15 g each, and the entire gland is hyperplastic, while atrophic areas may be present in ACTH-independent macronodular hyperplasia with marked adrenal enlargement.

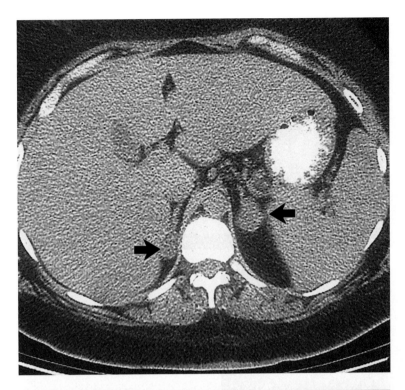

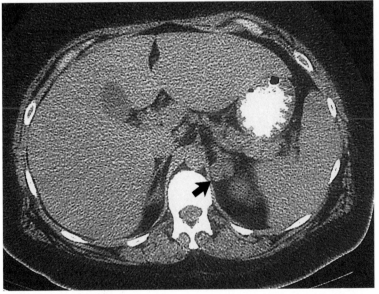

Figure 4-68

MACRONODULAR HYPERPLASIA WITH MARKED ADRENAL ENLARGEMENT

Unenhanced axial CT scans through the upper abdomen show multiple, small (1-2 cm), soft tissue density nodules in both adrenal glands (black arrows). On the top is a more cephalad image showing bilateral involvement, while the image on the bottom better displays the nodular appearance of the left-sided involvement.

Treatment and Prognosis. Bilateral adrenalectomy is the treatment of choice. Laparoscopic adrenalectomy is sometimes used in the treatment (301). Patients do not develop Nelson's syndrome after adrenalectomy. Of nine cases from the Mayo Clinic, no patient had recurrent disease after bilateral adrenalectomy up to 8.5 years after surgery (302).

Primary Pigmented Nodular Adrenocortical Disease

Definition. This form of pituitary-independent Cushing's syndrome is caused by bilateral micronodular hyperplasia of pigmented nodules in the adrenal cortex. Synonyms include *adrenocortical dysplasia* and *bilateral micronodular hyperplasia*.

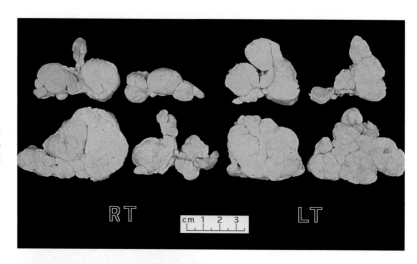

Figure 4-69

MACRONODULAR HYPERPLASIA
WITH MARKED ADRENAL
ENLARGEMENT

Transverse sections show marked
thickening and nodularity of the
adrenal cortex. Each gland weighed
more than 40 g.

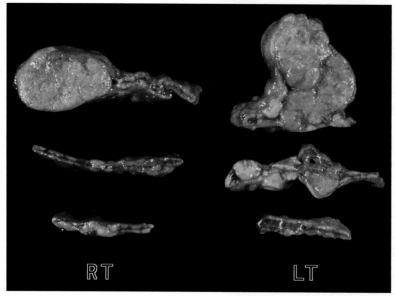

Figure 4-70

MACRONODULAR HYPERPLASIA
WITH MARKED ADRENAL
ENLARGEMENT

Transverse sections show marked
nodularity throughout most of the
adrenal gland. There is asymmetric
nodular hyperplasia, with the left gland
larger than the right.

Figure 4-71

MACRONODULAR HYPERPLASIA
WITH MARKED ADRENAL
ENLARGEMENT

This histologic section accentuates the
nodules and the distortion of the gland.

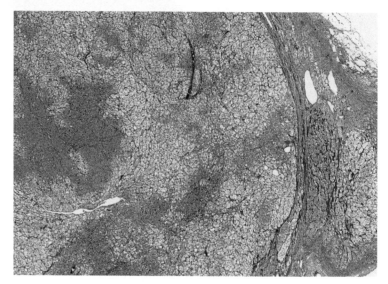

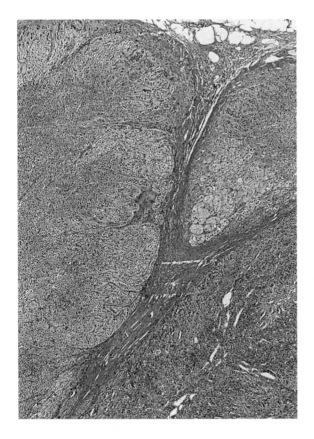

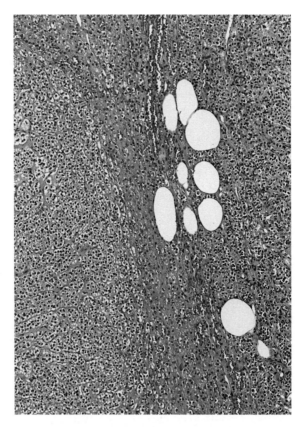

Figure 4-72

MACRONODULAR HYPERPLASIA
WITH MARKED ADRENAL ENLARGEMENT

The nodules are composed of lipid-rich fasciculata-type
cells and some lipid-depleted cells.

Figure 4-73

MACRONODULAR HYPERPLASIA
WITH MARKED ADRENAL ENLARGEMENT

There is atrophy between the lipid-rich nodules. Fatty
metaplasia is also present focally, which is usually associated
with hyperactivity.

General Remarks. The etiology of this disorder is unknown. It can occur in a familial form
that is inherited as an autosomal dominant trait
and associated with Carney's complex (pigmented lentigenes; blue nevi of the face, lips,
trunk, and other sites; atrial and cutaneous myxomas) (306,307,310–312,321). Patients with the
nonfamilial sporadic form of primary pigmented nodular adrenocortical disease (PPNAD)
are young (always less than 30 years of age) and
may be infants (307,313). The familial form of
the disorder has been linked to the short arm
of chromosome 2 (2p16) (318).

Carney's Complex. This complex consists
of myxomas, spotty pigmentation, and endocrine overactivity (307,321). The abnormalities
in decreasing frequency include: cutaneous abnormalities (80 percent) with lentigenes, ephelides (fig. 4-74), blue nevi and cutaneous myxomas; cardiac myomas (72 percent) including multiple myxomas; primary pigmented nodular
adrenocortisol disease (45 percent); testicular
tumors (56 percent) including Leydig cell tumor and Leydig cell calcifying Sertoli cell tumor;
mammary myxoid fibroadenoma in females (42
percent); pituitary macroadenoma (10 percent);
uterine myxomas in females (8 percent); oral
cavity myxomas (8 percent); and psammoma-
tous melanotic schwannoma (5 percent).

The complex has been designated by other
investigators with acronyms like the *LAMB syndrome* (lentigines, atrial myxomas, mucocutaneous myxomas, blue nevi) (314) and the
NAME syndrome (nevi, atrial myxomas, myxoid

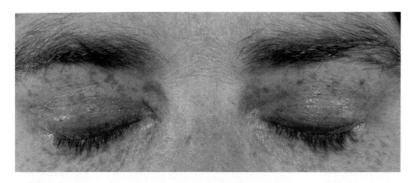

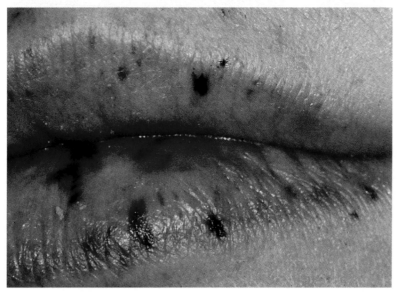

Figure 4-74

CARNEY'S COMPLEX

Top: A 38-year-old woman with the findings of Carney's complex: central facial lentigines and Cushing's syndrome due to primary pigmented nodular adrenal disease.

Bottom: Lentigines on the vermilion borders of the lips in a 19-year-old woman with Carney's complex. Her initial presentation was at age 17 with an embolic stroke associated with multiple cardiac myxomas (3 in left ventricle, 1 in left atrium, and 2 in right ventricle).

neurofibroma, ephelides) (305) or the *Swiss syndrome* (310). However, Carney's complex is the currently used designation (307,321). In addition to the other health risks for patients with Cushing's syndrome, the presence of atrial myxomas in multiple locations can be life threatening.

Clinical and Radiologic Findings. In the sporadic form of PPNAD, the median time from manifestation of symptoms until diagnosis is 1 year, but intervals of up to 18 years have been noted (319). PPNAD is associated with Cushing's syndrome in 32 percent of patients with Carney's complex. Clinically evident Cushing's syndrome is present in 84 percent of patients with PPNAD, while 6 percent have only biochemical evidence of adrenocortical autonomy (subclinical PPNAD), and 10 percent have latent PPNAD without a firm diagnosis.

Patients with Cushing's syndrome usually present during the second decade of life (317, 321). Short stature due to stunted growth occurs in about a third of patients due to the early onset of hypercortisolism. Radiologic examination shows normal adrenal glands in about half the cases. Adrenal macronodules may be detected radiologically. ^{131}I-iodomethyl-19-norcholesterol scans may show bilateral adrenal nuclide uptake which assists in the diagnosis (308).

Laboratory Findings. Plasma cortisol is usually moderately elevated but without a diurnal rhythm. Plasma ACTH is low or undetectable, and steroid production may be irregular or cyclic. The hypercortisolism is resistant to dexamethasone suppression, metyrapone stimulation, and corticotropin-releasing hormone stimulation.

Macroscopic Findings. The size of the adrenal glands is quite variable and ranges from 0.9 to 13.4 g, with an average of 4.0 g, which is within normal limits in an adult. The average

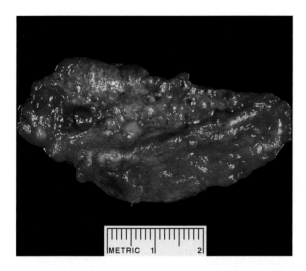

Figure 4-75

PRIMARY PIGMENTED NODULAR
ADRENOCORTICAL DISEASE

Pigmented black nodules are present over the dorsal surface of the adrenal glands.

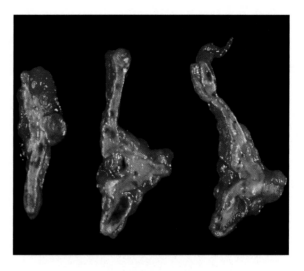

Figure 4-76

PRIMARY PIGMENTED NODULAR
ADRENOCORTICAL DISEASE

Transverse sections of the adrenal gland show pigmented micronodules, many of which are in the inner cortex.

combined weight is 9.6 g. The surface has scattered pigmented nodules ranging from 1 to 4 mm in diameter (figs. 4-75, 4-76). A wide range in the size and distribution of pigmented nodules is noted. Nodules are commonly black, but some may be tan or yellow. A few macronodules up to 3 cm in diameter may be present, and some of these may not be pigmented.

Microscopic Findings. The nodules are round to oval or irregularly shaped, and unencapsulated (figs. 4-77–4-80). Many nodules abut on the corticomedullary junction, extend into the periadrenal fat, or involve the entire thickness of the cortex. The intranodular cells are usually compact and eosinophilic. Larger vacuolated or balloon cells are often seen in the nodules.

The frequent lipomatous or myelolipomatous change may be associated with increased activity of the glands with Cushing's syndrome. Lymphocytic infiltrates of mixed, cytotoxic, and T-helper cells (319) are often present. Occasional binucleated or multinucleated cells are seen, but mitoses are uncommon.

Immunohistochemical Findings. Studies by Sasano et al. (304,316) with antibodies to steroid metabolizing enzymes showed a marked increase in immunoreactivity in the nodules, suggesting increased glucocorticoid synthesis. This may explain in part the Cushing's syndrome ob-

served with these relatively small adrenal glands and the adjacent areas of atrophy.

Ultrastructural Findings. Adrenal cortical cells with ultrastructural features of zona reticularis–type cells are admixed with zona fasciculata–type cells. Both types contain abundant lipofuscin-type bodies, which would explain the dark pigment noted grossly and microscopically (fig. 4-81) (320).

Differential Diagnosis. The findings in PPNAD are relatively pathognomonic. One source of potential confusion is a metastatic malignant melanoma, especially if both adrenal glands are involved. If necessary, immunohistochemical staining for S100 protein and HMB45 can readily separate these two diseases.

Myelolipomatous metaplasia with metaplastic fat and hematopoietic precursors can be seen in the adrenal glands of patients with Carney's complex, but are also seen in cases of ACTH-dependent and -independent Cushing's syndrome, suggesting that these changes may be dependent on increased glucocorticoid activity (figs. 4-82, 4-83). Myelolipomatous change should be distinguished from myelolipomas which consist of tumefactive masses of myeloid and fat cells occurring in varying proportions (fig. 4-84). Myelolipomas are not associated with increased glucocorticoid production.

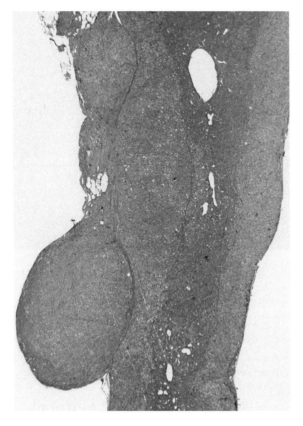

Figure 4-77

PRIMARY PIGMENTED NODULAR
ADRENOCORTICAL DISEASE

Cut section through the body of the adrenal gland
shows well-defined micronodules.

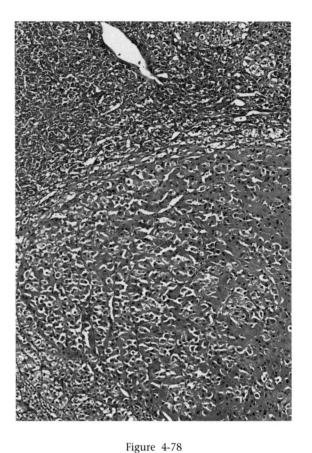

Figure 4-78

PRIMARY PIGMENTED NODULAR
ADRENOCORTICAL DISEASE

Histologic section shows micronodules adjacent to the
adrenal medulla.

Figure 4-79

PRIMARY PIGMENTED NODULAR
ADRENOCORTICAL DISEASE

Higher magnification of a micronodule composed of cells with
abundant eosinophilic cytoplasm and
pleomorphic nuclei.

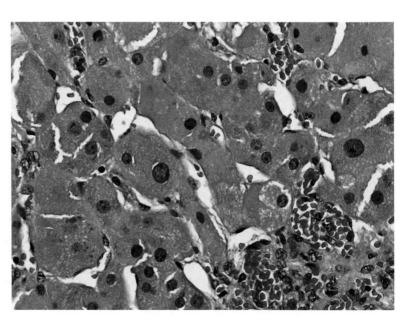

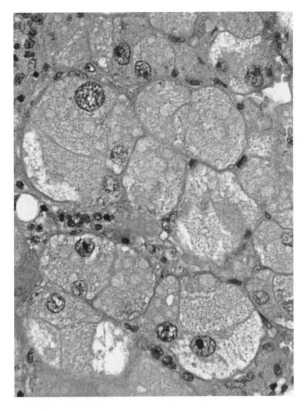

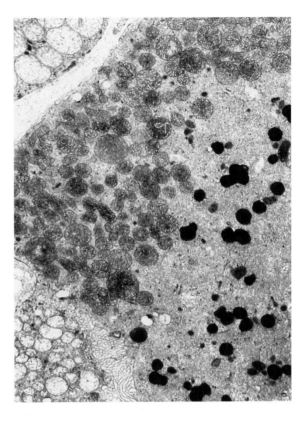

Figure 4-80

PRIMARY PIGMENTED NODULAR
ADRENOCORTICAL DISEASE

The pigmented nodule cells have pleomorphic nuclei and prominent nucleoli. The cells are reminiscent of zona reticularis-type cells but do not contain lipofuscin pigment.

Figure 4-81

PRIMARY PIGMENTED NODULAR
ADRENOCORTICAL DISEASE

Ultrastructural examination of the pigmented nodule cell shows abundant lipofuscin in the cytoplasm along with mitochondria with tubular-vesicular cristae similar to the cells of the zona reticularis (X5,000).

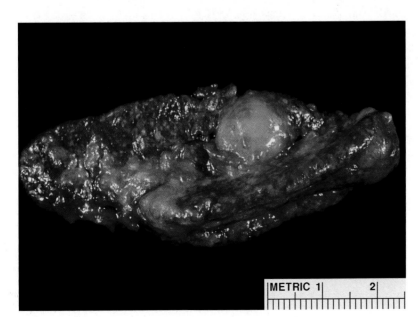

Figure 4-82

DIFFUSE HYPERPLASIA WITH
MYELOLIPOMATOUS METAPLASIA

An adrenal gland from a patient with diffuse cortical hyperplasia shows a yellow nodule of myelolipomatous metaplasia.

Figure 4-83

DIFFUSE HYPERPLASIA WITH MYELOLIPOMATOUS METAPLASIA

A histologic section of an adrenal gland with diffuse hyperplasia and myelolipomatous metaplasia. The mature adipose tissue and hemato-poietic precursor cells are associated with increased adrenocortical activity.

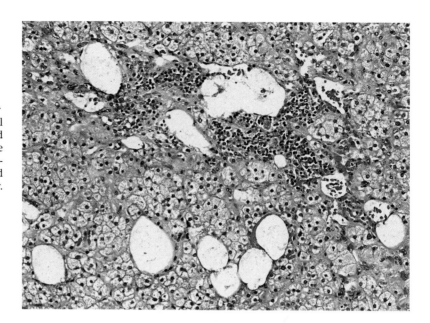

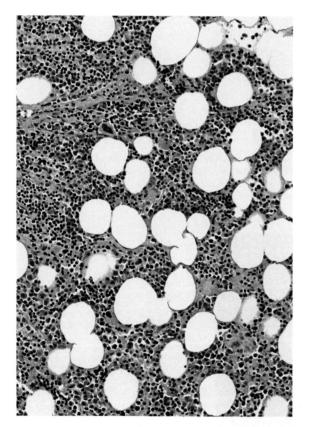

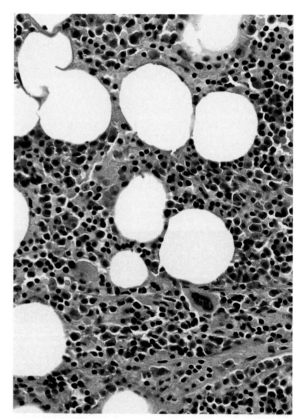

Figure 4-84

MYELOLIPOMA

Left: Myelolipoma is a tumor-like condition, developing commonly in the adrenal gland. It is composed of mature adipose tissue and hematopoietic precursor cells.

Right: Myelolipoma with hematopoietic precursor cells including megakaryocytes.

Treatment and Prognosis. Bilateral adrenalectomy is the treatment of choice for patients with PPNAD (309). Unilateral adrenalectomy can lead to recurrence of Cushing's syndrome (307) even many decades after treatment (315).

Aldosterone Excess Due to Adrenocortical Hyperplasia

Definition. This hyperplasia of the zona glomerulosa is associated with excessive production of aldosterone and low levels of plasma renin.

General Remarks. Although the pathogenesis of zona glomerulosa hyperplasia is uncertain, possible causes include other products from the pro-opiomelanocortin (POMC) gene including α-MSH, β-MSH, and β-endorphin (325, 331). There are some differences between hyperaldosteronism related to hyperplasia and that related to true adenomas, i.e., aldosterone levels are generally lower, and the hypokalemia and suppression of renin are not as severe in the former (322,329). The hypertension caused by bilateral hyperplasia is usually not cured by total bilateral adrenalectomy and should be treated medically (329). One type of bilateral adrenal hyperplasia has been described as primary hyperplasia, because unilateral or subtotal (75 percent) adrenalectomy results in permanent cure (325). Approximately 60 percent of cases of primary hyperaldosteronism are idiopathic and result in bilateral hyperplasia of the zona glomerulosa (334)

Secondary hyperaldosteronism results from activation of the renin-angiotensin system and increased secretion of aldosterone in response to increased levels of circulating renin and angiotensin, which are secondary to extraadrenal disease. Etiologies include hyperthyroidism, renal artery stenosis, and malignant hypertension. Patients have a low plasma sodium level, hyperplasia of the renal juxtaglomerular apparatus associated with renin, and increase in the width of the zona glomerulosa (330).

Tertiary aldosteronism (*Bartter's syndrome*) describes a disorder associated with elevated plasma renin, angiotensin II, and aldosterone. Patients may present in infancy or during adult life. Some cases are inherited as an autosomal recessive condition. It is not associated with hypertension (324). The adrenal changes in tertiary aldosteronism are not well characterized. Cases in which bilateral adrenalectomy was performed to control the hypokalemia show grossly normal adrenal glands and biopsy specimens reportedly show hyperplasia of the zona glomerulosa (323).

Clinical and Radiologic Findings. Clinical signs and symptoms include hypertension, spontaneous hypokalemia, frontal headache, muscular weakness, and flaccid paralysis caused by hypokalemia. The peak incidence is from 30 to 50 years of age. The screening test for primary aldosteronism is the activity ratio of plasma aldosterone to plasma renin. Primary aldosteronism is confirmed by a lack of suppression of aldosterone with volume expansion. High resolution CT can detect nodules as small as 5 mm in diameter (326). These nodules may be difficult to distinguish from small adenomas (fig. 4-85) (333).

Macroscopic Findings. The gross features of the adrenal glands are quite variable. They may be of normal size, weight, and appearance; less than normal weight; or of increased size and weight. Macronodular glands have nodules between 0.25 to 1.0 cm in diameter but may be up to 3.0 cm. Cut sections show yellow nodules intraglandularly and intracortically (fig. 4-86), including adjacent to the central vein. Larger nodules may be present at one pole or within the gland. Although the macronodules are usually multiple, a few may be single and simulate an adenoma (fig. 4-86).

Microscopic Findings. The most common findings are hyperplasia of the zona glomerulosa and micronodules (figs. 4-87, 4-88). The hyperplastic changes may be focal, so many sections are needed to make the correct diagnosis (327,328).

In patients treated with spironolactone, spironolactone bodies may be seen in the cells of the zona glomerulosa as well as in the zona fasciculata (fig. 4-89). Intermediate-type cells with eosinophilic and lipid-containing cytoplasm may be present below the hyperplastic zona glomerulosa. Columns of these cells extend through the fasciculata to the reticularis.

Differential Diagnosis. Distinguishing between adenomas and nodular hyperplasia may be very difficult. The presence of one nodule usually indicates an adenoma, which is often unilateral. Nodular hyperplasia is usually a bilateral disorder.

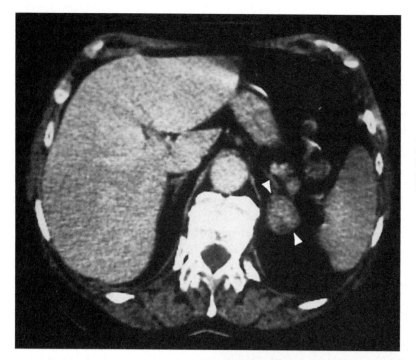

Figure 4-85

ADRENAL ALDOSTERONOMA

Contrast-enhanced CT scan of the abdomen shows a left adrenal aldosteronoma as a small low density mass. It may be difficult to distinguish an aldosteronoma from nodular hyperplasia with a dominant nodule.

Figure 4-86

ZONA GLOMERULOSA NODULAR HYPERPLASIA

Gross photograph of nodular hyperplasia in a patient with primary hyperaldosteronism shows a dominant pale yellow cortical nodule and several other smaller nodules.

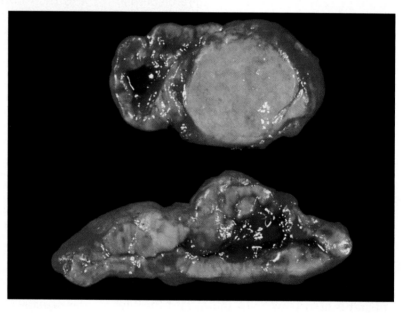

Treatment and Prognosis. The prognosis of patients with adenomas treated by unilateral adrenalectomy is usually much better than that for patients with hyperplasia. After adrenalectomy, 90 percent of patients with aldosterone excess and 50 percent of patients with long-term hypertension are cured. Some patients with primary bilateral hyperplasia may be treated with subtotal adrenalectomy. Laparoscopic adrenalectomy should be considered in patients with a unilateral hypodense macroadenoma detected on CT. In many cases, however, adrenal venous sampling is required to distinguish between unilateral and bilateral disease (332).

Medical therapy is usually indicated for patients with bilateral adrenal hyperplasia. Spironolactone and an additional antihypertensive agent are used for these patients. Amiloride,

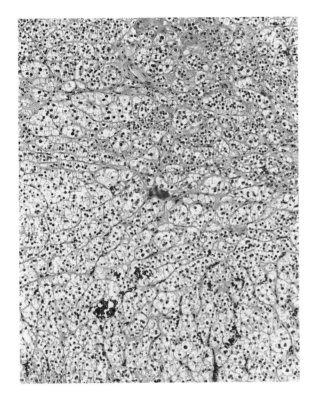

Figure 4-87

ZONA GLOMERULOSA NODULAR HYPERPLASIA

The histologic view shows diffusely hyperplastic glomerulosa- and fasciculata-type cells.

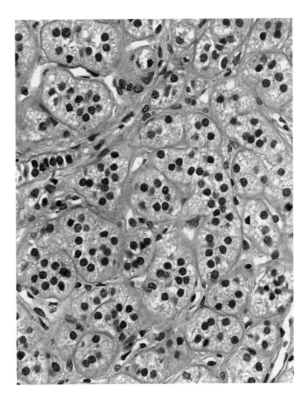

Figure 4-88

ZONA GLOMERULOSA HYPERPLASIA

The hyperplastic cells are arranged in nests and cords with a transition between glomerulosa- and fasciculata- or "hybrid-" type cells.

which is an inhibitor of distal tubular sodium transport, has been used in hyperaldosteronism, but does not usually control blood pressure in patients with hyperplasia (329).

Unilateral Adrenal Cortical Hyperplasia

There are a few reported cases of unilateral adrenal cortical hyperplasia in patients with Cushing's syndrome or with hyperaldosteronism (335–340). This disorder is extremely uncommon, and the possibility of bilateral disease with only a few microscopic nodules involving the other adrenal gland in an ACTH-independent manner must always be excluded. When unilateral nodular hyperplasia is diagnosed in the presence of low plasma ACTH levels, the most likely diagnosis is an adenoma (337,338). Careful examination of the attached adrenal tissue and contralateral adrenal gland for evidence of atrophy can usually help to determine if there is a functional

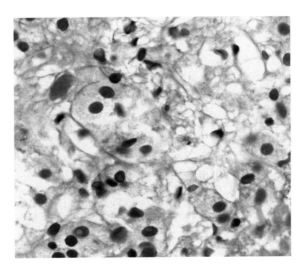

Figure 4-89

ZONA GLOMERULOSA HYPERPLASIA

A spironolactone body is seen as an eosinophilic inclusion in a patient treated with spironolactone before surgery.

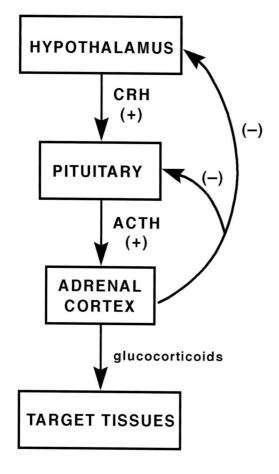

Figure 4-90

HYPOTHALAMIC-PITUITARY-ADRENAL AXIS

The schematic diagram shows the consequences of decreased cortisol production due to an enzyme deficit in the regulation of the hypothalamic-pituitary-adrenal axis. Increased production of pituitary ACTH leads to bilateral adrenal cortical hyperplasia.

adenoma. The periodic production of ACTH by some pituitary and ectopic tumors may cause a cyclically functional tumor to be missed. An exception to the existence of unilateral hyperplasia occurs when ectopic ACTH production and inhibition of pituitary ACTH production, due to a metastasis to one adrenal gland, results in atrophy of the contralateral adrenal gland (340).

Congenital Adrenal Hyperplasia

Definition. These are syndromes associated with adrenocortical hyperplasia caused by inherited defects in cortisol biosynthesis.

General Remarks. Various enzymes in adrenal steroidogenesis are involved in congenital adrenal hyperplasia. The resultant decrease in cortisol production negatively feeds back on pituitary ACTH secretion, leading to adrenal cortical hyperplasia (fig. 4-90). Although congenital adrenal hyperplasia was first described more than 135 years ago (345), its pathophysiology was uncovered much later (342). These disorders are inherited as an autosomal recessive trait causing inborn errors of metabolism.

The most common cause of congenital adrenal hyperplasia, which occurs in 90 percent of cases, is 21-hydroxylase (CYP21A2) deficiency (344,347,352,353,356,359). It occurs in 1 of 5,000 to 1 of 15,000 live births in most Western populations (350). The microsomal enzyme 21-hydroxylase is responsible for conversion of 17-alpha-hydroxyprogesterone to 11-deoxycortisol; with defects in enzymatic activity, there is decreased cortisol biosynthesis and accumulation of cortisol precursors, which are then converted to adrenal androgens. The gene for CYP21A2 is located in chromosome 6 within the major histocompatibility locus. Genetic alterations include deletions and other gene defects (357).

Deficiency of 11-beta-hydroxylase (CYP11B1) accounts for about 5 percent of adrenal steroidogenic defects and is seen in 1 of 100,000 live births. This deficiency inhibits the conversion of 11-deoxycortisol and deoxycorticosterone to cortisol and corticosteroid, resulting in excessive androgen production and virilization of female fetuses. The disorder is caused by a mutation in the gene on chromosome 8 (361).

Other less common deficiencies include: 17-alpha-hydroxylase (CYP17) deficiency in which many mutations are present in the CYP17 genes; 3-beta-hydroxysteroid dehydrogenase deficiency in which synthesis of all steroid hormone classes are impaired due to a mutation in the hydroxysteroid dehydrogenase 32 gene; and a deficiency of all adrenal and gonadal steroid hormones causing congenital lipoid adrenal hyperplasia, the rarest form of congenital hyperplasia. These patients have low cortisol and aldosterone secretion rates and increased activity of ACTH, follicle-stimulating hormone (FSH), luteinizing hormone (LH), and plasma renin. Multiple genetic mutations are present in a gene on chromosome 8.

Clinical and Radiologic Findings. With 21-hydroxylase deficiency infants or children present with salt wasting, ambiguous genitalia, or hypotension (fig. 4-91). There are elevated adrenal androgens such as dihydroepiandosterone and cortisol precursors. Prenatal diagnosis allows prenatal treatment to prevent marked masculinization of female fetuses (360).

Patients with 11-beta-hydroxylase deficiency present with androgen excess in the neonatal period, leading to ambiguous genitalia and later on to hypertension. In contrast, 17-alpha-hydroxylase deficiency is diagnosed at the time of puberty because of hypertension, hypokalemia, and hypogonadism. Females usually have primary amenorrhea and absent secondary sexual characteristics, while males have pseudohermaphrodism with female external genitalia and intra-abdominal testes (355). Patients with 17-alpha-hydroxylase deficiency have increased levels of corticosteroid and deoxycorticosteroid. Patients with 3-beta-hydroxysteroid dehydrogenase deficiency present in early infancy with adrenal insufficiency, varying degrees of virilization in females, and problems with genital development. With congenital lipoid adrenal hyperplasia, patients have severe adrenal insufficiency during the neonatal period with hyponatremia, hypokalemia, vomiting, and diarrhea.

Radiologic studies show enlarged adrenal glands. High resolution CT scans and MRI studies can detect even slightly enlarged glands in patients with the milder forms of congenital adrenal hyperplasia (341,351).

Laboratory Findings. Patients with 21-hydroxylase deficiency have elevated plasma levels of ACTH and adrenal androgens including dihydroepiandosterone and androstenedione. Patients with 11-beta-hydroxylase deficiency also have increased adrenal androgens. With 17-alpha-hydroxylase deficiency, there are increased plasma levels of corticosteroid and deoxycorticosteroid and decreased levels of cortisol, adrenal androgens, and gonadal steroids (358).

Macroscopic Findings. Most of the histologic studies of adrenal glands of patients with congenital adrenal hyperplasia have come from those with 21-hydroxylase deficiency, since these patients constitute 90 to 95 percent of those with congenital adrenal hyperplasia. The mean weight of the adrenal gland at autopsy in

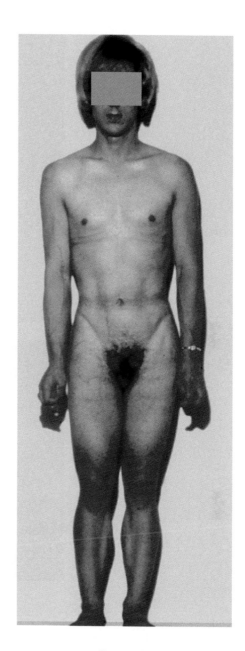

Figure 4-91

CONGENITAL ADRENAL HYPERPLASIA

A 21-year-old genetic female with 21-hydroxylase deficiency. Male body habitus and virilization are shown.

untreated children is 15 g compared to the normal 1 to 4 g seen from the neonatal period to age 12. Single gland weight may reach as much as 30 g. The gland has a cerebriform convoluted appearance (fig. 4-92). The cut surface is dusky brown and irregular.

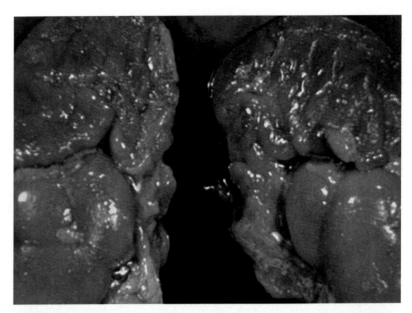

Figure 4-92

CONGENITAL ADRENAL
HYPERPLASIA

Top: The marked enlargement of
the adrenal glands due to 21-hydroxy-
lase deficiency gives the glands a
cerebriform appearance.

Bottom: Resected adrenal glands
from a patient with congenital hyperplasia secondary to 21-hydroxylase
deficiency weigh 11 g (left gland) and
14 g (right gland).

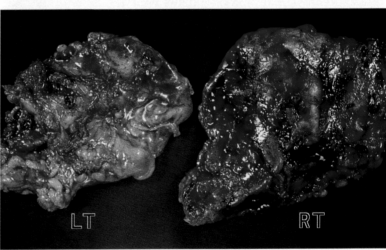

Microscopic Findings. In older children
and adults, the cortex consists of compact cells,
some of which contain lipofuscin granules, and
extends from the medulla to the zona
glomerulosa (figs. 4-93, 4-94). A thin layer of clear
cells from the outer zona fasciculata is usually
next to the zona glomerulosa. In children, the
zona glomerulosa is often hyperplastic, especially
when the enzyme defect leads to decreased aldosterone secretion and the renin-angiotensin
system is activated (354). Hyperplasia of the zona
glomerulosa is not prominent in cases of 11-
hydroxylase deficiency, although the remainder of the gland may be enlarged.

Glands from neonates and infants usually
have a hyperplastic definitive zone consisting
of compact cells with lipid-poor eosinophilic
cytoplasm. In addition, these glands also show
the predictable degeneration and involution of
the fetal zone.

**Testicular Involvement with 21-Hy-
droxylase Deficiency.** Patients with congenital adrenal hyperplasia usually have hyperplasia of testicular hilar cells and extratesticular
Leydig cells (figs. 4-95, 4-96) (343,346,348–
350). The cell of origin of these nodules is uncertain, but they have been shown to be dependent on ACTH for growth, and cases of malignant

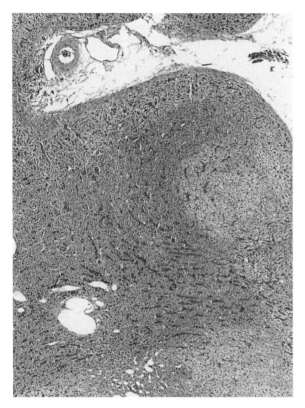

Figure 4-93

CONGENITAL ADRENAL HYPERPLASIA

The diffuse enlargement of the cortex is predominantly of compact cells, with focal areas of lipid-rich clear cells.

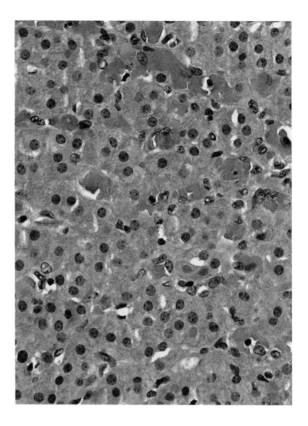

Figure 4-94

CONGENITAL ADRENAL HYPERPLASIA

Diffuse hyperplasia of the adrenal cortex with a predominance of compact cells.

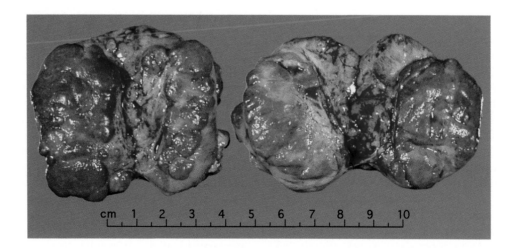

Figure 4-95

BILATERAL ORCHIECTOMY SPECIMENS FROM A 25-YEAR-OLD MALE WITH
SALT-LOSING FORM OF 21-HYDROXYLASE DEFICIENCY

Both testes on cross section are almost completely replaced by bulging nodules of tan tumor. The testicular tumor was shown to be ACTH dependent. (Fig. 2-13 from Fascicle 19, 3rd Series.)

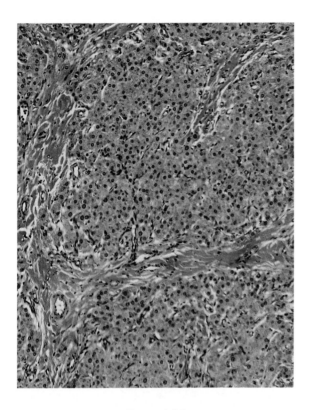

Figure 4-96

TESTICULAR TUMOR IN PATIENT
WITH SALT-LOSING FORM OF
21-HYDROXYLASE DEFICIENCY

The tumor cells grow in lobules and solid sheets with some intervening fibrous stroma. (Fig. 2-14 left, from Fascicle 19, 3rd Series.)

tumors with metastases have not been reported (350), suggesting that they represent hyperplastic foci. A striking difference between these lesions and true Leydig cell tumors is that the Reinke crystalloids seen in up to 35 percent of Leydig cell tumors (348) are not present in testicular tumors arising in patients with congenital adrenal hyperplasia.

Differential Diagnosis. The diagnosis of congenital adrenal hyperplasia is usually made clinically. In a few instances, if a clinical history is not available, the histopathologic appearance of the glands may be confused with bilateral hyperplasia secondary to ectopic ACTH production. The cerebriform appearance of the glands is more in keeping with congenital adrenal hyperplasia. Both disorders have prominent compact cells extending from the medulla to the zona glomerulosa. However, foci of clear cells are more commonly seen in ectopic ACTH hyperplasia. The presence of microscopic deposits of metastatic carcinoma in ectopic ACTH hyperplasia can help to confirm that diagnosis.

Treatment and Prognosis. Patients with 21-hydroxylase deficiency are treated by replacement of glucocorticoids and mineralocorticoids, suppressing ACTH secretion and the hyperandrogenemia and allowing normal growth and skeletal maturation. Reconstructive surgery is usually required for females with ambiguous genitalia. Once the diagnosis is established, initiation of treatment in utero by second-trimester amniocentesis or chorionic villi biopsy at 8 to 10 weeks is effective (358). The prognosis is good with treatment (358). Reproductive function in women is impaired in untreated cases. Strict adherence to glucocorticoid therapy can correct the dysregulation of cyclic ovulatory function.

Treatment of 11-beta-hydroxylase deficiency is by replacement of glucocorticoids. Genital malformation in females must be surgically corrected. 17-beta-hydroxylase and 3-beta-hydroxysteroid dehydrogenase deficiencies are also treated by replacement therapy.

Most patients with congenital lipoid adrenal hyperplasia do not survive infancy, but the glucocorticoid and mineralocorticoid deficiencies in some survivors have been successfully treated by replacement therapy (358).

Beckwith-Wiedemann Syndrome

Definition. Beckwith-Wiedemann syndrome is a complex disorder that is manifested by visceromegaly, gigantism, macroglossia, abdominal wall defects, craniofacial abnormalities, midfacial hypoplasia, and adrenal cortical hyperplasia. This syndrome is also referred to as the *exophthalmus, macroglossia, gigantism syndrome.*

General Remarks. The estimated frequency is 1 in 13,000 births (364). Most cases are sporadic, while a small percentage are part of a familial syndrome. The complication of hypoglycemia can lead to brain damage with mental retardation or even death (366). A small percentage of children with the syndrome develop malignant tumors which include nephroblastoma (Wilm's tumor), adrenal cortical carcinoma, neuroblastoma, pancreatoblastoma, and pheochromocytoma. The genetic abnormality associated with adrenal cortical neoplasia has been

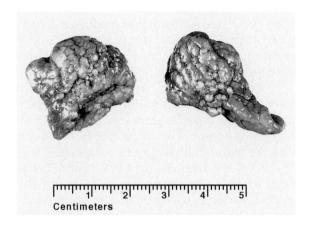

Figure 4-97

BECKWITH-WIEDEMANN SYNDROME

Adrenal glands from a 3-week-old infant with Beckwith-Wiedemann syndrome showing enlargement of both glands with excessive cortical nodularity and redundant folds on the external aspect. (Fig. 2-20 left, from Fascicle 19, 3rd Series.)

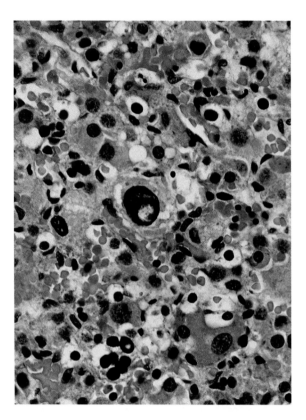

Figure 4-98

BECKWITH-WIEDEMANN SYNDROME

There is marked adrenal cytomegaly with nuclear enlargement and hyperchromasia. A nuclear "pseudo-inclusion" is near the center of the field. Mitotic figures were not identified. (Fig. 2-21 right, from Fascicle 19, 3rd Series.)

mapped to chromosome 11p15.5 (363). Mice lacking the cyclin-dependent kinase inhibitor p57^{kip2}, which is located on chromosome 11p15, develop abdominal muscle defects, renal medullary dysplasia, adrenal cortical hyperplasia, and cytomegaly. Since these phenotypes are seen in patients with Beckwith-Wiedemann syndrome, loss of p57^{kip2} expression may play an important role in this syndrome (367).

Macroscopic Findings. The adrenal glands are enlarged and have a combined weight of up to 16 g. They are nodular and may have a cerebriform appearance (364).

Microscopic Findings. Adrenal cortical cytomegaly involving both adrenal glands, usually in the fetal cortex, is a common finding. The nuclei are large and pleomorphic, and cytoplasmic nuclear pseudoinclusions are present (figs. 4-97, 4-98). There may be hemorrhagic macrocysts (365,366). The chromaffin cells are also hyperplastic in the gland and at extra-adrenal sites (362,364).

ADRENAL MEDULLARY HYPERPLASIA

Definition. This is an increase in the mass of the adrenal medullary cells and expansion of these cells into areas of the gland where they are not normally present, such as the tail.

General Remarks. The adrenal medulla normally comprises about 10 percent of the adrenal volume (377). This percentage is increased in sporadic and familial medullary hyperplasia. Sporadic medullary hyperplasia may develop in different settings (Table 4-4). Patients with cystic fibrosis and elevated catecholamine levels have been reported to have adrenal medullary hyperplasia (371). Some infants dying of sudden infant death syndrome (SIDS) have been reported to have adrenal medullary hyperplasia (388). Medullary hyperplasia has been associated with Cushing's syndrome in which the patient also had an adrenal cortical adenoma (388), and has been postulated as a cause of hypertension in young patients (370). The sporadic form of Beckwith-Wiedemann syndrome, which includes most cases of this disorder, has

Table 4-4

CAUSES OF AND CONDITIONS ASSOCIATED WITH ADRENAL MEDULLARY HYPERPLASIA

Sporadic
Cystic fibrosis
Sudden infant death syndrome
Beckwith-Wiedemann syndrome
Idiopathic

Familial
Multiple endocrine neoplasia 2a
Multiple endocrine neoplasia 2b
Familial Beckwith-Wiedemann syndrome
Von Hippel-Lindau disease
Neurofibromatosis (von Recklinghausen's disease)

been associated with adrenal medullary hyperplasia (368,369). Other unusual causes of sporadic adrenal medullary hyperplasia have also been reported (376,404,405,407).

Familial medullary hyperplasia is most commonly associated with multiple endocrine neoplasia (MEN) types 2a and 2b (Tables 4-4–4-6). MEN 2a is inherited as an autosomal dominant disorder with a high degree of penetrance (381, 382,391–393). The gene for MEN 2a and 2b has been localized to chromosome 10q, and the molecular defect involves an activating mutation of the tyrosine kinase receptor (379,384, 387). While the thyroid C cells and adrenal medullary cells are involved in both MEN 2a and 2b, parathyroid hyperplasia/adenoma is usually associated with MEN 2a while mucosal neuromas and ganglioneuromas are associated only with MEN 2b (401,403). MEN 2b is also inherited in

Table 4-5

MULTIPLE ENDOCRINE NEOPLASIA SYNDROME

Syndrome	Chromosome Location	Gene	Abnormality
MEN 1	11q	Menin	Tumor suppressor gene
MEN 2a	10q	RET proto-oncogene	Activating mutation of tyrosine kinase receptor
MEN 2b	10q	RET proto-oncogene	Activating mutation of tyrosine kinase receptor

Table 4-6

MULTIPLE ENDOCRINE NEOPLASIA SYNDROME

Abnormality	MEN 1	MEN 2a	MEN 2b
Pituitary tumors	+		
Parathyroid hyperplasia/adenoma	+	+	
Pancreatic hyperplasia/adenoma	+		
Carcinoid tumors	±		
C-cell hyperplasia/medullary thyroid carcinomas		+	+
Adrenal medullary hyperplasia/pheochromocytoma		+	+
Mucosal neuromas			+
Ganglioneuromas			+

an autosomal dominant mode of inheritance, but sporadic development of this disorder is more common than with MEN 2a (372,389).

Analysis of the specific mutations of the RET proto-oncogene in medullary carcinoma of the thyroid in patients with MEN 2a, MEN 2b familial medullary thyroid carcinoma (C-cell tumors not associated with the other stigmata of MEN 2a or 2b), and sporadic medullary thyroid carcinoma has provided insight into the relationship of these conditions with respect to the location of the mutations. Exon 10 mutations of the RET proto-oncogene are most common in both MEN 2a and familial medullary carcinoma. Mutations in MEN 2a occur in exon 11. Exon 15 mutations of RET proto-oncogenes are most common in MEN 2b and in sporadic medullary thyroid carcinoma (380).

Proliferative lesions of the adrenal medulla have been studied in experimental models, especially in rats (395–399,402). Specific drugs such as nicotine, hormones such as estrogen and growth hormone, and physical agents such as radiation can lead to diffuse and nodular medullary hyperplasia. Some species of rats have a greater propensity to develop medullary hyperplasia than others, with Wistar rats showing the highest prevalence (396). As in humans, it may be difficult to distinguish between medullary hyperplasia and pheochromocytoma in rats (399).

Clinical and Radiologic Findings. The clinical features of patients with pheochromocytoma are well defined, while those of adrenal medullary hyperplasia are less clear, except in patients with familial diseases such as MEN 2a and 2b. The most common findings in patients with pheochromocytoma are headaches (80 percent), excessive perspiration (71 percent), palpitation with or without tachycardia (64 percent), pallor (42 percent), followed by nausea, tremor, weakness, and exhaustion (394). Some of these signs and symptoms may be present in patients with familial adrenal medullary hyperplasia, especially those with larger nodules approaching the size of true pheochromocytomas; however, it is often difficult to make the distinction between small pheochromocytomas and extensive nodular medullary hyperplasia with familial disease (374,375,400).

Radiologic studies of both adrenal medullary hyperplasia and pheochromocytoma have been enhanced by radionuclide scanning with iodinated meta-iodobenzylguanidine (MIBG) (386,406). CT and MRI are also very useful techniques since nodular hyperplasia can be readily detected, especially by high resolution MRI. The localization technique should be done after biochemical diagnosis of the hyperplasia or pheochromocytoma (390). When evaluating a patient with previous surgery, MIBG scintigraphy is the preferred technique, since it is more sensitive than CT and is as sensitive as MRI but more specific with recurrent disease (386). The diagnosis of medullary hyperplasia may be suggested by the increased concentration of ^{131}I-MIBG in both glands when the abdominal CT is normal (406).

Laboratory Findings. The diagnosis of pheochromocytoma is usually made by demonstrating increased urinary excretion of catecholamines or catecholamine metabolites, including epinephrine, norepinephrine, vanillylmandelic acid (VMA), and metanephrines (Table 4-7). An elevated ratio of epinephrine to norepinephrine in the urine (371,377) and increased levels of tissue epinephrine have been associated with medullary hyperplasia.

Macroscopic Findings. The use of morphometric analysis may be required to diagnose adrenal medullary hyperplasia in subtle cases. Occasionally, the diagnosis is easily made on gross examination of the adrenal glands. Patients with MEN 2a and 2b usually have diffuse or nodular hyperplasia, with multiple nodules involving both adrenal glands (figs. 4-99–4-104). In a study of 19 patients with MEN 2a and 2b, most had bilateral gland involvement with diffuse or nodular hyperplasia, but surprisingly normal glands or unilateral changes were present in some (373, 374,383,385). The nodules and hyperplastic medulla often extend to both alae and the tail of the adrenal gland, a finding that is usually not present in the normal gland. The nodules are gray to tan, and they may compress the adjacent cortex (fig. 4-103). They do not have a capsule. In patients with MEN 2b, these nodules have been shown to be monoclonal (378).

Microscopic Findings. The hyperplastic medullary cells may show various growth patterns: alveolar, trabecular, or solid (figs. 4-101, 4-102). There may be progression from diffuse to nodular hyperplasia, with nodules of varying size evident. Some cases of diffuse hyperplasia may

Table 4-7

NORMAL VALUES FOR ADRENAL HORMONES[a]

Hormone	SI[b]	Conventional
Adrenal cortex steroids, plasma		
Aldosterone, supine, saline suppression	<240 pmol/L	<8.5 ng/dL
Aldosterone, upright, normal diet	140-560 pmol/L	5-20 ng/dL
Cortisol - 8 AM	140-690 nmol/L	5-25 µg/dL
- 4 PM	80-330 nmol/L	3-12 µg/dL
- overnight dexamethasone suppression	<140 nmol/L	<5 µg/dL
Dehydroepiandrosterone (DHEA)	7-31 nmol/L	2-9 µg/dL
Dehydroepiandrosterone sulfate (DHEAS)	1.3-6.8 µmol/L	500-2500 µg/ml
17-hydroxyprogesterone		
Women, follicular phase	0.6-3.0 nmol/L	0.2-1.0 µg/L
Women, luteal phase	1.5-10.6 nmol/L	0.5-3.5 µg/L
Men	1.8-9.0 nmol/L	0.6-3.0 µg/L
Adrenal steroids, urine		
Aldosterone	14-53 nmol/d	5-19 µg/d
Cortisol, free	55-276 nmol/d	20-100 µg/d
17-hydroxycorticosteroid	5.4-27.5 µmol/d	2-10 mg/d
17-ketosteroids		
Men	25-88 µmol/d	7-25 mg/d
Women	14-53 µmol/d	4-16 mg/d
Adrenal medulla catecholamines, urine		
Free catecholamines	<590 nmol/d	<100 µg/d
Epinephrine	<275 nmol/d	<50 µg/d
Metanephrine	<7 µmol/d	<1.3 mg/d
Norepinephrine	89-473 mmol/d	15-89 µg/d
Vanillylmandelic acid (VMA)	<40 µmol/d	<8 mg/d

[a]Wilson JD, Foster DW, Kronenberg DW, Larsen PR, eds. Williams textbook of endocrinology, 9th ed. Philadelphia: WB Saunders, 1998:back cover.

[b]SI - System of international units.

Figure 4-99

ADRENAL MEDULLARY
HYPERPLASIA

Transverse section of an adrenal gland from a patient with MEN 2a showing nodular adrenal medullary hyperplasia.

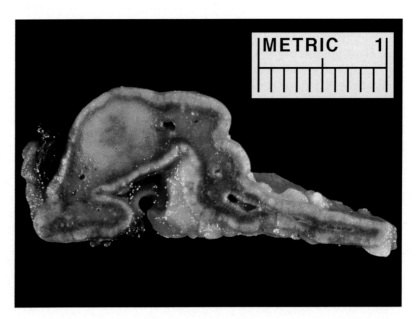

Figure 4-100

ADRENAL MEDULLARY
HYPERPLASIA

Histologic section of an adrenal
gland from an MEN 2a patient showing
several hyperplastic medullary nodules.

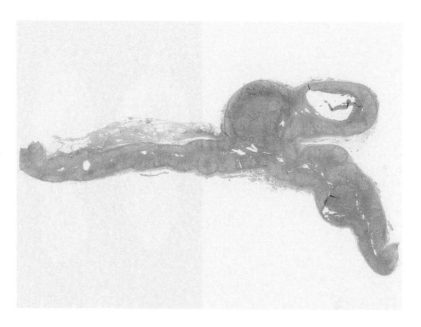

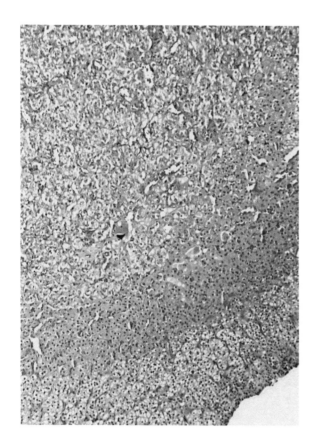

Figure 4-101

ADRENAL MEDULLARY HYPERPLASIA

The hyperplastic medullary cells from a patient with
MEN 2a have abundant cytoplasm.

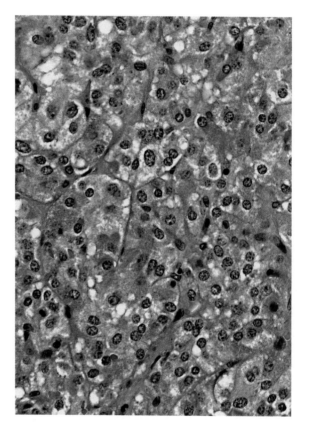

Figure 4-102

ADRENAL MEDULLARY HYPERPLASIA

This adrenal medulla from a MEN 2a patient has cells
with abundant basophilic cytoplasm.

Figure 4-103

ADRENAL MEDULLARY
HYPERPLASIA

This adrenal gland from a patient
with MEN 2a shows a mixed picture of
hyperplastic nodules and early
development of pheochromocytomas.

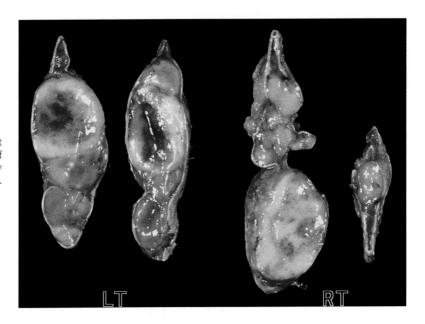

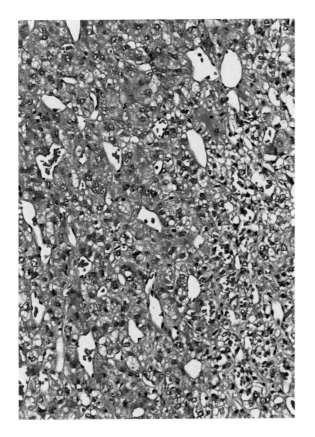 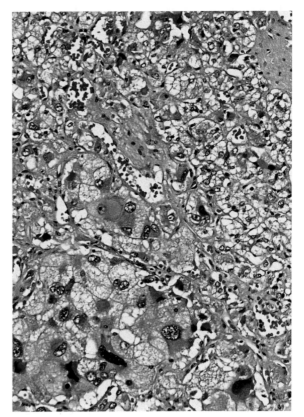

Figure 4-104

ADRENAL MEDULLARY HYPERPLASIA

Left: A mixture of normal and hyperplastic medullary cells are present in a patient with MEN 2a.
Right: Hyperplastic medullary cells with transition to a pheochromocytoma in a patient with MEN 2a.

be very subtle. The presence of medullary tissue in both alae (normally present in only one) or in the tail of the gland (normally present only in the head and body), and a medullary volume greater than the normal 10 percent, point to medullary hyperplasia (377,408). Mixed cell types are common (fig. 4-104). The nodules may show nuclear atypia, but this is not associated with neoplasia or malignancy.

Differential Diagnosis. The distinction between nodular medullary hyperplasia and pheochromocytoma can be difficult. The use of a 1 cm cut-off size to separate nodular hyperplasia from small pheochromocytoma is arbitrary (374), since some pheochromocytomas may be smaller than 1 cm. This is confounded by recent findings that benign adrenal nodules in patients with MEN 2b can be monoclonal (378). It is probably best to consider nodular

hyperplasia and small pheochromocytomas as part of a continuum of the same disease process, especially in patients with MEN 2a and 2b.

The presence of unilateral versus bilateral disease has been suggested as a helpful distinguishing feature. However, unilateral medullary hyperplasia has been reported in isolated as well as familial adrenal medullary hyperplasia (383,385).

Treatment and Prognosis. Bilateral adrenalectomy is the recommended treatment for adrenal medullary hyperplasia (374). Although the prognosis differs for patients with pheochromocytoma with MEN 2a or 2b and sporadic tumors (373,389), there are no data to evaluate these differences. Some patients with von Recklinghausen's disease may have adrenal medullary hyperplasia (407), and these patients are at increased risk for malignant tumors such as malignant nerve sheath tumors.

REFERENCES

Embryology

1. Beckwith JB, Perrin EV. In situ neuroblastomas: a contribution to the natural history of neural crest tumors. Am J Pathol 1963;43:1089–104.

2. Crowder RE. The development of the adrenal gland in man with special reference to origin and ultimate location of cell types and evidence in favor of the "cell migration" theory. Contributions to embryology, vol. 36, publication no. 251. Carnegie Institute of Washington, 1957: 193–210.

3. Elliot TR, Armoy RG. The development of the cortex in the human suprarenal gland and its condition in hemicephaly. J Pathol Bacterial 1911;15:481–8.

4. Neville AM. The adrenal medulla. In: Symington T, ed. Functional pathology of the adrenal gland. Baltimore: Williams & Wilkins, 1969:219–324.

5. Turkel SB, Itabashi HH. The natural history of neuroblastic cells in the fetal adrenal glands. Am J Pathol 1974;76:225–44.

6. Zajicek G, Ariel I, Arber N. The streaming adrenal cortex: direct evidence of centripetal migration of adrenocytes by estimation of cell turnover rate. J Endocr 1986;111:477–82.

Anatomy

7. Bartman J, Driscoll SG. Fetal adrenal cortex in erythroblastosis fetalis. Arch Pathol 1969;87: 343–6.

8. Black J, Williams DI. Natural history of adrenal haemorrhage in the newborn. Arch Dis Child 1973;48:183–90.

9. Bocian-Sobkowska J, Wozniak W, Malendowicz LK. Postnatal involution of the human adrenal fetal zone: stereologic description and apoptosis. Endocrine Res 1998;24:969–73.

10. Carney JA. Adrenal gland. In: Sternberg SS, ed. Histology for pathologist. New York: Raven Press, 1992:321–46.

11. Chester Jones I. The adrenal cortex. Cambridge: University Press, 1957.

12. DeLellis RA, Wolfe HJ, Gagel RF, et al. Adrenal medullary hyperplasia. A morphometric analysis in patients with familial medullary thyroid carcinoma. Am J Pathol 1976;83:177–96.

13. Dhom G. Die Nebennierenriride im kindsalter. Berlin, New York: Springer Verlag, 1965.

14. Dhom G. The prepubertal and pubertal growth of the adrenal (adrenarche). Beitr Pathol 1973;150:357–77.

15. Dhom G, Ross W, Widok K. Die Nebennieren des Feten und des Neugeborenen. Ein quantitative und qualitative Analyze. Beitr Pathol Anat 1958;119:177–216.

16. Dobbie JW, Mackay AM, Symington T. The structure and functional zonation of the human adrenal cortex. Proceedings of the Royal Society of Medicine 1967;60:706.

17. Holmes RO, Moon HD, Rinehart JF. A morphologic study of adrenal glands with correlation of body size and heart size. Am J Pathol 1951;27:724.

18. Lack EE. Tumors of the adrenal gland and extra-adrenal paraganglia. Atlas of Tumor Pathology, 3rd Series, Fascicle 19. Washington, DC: Armed Forces Institute of Pathology, 1997.

19. Lack EE, Kozakewich HP. Embryology, developmental anatomy and selected aspects of non-neoplastic pathology. In: Lack EE, ed. Pathology of the adrenal gland. New York: Churchill, Livingstone 1990:1–74.

20. Mikhail Y, Amin F. Intrinsic innervation of the human adrenal gland. Acta Anat (Basal) 1969;72:25–32.

21. Neville AM, O'Hare MJ. The human adrenal cortex. Pathology and biology—an integrated approach. New York: Springer-Verlag, 1982.

22. Oppenheimer EH. Cyst formation in the outer adrenal cortex. Studies in the human fetus and newborn. Arch Pathol 1969;87:653–9.

23. Quinan C, Berger AA. Observations on human adrenals with especial reference to the relative weight of the normal medulla. Ann Int Med 1933;6:1180–92.

24. Spencer SJ, Mesiano S, Lee JY, Jaffe RB. Proliferation and apoptosis in the human adrenal cortex during the fetal and perinatal periods: implications for growth and remodeling. J Clin Endocrinol Metab 1999;84:1110–5.

25. Symington T. Functional pathology of the human adrenal gland. Edinburgh: Livingstone, 1969.

26. Tahka H. On the weight and structure of the adrenal glands and the factors affecting them in children 0-2 years. Acta Paediatr Scan [Suppl] 1951;81:401–95.

27. Tanimura T, Nelson T, Hollingsworth RR, Shepard TH. Weight standards for organs from early human fetuses. Anat Rec 1971;171:227–36.

Ultrastructure

28. Brown WJ, Barajas L, Latta H. The ultrastructure of the human adrenal medulla with comparative studies of white rat. Anat Rec 1971;169:173–83.

29. Lauriola L, Maggiano N, Sentinelli S, Michetti F, Cocchia D. Satellite cells in the normal human adrenal gland and in pheochromocytomas. Virchows Arch [Cell Pathol] 1985;49:13–21.

30. Long JA, Jones AL. Observations on the fine structure of the adrenal cortex of man. Lab Invest 1967;17:355–70.

31. McNutt NS, Jones AL. Observations on the ultrastructure of cytodifferentiation in the human fetal adrenal cortex. Lab Invest 1970;22:513–27.

32. Tannebaum M. Ultrastructural pathology of the adrenal cortex. Pathol Ann 1973;8:109–56.

Immunohistochemistry and In Situ Hybridization

33. Cocchia D, Michetti F. S-100 antigen in satellite cells of the adrenal medulla and the superior cervical ganglion of the rat. An immunochemical and immunocytochemical study. Cell Tissue Res 1981;215:103–12.

34. Cote RJ, Cordon-Cardo C, Reuter VE, Rosen PP. Immunopathology of adrenal and renal cortical tumors. Coordinated change in antigen expression is associated with neoplastic conversion in the adrenal cortex. Am J Pathol 1990;136:1077–84.

35. Fogt F, Vortmeyer AO, Poremba C, Minda M, Harris CA, Tomaszewski JE. bcl-2 expression in normal adrenal glands and in adrenal neoplasms. Mod Pathol 1998;11:716–20.

36. Gaffey MJ, Traweek ST, Mills SE, et al. Cytokeratin expression in adrenocortical neoplasia: an immunohistochemical and biochemical study with implications for the differential diagnosis of adrenocortical, hepatocellular, and renal cell carcinoma. Hum Pathol 1992;23:144–53.

37. Gonzalez-Hernandez JA, Bornstein SR, Ehrhart-Bornstein M, Späth-Schwalbe E, Jirikowski G, Scherbaum WA. Interleukin-6 messenger ribonucleic acid expression in human adrenal gland in vivo: new clue to a paracrine or autocrine regulation of adrenal function. J Clin Endocrinol Metab 1994;79:1492–7.

38. Guo W, Burris TP, McCabe ER. Expression of the DAX-1, the gene responsible for x-linked adrenal hypoplasia congenita and hypogonadotropic hypogonadism in the hypothalamic-pituitary-adrenal/gonadal axis. Biochem Mol Med 1995;56:8–13.

39. Jungbluth AA, Bunsan KJ, Gerald WL, et al. A103: an anti-melan-A monoclonal antibody for the detection of malignant melanoma in paraffin-embedded tissues. Am J Surg Pathol 1998;22:595–602.

40. Khoury EL, Greenspan JS, Greenspan FS. Adrenocortical cells of the zona reticularis normally express HLA-DR antigenic determinants. Am J Pathol 1987;127:580–91.

41. Lehto VP, Virtanen I, Miettinen M, Dahl D, Kahri A. Neurofilaments in adrenal and extra-adrenal pheochromocytoma. Demonstration using immunofluorescence microscopy. Arch Lab Med Pathol 1983;107:492–4.

42. Lloyd RV, Blaivas M, Wilson BS. Distribution of chromogranin and S-100 protein in normal and abnormal adrenal medullary tissues. Arch Pathol Lab Med 1985;109:633–5.

43. Lloyd RV, Shapiro B, Sisson JC, Kalff V, Thompson NW, Beierwaltes WA. An immunohistochemical study of pheochromocytomas. Arch Pathol Lab Med 1984;108:541–4.

44. Lloyd RV, Sisson JC, Shapiro B, Verhofstad AA. Immunohistochemical localization of epinephrine, norepinephrine, catecholamine-synthesizing enzymes and chromogranin in neuroendocrine cells and tumors. Am J Pathol 1986;125:45–54.

45. McCluggage WG, Burton J, Maxwell P, Sloan JM. Immunohistochemical staining of normal, hyperplastic and neoplastic adrenal cortex with a monoclonal antibody against alpha inhibin. J Clin Pathol 1998;51:114–6.

46. Miettinen M, Lehto VP, Virtanen I. Immunofluorescence microscopic evaluation of the intermediate filament expression of the adrenal cortex and medulla and their tumors. Am J Pathol 1985;118:360–6.

47. Morohashi K, Honda S, Inomata Y, Handa H, Omura T. A common transacting factor, Ad4-binding protein, to the promoters of steroidogenic P-450s. J Biol Chem 1992;267:17913–9.

48. Muscatelli F, Strom TM, Walker AP, et al. Mutations in the DAX-1 gene give rise to both x-linked adrenal hypoplasia congenita and hypogonadotropic hypogonadism. Nature 1994;372:672–6.

49. Pelkey TJ, Frierson HF Jr, Mills SE, Stoler MH. The alpha subunit of inhibin in adrenal cortical neoplasia. Mod Pathol 1998;11:516–24.

50. Sasano H. New approaches in human adrenocortical pathology. Assessment of adrenocortical function in surgical specimen of human adrenal glands. Endocr Pathol 1992;3:4–13.

51. Sasano H, Miyazaki S, Sawai T, et al. Primary pigmented nodular adrenocortical disease (PPNAD): immunohistochemical and in situ hybridization analysis of steroidogenic enzymes in eight cases. Mod Pathol 1992;5:23–9.

52. Sasano H, Nose M, Sasano N. Lectin histochemistry in adrenocortical hyperplasia and neoplasms with emphasis on carcinoma. Arch Pathol Lab Med 1989;113:68–72.

53. Sasano N, Sasano H. The adrenal cortex. In: Kovacs K, Asa SL, eds. Functional endocrine pathology. London: Blackwell Scientific, 1991:546–84.

54. Sasano H, Sasano N, Okamoto M, et al. Immunohistochemical demonstration of adrenodoxin reductase in bovine and human adrenals. Pathol Res Pract 1989;184:473–9.

55. Sasano H, Shizawa S, Suzuki T, et al. Ad4BP in the human adrenal cortex and its disorders. J Clin Endocrinol Metab 1995;80:2378–80.

56. Sasano H, Suzuki T, Nagura H, Nishikawa T. Steroidogenesis in human adrenocortical carcinoma: biochemical activities, immunohistochemistry and in situ hybridization of steroidogenic enzymes and histopathologic study in nine cases. Human Pathol 1993;24:397–404.

57. Sasano H, Suzuki T, Shizawa S, Kato K, Nagura H. Transforming growth factor alpha, epidermal growth factor and epidermal growth factor receptor expression in normal and diseased human adrenal cortex by immunohistochemistry and in situ hybridization. Mod Pathol 1994;7:741–6.

Molecular Biology and Physiology

58. Bohen SP, Kralli A, Yamamoto KR. Hold em and fold em: chaperones and signal transduction. Science 1995;268:1303–4.

59. Lloyd RV, Jin L, Kulig E, Fields K. Molecular approaches for the analysis of chromogranins and secretogranins. Diagn Mol Pathol 1992;1:2–15.

60. Orth DN, Kovacs WJ. The adrenal cortex. In: Wilson JD, Foster DW, Kronenberg HM, Larsen PR, eds. Williams textbook of endocrinology, 9th ed. Philadelphia: WB Saunders, 1998:517–664.

61. Vaughan GM, Becker RA, Allen JP, et al. Cortisol and corticotrophin in burned patients. J Trauma 1982;22:263–72.

62. Yaswen L, Diehl N, Brennan MB, Hochgeschewender U. Obesity in the mouse model of pro-opiomelanocortin deficiency responds to peripheral melanocortin. Nat Med 1999;5:1066–70.

63. Young JB, Landsberg L. Catecholamines and the adrenal medulla. In: Wilson JD, Foster DW, Kronenberg HM, Larsen PR, eds. Williams textbook of endocrinology, 9th ed. Philadelphia: WB Saunders, 1998:665–728.

Reactive, Hereditary, and Developmental Disorders

64. Aimone V, Campagnoli C. Severe adrenal hypoplasia in a live-born normocephalic infant with neurohypophyseal aplasia. Am J Obstet Gynecol 1970;107:327.

65. Ashley DJ, Mostofi FK. Renal agenesis and dysgenesis. J Urology 1960;83:211–8.

66. Aterman K, Kerenyi N, Lee M. Adrenal cytomegaly. Virchows Arch [A] 1972;355:105–22.

67. Carney JA. Unusual tumefactive spindle-cell lesions in the adrenal glands. Hum Pathol 1987;18:980–5.

68. Craig JM, Landing BH. Anaplastic cells of fetal adrenal cortex. Am J Clin Pathol 1951;21:940–9.

69. Favara BE, Steele A, Grant JH, Steele P. Adrenal cytomegaly: quantitative assessment by image analysis. Pediatr Pathol 1991;11:521–36.

70. Fidler WJ. Ovarian thecal metaplasia in adrenal glands. Am J Clin Pathol 1977;67:318–23.

71. Krude H, Biebermann H, Luck W, Horn R, Brabant G, Grüters A. Severe early-onset obesity, adrenal insufficiency and red hair pigmentation caused by POMC mutations in humans. Nat Gen 1998;19:155–7.

72. Lack EE. Tumors of the adrenal gland and extra-adrenal paraganglia. Atlas of Tumor Pathology, 3rd Series, Fascicle 19. Washington, DC: Armed Forces Institute of Pathology, 1997.

73. Moncrieff MW, Hill DS, Archer J, Arthur LJ. Congenital absence of pituitary gland and adrenal hypoplasia. Arch Dis Child 1972;47:136–7.

74. Neville AM, O'Hare MJ. The human adrenal cortex: pathology and biology—an integrated approach. New York: Springer-Verlag, 1982.

75. Orth DN, Kovacs WJ. The adrenal cortex. In: Wilson JD, Foster DM, Kronenberg HM, Larsen PR, eds. Williams textbook of endocrinology, 9th ed. Philadelphia: WB Saunders, 1998:517–664.

76. Osamura RY. Functional prenatal development of anencephalic and normal anterior pituitary glands. In human and experimental animals studied by peroxidase-labeled antibody method. Acta Pathol Jpn 1977;27:495–509.

77. Pakravan P, Kenny FM, Depp R, Allen AC. Familial congenital absence of adrenal glands: evaluation of glucocorticoid, mineralocorticoid and estrogen metabolism in the perinatal period. J Pediatr 1974;84:74–8.

78. Reed RJ, Pabic JT. Nodular hyperplasia of the adrenal cortical blastema. Bull Tulane Univ Med Fac 1967;26:151–7.

79. Rimoin DL, Schimke RN. Genetic disorders of the endocrine glands. St. Louis: CV Mosby Co., 1971:281.

80. Salazar H, MacAulay MA, Charles D, Pardo M. The human hypophysis in anencephaly. I. Ultrastructure of the pars distalis. Arch Pathol 1969;87:201–11.

81. Wont TW, Warner NE. Ovarian thecal metaplasia in the adrenal gland. Arch Pathol 1971;92:319–28.

82. Yamashina M. Focal adrenocortical cytomegaly observed in two adult cases. Arch Pathol Lab Med 1986;110:1072–5.

Malformations and Heterotopias

83. Bell JE. Fused suprarenal glands in association with central nervous system defects in the first half of fetal life. J Pathol 1979;127:191–4.

84. Dolan MF, Jonovski NA. Adreno-hepatic union (adrenodystopia). Arch Pathol 1968;86:22–4.

Adrenal Rests and Accessory Adrenal Tissues

85. Albores-Saavedra J. The pseudometastasis. Patologia 1994;32:63–71.

86. Armin A, Castelli M. Congenital adrenal tissue in the lung with adrenal cytomegaly. Case report and review of the literature. Am J Clin Pathol 1984;82:225–8.

87. Culp OS. Adrenal heterotopia. A survey of the literature and report of a case. J Urol 1939;41:303–9.

88. Graham LS. Celiac accessory adrenal glands. Cancer 1953;6:149–52.

89. Honoré LH. Intra-adrenal hepatic heterotopia. J Urol 1985;133:652–4.

90. Mares AJ, Shkolnik A, Sacks M, Feuchtwanger MM. Aberrant (ectopic) adrenocortical tissue along the spermatic cord. J Pediatr Surg 1980;15:289–92.

91. Mitchell N, Angrist A. Adrenal rests in the kidney. Arch Pathol 1943;35:46–52.

92. Morimoto Y, Hiwada K, Nanahoshi M, et al. Cushing's syndrome caused by malignant tumor in the scrotum: clinical, pathologic and biochemical studies. J Clin Endocr Metab 1971;32:201–10.

93. Nelson AA. Accessory adrenal cortical tissue. Arch Pathol 1939;27:955–65.

94. Symonds DA, Driscoll SG. An adrenal cortical rest within the fetal ovary: report of a case. Am J Clin Pathol 1973;60:562–4.

95. Wallace EZ, Leonidas JR, Stanek AE, Avramides A. Endocrine studies in a patient with functioning adrenal rest tumor of the liver. Am J Med 1981;70:1122–5.

96. Wiener MF, Dallgaard SA. Intracranial adrenal gland: a case report. Arch Pathol 1959;67:228–33.

Congenital Adrenal Hypoplasia

97. Hay ID, Smail PJ, Forsyth CC. Familial cytomegalic adrenocortical hypoplasia: an X-linked syndrome of pubertal failure. Arch Dis Child 1981;56:715–21.

98. Mortin MM, Mortin AL. The syndrome of congenital hereditary adrenal hypoplasia and hypogonadotropic hypogonadism. Int J Adolesc Med Health 1985;1:119–37.

99. Prader A, Zachmann M, Illig R. Luteinizing hormone deficiency in hereditary congenital adrenal hypoplasia. J Pediatr 1975;86:421–2.

Hereditary Adrenal Cortical Unresponsiveness to ACTH

100. Migeon CJ, Kenny EM, Kowarski A, et al. The syndrome of congenital adrenocortical unresponsiveness to ACTH. Report of six cases. Pediatr Res 1968;2:501–13.

101. Shepard TH, Landing BH, Mason DG. Familial Addison's disease. Case reports of two sisters with corticoid deficiency unassociated with hypo-aldosternism. Am J Dis Child 1959;97:154–62.

102. Yamaoka T, Kudo T, Takuwa Y, et al. Hereditary adrenocortical unresponsiveness to adrenocorticotropin with a postreceptor defect. J Clin Endocrinol Metab 1992;75:270–4.

Exogenous Injury

103. Bergenstal DM, Hertz R, Lipsett MB, et al. Chemotherapy of adrenocortical cancer with o,p'-DDD. Ann Intern Med 1966;53:672–82.

104. Costin G, Kogut MD, Hyman CB, Ortega JA. Endocrine abnormalities in thalassemia major. Am J Dis Child 1979;133:497–502.

105. Dexter RN, Fishman LM, Ney RL, Liddle GW. Inhibition of adrenal corticosteroid synthesis by aminoglutethimide: studies of the mechanism of action. J Clin Endocrinol Metab 1967;27:473–80.

106. James VH, Few JD. Adrenocorticosteroids: chemistry, synthesis and disturbances in disease. Clin Endocrinol Metab 1985;14:867–92.

107. Liddle GW, Island D, Lance EM, et al. Alterations of adrenal steroid patterns in man resulting from treatment with a chemical inhibitor of 11-hydroxylation. J Clin Endocrinol Metab 1958;18:906–12.

108. Sommers SC, Carter ME. Adrenocortical postirradiation fibrosis. Arch Pathol 1975;99:421–3.

109. Southren AL, Tochimoto S, Strom L, et al. Remission in Cushing's syndrome with o,p'-DDD. J Clin Endocrinol Metab 1966;26:268–78.

110. Vilar O, Tullner WW. Effects of o,p'DDD on histology and 17-hydroxycorticosteroid output of the dog adrenal cortex. Endocrinology 1959;65:80–6.

Infectious Diseases and Miscellaneous Conditions

111. Abad A, Gomez I, Velez P, et al. Adrenal function in paracoccidioidomycosis: a prospective study in patients before and after ketoconazole therapy. Infection 1986;14:22–6.

112. Barker NW. Pathologic anatomy in twenty-eight cases of Addison's disease. Arch Pathol 1928; 8:432–50.

113. Del Negro G, Melo EH, Rodbard D, Melo MR, Layton J, Wachslicht-Rodband H. Limited adrenal reserve in paracoccidiomycosis: cortical and aldosterone responses to 1-24 ACTH. Clin Endocrinol 1980;13:553–9.

114. Frenkel JK. Pathogenesis of infections of the adrenal gland leading to Addison's disease in man: the role of corticoids in adrenal and generalized infection. Ann NY Acad Sci 1960;84:391–439.

115. Guttman PH. Addison's disease: statistical analysis of 566 cases and a study of the pathology. Arch Pathol 1930;10:742-895.

116. Kamp P, Platz P, Nerup J. "Steroid-cell" antibody in endocrine diseases. Acta Endocrinol 1974; 76:729–40.

117. Marsigli I, Pinto J. Adrenal cortical insufficiency associated with paracoccidioidomycosis (South American blastomycosis). Report of four patients. J Clin Endocrinol Metab 1966;26:1109.

118. Osa SR, Peterson RE, Roberts RB. Recovery of adrenal reserve following treatment of disseminated South American blastomycosis. Am J Med 1981;71:298–301.

119. Penrice J, Nussey SS. Recovery of adrenocortical function following treatment of tuberculous Addison's disease. Postgrad Med J 1992;68:204–5.

120. Salyer WR, Moravec CL, Salyer DC, Guerin PF. Adrenal involvement in cryptococcosis. Am J Clin Pathol 1973;60:559–61.

121. Sanoni N. The use of ketoconazole as an inhibitor of steroid production. N Engl J Med 1987;317:812–8.

122. Sarosi GA, Voth DW, Dahl BA, Doto IL, Tosh FE. Disseminated histoplasmosis: results of long-term follow-up. A center for disease control cooperation mycosis study. Ann Intern Med 1971;75:511–6.

123. Sloper JC. The pathology of the adrenals, thymus and certain other endocrine glands in Addison's disease. An analysis of 37 necropsies. Proc R Soc Med 1955;48:625–8.

124. Walker BF, Gunthel CJ, Bryan JA, Watts NB, Clark RV. Disseminated cryptococcosis in an apparently normal host presenting as primary adrenal insufficiency: diagnosis by fine needle aspiration. Am J Med 1989;86:715–7.

Acquired Immunodeficiency Syndrome Adrenalitis

125. Dluhy RG. The growing spectrum of HIV-related endocrine abnormalities. J Clin Endocrinol Metab 1990;70:563–5.

126. Dobs AS, Dempsey MA, Landenson PW, Polk BF. Endocrine disorders in men infected with human immunodeficiency virus. Am J Med 1988;84:611–6.

127. Glasgow BJ, Steinsapir KD, Anders K, et al. Adrenal pathology in the acquired immune deficiency syndrome. Am J Clin Pathol 1985;84:594–7.

128. Greene LW, Cole W, Greene JB, et al. Adrenal insufficiency as a complication of the acquired immunodeficiency syndrome. Ann Intern Med 1984;101:497–8.

129. Membreno L, Irony I, Dere W, Klein R, Biglieri EG, Cobb E. Adrenocortical function in acquired immunodeficiency syndrome. J Clin Endocrinol Metab 1987;65:482–7.

130. Norbiato G, Bevilacqua M, Vago T, et al. Cortisol resistance in acquired immunodeficiency syndrome. J Clin Endocrinol Metab 1992;74:608–13.

131. Rotterdam H, Dembitzer F. The adrenal gland in AIDS. Endocr Pathol 1993;4:4–14.

Miscellaneous Infections

132. Guttman PH. Addison's disease: statistical analysis of 566 cases and study of the pathology. Arch Pathol 1930;10:742–895.

133. Heppner C, Petzke F, Arlt W, et al. Adrenocortical insufficiency in Rhodesian sleeping sickness is not attributable to suramin. Trans R Soc Trop Med Hyg 1995;89:65–8.

134. Joeseph TJ, Vogt PJ. Disseminated herpes with hepatoadrenal necrosis in an adult. Am J Med 1974;56:735–9.

135. Ruiz-Palacios G, Pickering LK, van Eys J, Conklin R. Disseminated herpes simplex with hepatoadrenal necrosis in a child with acute leukemia. J Pediatr 1977;91:757–9.

Adrenal Cortical Hypofunction

136. Betterle C, Scalici C, Presotto F, et al. The natural history of adrenal function in autoimmune patients with adrenal autoantibodies. J Endocrinol 1988;117:467–75.

137. Blizzard RM, Chee D, Davis W. The incidence of parathyroid and other antibodies in the sera of patients with idiopathic hypoparathyroidism. Clin Exp Immunol 1966;1:119–28.

138. Boscaro M, Betterle C, Sonino N, et al. Early adrenal hypofunction in patients with organ-specific autoantibodies and no clinical adrenal insufficiency. J Clin Endocrinol Metab 1994;79:452–5.

139. Butler MG, Hodes ME, Conneally PM, et al. Linkage analysis in a large kindred with autosomal dominant transmission of polyglandular autoimmune disease type II (Schmidt syndrome). Am J Med Genet 1984;18:61–5.

140. Buxi TB, Vohra RB, Sujatha S, et al. CT in adrenal enlargement due to tuberculosis: a review of the literature with five new cases. Clin Imaging 1992;16:102–8.

141. Dunlop D. Eighty-six cases of Addison's disease. BMJ 1963;5362:887–91.

142. Fairchild RS, Schimke RN, Abdou NI. Immunoregulation abnormalities in familial Addison's disease. J Clin Endocrinol Metab 1980;51:1074–7.

143. Florkowski CM, Holmes SJ, Elliot JR, et al. Bone mineral density is reduced in female but not male subjects with Addison's disease. N Z Med J 1994;107:52–3.

144. Irvine WJ, Barnes EW. Adrenocortical insufficiency. Clin Endocrinol Metab 1972;1:1549–94.

145. Jackson R, McNicol AM, Farquharson M, Foulis AK. Class II MHC expression in normal adrenal cortex and cortical cells in autoimmune Addison's disease. J Pathol 1988;155:113–20.

146. Jarvis JL, Jenkins D, Sosman MC, et al. Roentgenologic observations in Addison's disease: a review of 120 cases. Radiology 1954;62:16–29.

147. Jensen MD, Handwerger BS, Scheithauer BW, et al. Lymphocytic hypophysitis with isolated corticotropin deficiency. Ann Intern Med 1986;105:200–3.

148. Knowlton AI, Baer L. Cardiac failure in Addison's disease. Am J Med 1983;74:829–36.

149. Kubota T, Hayashi M, Kabuto M, et al. Corticotroph cell hyperplasia in a patient with Addison's disease: case report. Surg Neurol 1992;37:441–7.

150. Leshin M. Polyglandular autoimmune syndromes. Am J Med Sci 1985;290:77–88.

151. Margaretten W, Nakai H, Landing BH. Septicemic adrenal hemorrhage. Am J Dis Child 1963;105:346–51.

152. McHardy-Young S, Lessof MH, Maisey MN. Serum TSH and thyroid antibody studies in Addison's disease. Clin Endocrinol (Oxf) 1972;1:45–56.

153. Mineura K, Goto T, Yoneya M, et al. Pituitary enlargement associated with Addison's disease. Clin Radiol 1987;38:435–7.

154. Nakahara M, Shibasaki T, Shizume K, et al. Corticotropin-releasing factor test in normal subjects and patients with hypothalamic-pituitary-adrenal disorders. J Clin Endocrinol Metab 1983;57:963–8.

155. Nerup J. Addison's disease: clinical studies. A report of 108 cases. Acta Endocrinol 1974;76:127–41.

156. Nerup J. Addison's disease—serological studies. Acta Endocrinol 1974;76:142–58.

157. Neufeld M, Maclaren NK, Blizzard RM. Two types of autoimmune Addison's disease associated with different polyglandular autoimmune (PGA) syndromes. Medicine 1981;60:355–62.

158. Nussey SS, Soo SC, Gibson S, et al. Isolated congenital ACTH deficiency: a cleavage enzyme defect? Clin Endocrinol (Oxf) 1993;39:381-5.

159. Orth DN, Kovacs WJ. The adrenal cortex. In: Wilson JD, Foster DW, Kronenberg HM, Larsen PR, eds. Williams textbook of endocrinology, 9th ed. Philadelphia: WB Saunders, 1998:517–664.

160. Otabe S, Muto S, Asano Y, et al. Hyperreninemic hypoaldosteronism due to hepatocellular carcinoma metastatic to the adrenal gland. Clin Nephrol 1991;35:66-71.

161. Partanen J, Peterson P, Westman P. Major histo-compatibility complex class II and III in Addison's disease. MHC alleles do not predict autoantibody specificity and 21-hydroxylase gene polymorphism has no independent role in disease susceptibility. Hum Immunol 1994;41:135–40.

162. Peterson P, Krohn KJ. Mapping of B cell epitopes on steroid 17-alpha-hydroxylase, an autoantigen in autoimmune polyglandular syndrome type I. Clin Exp Immunol 1994;98:104–9.

163. Rabinowe SL, Jackson RA, Dluhy RG, et al. Ia-positive T lymphocytes in recently diagnosed idiopathic Addison's disease. Am J Med 1984;77:597–601.

164. Rao RH, Vagnucci AH, Amico JA. Bilateral massive adrenal hemorrhage—early recognition and treatment. Ann Intern Med 1989;110:227–35.

165. Schambelan M, Stockigt JR, Biglieri EG. Isolated hypoaldosteronism in adults. A renin-deficiency syndrome. N Engl J Med 1972;287:573–8.

166. Sloper JC. The pathology of the adrenals, thymus and certain other endocrine glands in Addison's disease: an analysis of 37 necropsies. Proc R Soc Med 1955;48:625–8.

167. Song YH, Connor EL, Muir A, et al. Autoantibody epitope mapping of the 21-hydroxylase antigen in autoimmune Addison's disease. J Clin Endocrinol Metab 1994;78:1108–12.

168. Stacpoole PW, Interlandi JW, Nicholson WE, et al. Isolated ACTH deficiency: a heterogeneous disorder. Critical review and report of four new cases. Medicine 1982;61:13–24.

169. Symington T. Functional pathology of the human adrenal gland. Edinburgh: Livingstone, 1969.

170. Ulick S. Diagnosis and nomenclature of the disorders of the terminal portion of the aldosterone biosynthetic pathway. J Clin Endocrinol Metab 1976;43:92–6.

171. Villabona CM, Sahun M, Ricart W, et al. Tuberculous Addison's disease. Utility of CT in diagnosis and follow-up. Eur J Radiol 1993;17:210–3.

172. Vita JA, Silverberg SJ, Goland RS, Austin JH, Knowlton AI. Clinical clues to the cause of Addison's disease. Am J Med 1985;78:461–6.

173. Wedlock N, Asawa T, Baumann-Antczak A, Smith BR, Furmaniak J. Autoimmune Addison's disease. Analysis of autoantibody binding sites on human steroid 21-hydroxylase. FEBS Lett 1993;332:123–6.

174. Weetman AP. Autoimmunity to steroid-producing cells and familial polyendocrine autoimmunity. Baillieres Clin Endocrinol Metab 1995;9:157–74.

175. Yaswen L, Diehl N, Brennan MB, Hochgeschwender U. Obesity in the mouse model of pro-opiomelanocortin deficiency responds to peripheral melanocortin. Nat Med 1999;5:1066–70.

176. Yoshida T, Arai T, Sugano J, Yarita H, Yanagisawa H. Isolated ACTH deficiency accompanied by "primary hypothyroidism" and hyperprolactinemia. Acta Endocrinol 1983;104:397–401.

177. Zelissen PM, Bast EJ, Croughs RJ. Associated autoimmunity in Addison's disease. J Autoimmun 1995;8:121–30.

Adrenal Hemorrhage and Necrosis

178. Black J, Williams DI. Natural history of adrenal haemorrhage in the newborn. Arch Dis Child 1973;48:183–90.

179. Brown BS, Dunbar JS, MacEwan DW. The radiologic features of acute massive adrenal hemorrhage of the newborn. J Can Assoc Radiol 1962;13:100–7.

180. Fox B. Venous infarction of the adrenal glands. J Pathol 1976;119:65–89.

181. Friderichsen C. Waterhouse-Friderichsen syndrome. Acta Endocrinol (Copenh) 1955;18:482–92.

182. Lawson DW, Corry RJ, Patton AS, Daggett WM, Austen WG. Massive retroperitoneal adrenal hemorrhage. Surg Gynecol Obstet 1969;129:989–94.

183. Waterhouse R. A case of supraneural apoplexy. Lancet 1911;I:577–8.

184. Xarli VP, Steele AA, Davis PJ, Buescher ES, Rios CN, Garcia-Bunuel R. Adrenal hemorrhage in the adult. Medicine 1978;57:211–21.

Metastatic Tumors Causing Adrenal Insufficiency

185. Allard P, Yankaskas BC, Fletcher RH, Parker LA, Halvorsen RA Jr. Sensitivity and specificity of computed tomography for the detection of adrenal metastatic lesions among 91 autopsied lung cancer patients. Cancer 1990;66:457–62.

186. Campbell CM, Middleton RG, Rigby OF. Adrenal metastasis in renal cell carcinoma. Urology 1983;21:403–5.

187. Cedermark BJ, Sjöberg HE. The clinical significance of metastases to the adrenal glands. Surg Gynecol Obstet 1981;152:607–10.

188. Kung AW, Punn KK, Lam K, Wang C, Leung CY. Addisonian crisis as presenting feature in malignancies. Cancer 1990;65:177–9.

189. Omoigui NA, Cave WT Jr, Chang AY. Adrenal insufficiency. A rare initial sign of metastatic colon carcinoma. J Clin Gastroenterol 1987;9:470–4.

190. Prayson RA, Segal GH, Stoler MH, Licata AA, Tubbs RR. Angiotropic large-cell lymphoma in a patient with adrenal insufficiency. Arch Pathol Lab Med 1991;115:1039–41.

191. Redman BG, Pazdur R, Zingas AP, Loredo R. Prospective evaluation of adrenal insufficiency in patients with adrenal metastasis. Cancer 1987;60:103–7.

192. Seidenwurm DJ, Elmer EB, Kaplan LM, Williams EK, Morris DG, Hoffman AR. Metastases to the adrenal glands and the development of Addison's disease. Cancer 1984;54:552–7.

193. Selli C, Corini M, Barbanti G, Barbadgli G, Turin D. Simultaneous bilateral adrenal involvement by renal cell carcinoma: experience with three cases. J Urol 1987;137:480–2.

194. Serrano S, Tejedor L, Garcia B, Hallal H, Polo JA, Algucil G. Addisonian crisis as the presenting feature of bilateral primary adrenal lymphoma. Cancer 1993;71:4030–3.

195. Sheeler LR, Myers JH, Eversman JJ, Taylor HC. Adrenal insufficiency secondary to carcinoma metastatic to the adrenal gland. Cancer 1983;52:1312–6.

Adrenal Amyloid

196. Arik N, Tasdemir I, Karaaslan Y, Yasavul U, Turgan C, Caglar S. Subclinical adrenocortical insufficiency in renal amyloidosis. Nephron 1990;56:246–8.

197. el-Reshaid KA, Hakim AA, Hourani HA, Seshadri MS. Endocrine abnormalities in patients with amyloidosis. Ren Fail 1994;16:725–30.

198. Ericksson L, Westermark P. Age-related accumulation of amyloid inclusions in adrenal cortical cells. Am J Pathol 1990;136:461–6.

199. Guttman PH. Addison's disease: a statistical analysis of 566 cases and study of the pathology. Arch Pathol 1930;10:742–895.

200. Neville AM, O'Hare MJ. The human adrenal cortex: pathology biology, an integrated approach. New York: Springer-Verlag, 1982:263–4.

201. Rocken C, Eick B, Saeger W. Senile amyloidoses of the pituitary and adrenal glands. Morphological and statistical investigations. Virchows Arch 1996;429:293–9.

202. Sasaki M, Kono M, Nakamura Y, Ishiura Y. Multinodular deposition of AA-type amyloid localized in the adrenal glands of an old man. Acta Pathol Jap 1992;42:893–6.

Adrenoleukodystrophy

203. Griffin JW, Goren E, Schaumburg H, et al. Adrenomyeloneuropathy: a probable variant of adrenoleukodystrophy. I. Clinical and endocrinologic aspects. Neurology 1977;27:1107–13.

204. Moser AB, Borel J, Odone A, et al. A new dietary therapy for adrenoleukodystrophy: biochemical and preliminary clinical results in 36 patients. Ann Neurol 1987;21:240–9.

205. Moser HW. Adrenoleukodystrophy. Curr Opin Neurol 1995;8:221–6.

206. Moser HW, Moser AE, Singh I, et al. Adrenoleukodystrophy: survey of 303 cases. Biochemistry, diagnosis, and therapy. Ann Neurol 1984;16:628–41.

207. Mosser J, Lutz Y, Stoeckel ME, et al. The gene responsible for adrenoleukodystrophy encodes a paroxysomal membrane protein. Hum Mol Genetics 1994;3:265–71.

208. Orth DN, Kovacs WJ. The adrenal cortex. In: Wilson JD, Foster DW, Kronenberg HM, Larsen PR, eds. Williams textbook of endocrinology, 9th ed. Philadelphia: WB Saunders, 1998:517–664.

209. Powers JM, Schaumberg HH. The adrenal cortex in adreno-leukodystrophy. Arch Pathol 1973;96:305–10.

210. Powers JM, Schaumberg HH. Adrenoleukodystrophy. Similar ultrastructural changes in adrenal cortical cells and Schwann cells. Arch Neurol 1974;30:406–8.

211. Powers JM, Schaumberg HH. The testis in adrenoleukodystrophy. Am J Pathol 1981;102:90–8.

212. Sarde CO, Mosser J, Kioschis P, et al. Genomic organization of the adrenoleukodystrophy gene. Genomics 1994;22:13–20.

213. Schaumberg HH, Powers JM, Raine CS, Suzuki K, Richardson EP. Adrenoleukodystrophy. A clinical and pathological study of 17 cases. Arch Neurol 1975;32:577–91.

Wolman's Disease

214. Crocker AC, Vawter GF, Neuhauser EB. Wolman's disease: three new patients with a recently described lipidosis. Pediatrics 1965;35:627–40.

215. Raafat F, Hashemian MP, Abrishami MA. Wolman's disease: report of two new cases with a review of the literature. Am J Clin Pathol 1973;59:490–7.

216. Wolman M, Sterk VV, Gratt S, Frenkel M. Primary familial xanthomatosis with involvement and calcification of adrenal. Report of two more cases in siblings of a previously described infant. Pediatrics 1961;28:742–57.

Adrenal Cysts

217. Abeshouse GA, Goldstein RB, Abeshouse BS. Adrenal cysts: review of the literature and report of three cases. J Urol 1959;81:711–9.

218. Barron SH, Emanuel B. Adrenal cyst. A case report and review of the pediatric literature. J Pediatr 1961;59:592–9.

219. Foster DG. Adrenal cysts. Review of the literature and report of a case. Arch Surg 1966;92:131–43.

220. Gaffey MJ, Mills SE, Fechner RE, Bertholf MF, Allen MS Jr. Vascular adrenal cysts. A clinicopathologic and immunohistochemical study of endothelial and hemorrhagic (pseudocystic) variants. Am J Surg Pathol 1989;13:740–7.

221. Ghandur-Mnaymneh L, Slim M, Muakassa K. Adrenal cysts: pathogenesis and histological identification with a report of six cases. J Urol 1979;122:87–91.

222. Gigax JH, Bucy JG, Troxler G, Chunn SP. Cystic hamartoma of the adrenal gland associated with hypertension. J Urol 1972;107:161–3.

223. Groben PA, Roberson JB, Anger SR, Askin FB, Price WG, Siegal GP. Immunohistochemical evidence for the vascular origin of primary adrenal pseudocysts. Arch Pathol Lab Med 1986;110:121–3.

224. Hodges FV, Ellis FR. Cystic lesions of the adrenal glands. Arch Pathol Lab Med 1958;66:53–8.

225. Incze JS, Lui PS, Merriam JC, Austen G, Widrich WC, Gerzof SG. Morphology and pathogenesis of adrenal cysts. Am J Pathol 1979;95:423–32.

226. Kearney GP, Mahoney EM, Maher E, Harrison JH. Functioning and nonfunctioning cysts of the adrenal cortex and medulla. Am J Surg 1977;134:363–8.

227. Lack EE. Tumors of the adrenal gland and extra-adrenal paraganglia. Atlas of Tumor Pathology. 3rd Series, Fascicle 19. Washington, DC: Armed Forces Institute of Pathology, 1997:172–4.

228. Levin SE, Collins DL, Kaplan GW, Weller MH. Neonatal adrenal pseudocysts mimicking metastatic disease. Ann Surg 1974;179:186–9.

229. Lynn RB. Cystic lymphangioma of the adrenal associated with arterial hypertension. Can J Surg 1965;15:92–5.

230. Medeiros LJ, Lewandrowski KB, Vickery AL Jr. Adrenal pseudocyst: a clinical and pathologic study of eight cases. Human Pathol 1989;20:660–5.

231. Medeiros LJ, Weiss LM, Vickery AL Jr. Epithelial-lined (true) cyst of the adrenal gland: a case report. Hum Pathol 1989;20:491–2.

232. Oppenheimer EH. Cyst formation in the outer adrenal cortex. Studies in the human fetus and newborn. Arch Pathol 1969;87:653–9.

233. Rodin AE, Hsu FL, Whorton EB. Microcysts of the permanent adrenal cortex in perinates and infants. Arch Pathol 1976;100:499–502.

234. Symington T. The adrenal cortex. In: Bloodworth JM, ed. Endocrine pathology, 2nd ed. Baltimore: William & Wilkins, 1982:437.

235. Thompson GB, Grant CS, van Heerden JA, et al. Laparoscopic versus open posterior adrenalectomy: a case-control study of 100 patients. Surgery 1997;122:1132–6.

236. Wahl HR. Adrenal cysts [Abstract]. Am J Pathol 1951;27:758.

237. Wells SA, Merke DP, Cutler GB Jr, Norton JA, Lacroix A. Therapeutic controversy. The role of laparoscopic surgery in adrenal disease. J Clin Endocrinol Metab 1998;83:3041–9.

Incidental, Nonfunctional Adrenal Cortical Nodules

238. Abecassis M, McLoughlin MJ, Langer B, Kudlow JE. Serendipitous adrenal masses: prevalence, significance and management. Am J Surg 1985;149:783–8.

239. Commons RR, Callaway CP. Adenomas of the adrenal cortex. Arch Intern Med 1984;81:37–41.

240. Damron TA, Schelper RL, Sorensen L. Cytochemical demonstration of neuromelanin in black pigmented adrenal nodules. Am J Clin Pathol 1987;87:334–41.

241. Dobbie JW. Adrenocortical nodular hyperplasia: the ageing adrenal. J Pathol 1969;99:1–18.

242. Gicquel C, Bertagna X, LeBouc Y. Recent advances in the pathogenesis of adrenocortical tumors. Eur J Endocrinol 1995;133:133–44.

243. Gicquel C, Leblond-Francillard M, Bertagna X, et al. Clinical analysis of human adrenocortical carcinomas and secreting adenomas. Clin Endocrinol 1994;40:465–77.

244. Glazer GM, Woolsey EJ, Borrello J, et al. Adrenal tissue characterization using MR imaging. Radiology 1986;158:73–9.

245. Hedeland H, Ostberg G, Hokfelt B. On the prevalence of adrenocortical adenomas in an autopsy material in relation to hypertension and diabetes. Acta Med Scan 1968;184:211–4.

246. Herrera MF, Grant CS, van Heerden JA, Sheedy PF II, Ilstrup DM. Incidentally discovered adrenal tumors: an institutional perspective. Surgery 1991;110:1014–21.

247. Kokko JP, Brown TC, Berman MM. Adrenal adenoma and hypertension. Lancet 1967;1:468–70.

248. Neville AM. The nodular adrenal. Invest Cell Pathol 1978;1:99–111.

249. O'Leary TJ, Ooi TC. The adrenal incidentaloma. Can J Surg 1986;29:6–8.

250. Prinz RA, Brooks MH, Churchill R, et al. Incidental asymptomatic adrenal masses detected by computed tomographic scanning. Is operation required? JAMA 1982;248:701–4.

251. Robinson MJ, Pardo V, Rywlin AM. Pigmented nodules (black adenomas) of the adrenal. An autopsy study of incidence, morphology, and function. Hum Pathol 1972;3:317–25.

252. Russi S, Blumenthol HT, Gray SH. Small adenomas of the adrenal cortex in hypertension and diabetes. Arch Intern Med 1945;76:284–91.

253. Shamnan AH, Goddard JW, Sommen SC. A study of the adrenal states in hypertension. J Chronic Dis 1958;8:587–95.

254. Spain DM, Weinsaft P. Solitary adrenal cortical adenoma in an elderly female. Arch Pathol 1964;78:231–3.

255. Suzuki T, Sasano H, Sawai T, et al. Small adrenocortical tumors without apparent clinical endocrine abnormalities: immunolocalization of steroidogenic enzymes. Path Res Pract 1992;188:883–9.

256. Witkiewicz AK, Blaszyk H, Kulig E, Carnes JA, Lloyd RV. Laser captured microdissection in the clonality evaluation of benign multicentric adrenal cortical proliferations [Abstract]. Modern Pathol 1999;12:71A–401.

257. Woodruff MF. Tumor clonality and its biological significance. Adv Cancer Res 1988;50:197–229.

Adrenal Cortical Hyperplasia

258. Anderson DC, Child DF, Sutcliffe CH, Buckley CH, Davies D, Longson D. Cushing's syndrome, nodular adrenal hyperplasia and virilizing carcinoma. Clin Endocrinol 1978;9:1–14.

259. Aron DC, Schnall AM, Sheeler LR. Cushing's syndrome and pregnancy. Am J Obstet Gynecol 1990;162:244–52.

260. Axiotis CA, Lippes HA, Merino MJ, de Lanerolle NC, Stewart AF, Kinder B. Corticotroph cell pituitary adenoma within an ovarian teratoma. A new cause of Cushing's syndrome. Am J Surg Pathol 1987;11:218–24.

261. Doppman JL, Miller DL, Dwyer AJ, et al. Macronodular adrenal hyperplasia in Cushing disease. Radiology 1988;166:347–52.

262. Drasin GF, Lynch T, Temes GP. Ectopic ACTH production and mediastinal lipomatosis. Radiology 1978;127:610.

263. Dupont AG, Somers G, van Steistegheim AC, Warson F, Vanhaelot L. Ectopic adrenocorticotropin production: disappearance after removal of inflammatory tissue. J Clin Endocrinol Metab 1984;58:654–8.

264. Gagner M, Lacroix A, Prinz RA, et al. Early experience with laparoscopic approach for adrenalectomy. Surgery 1993;114:1120–4.

265. Grua JR, Nelson DH. ACTH-producing tumors. Endocrinol Metab Clin N Am 1991;20:319–62.

266. Josse RG, Bear R, Kovacs K, Higgins HP. Cushing's syndrome due to unilateral nodular adrenal hyperplasia. A new pathophysiological entity. Acta Endocrinol (Copenh) 1980;93:495–504.

267. Kay S. Hyperplasia and neoplasia of the adrenal gland. Pathol Ann 1976;11:103–39.

268. Lam KY, Lu CY. The clinicopathologic significance of unilateral adrenal cortical hyperplasia: report of an unusual case and a review of the literature. Endocr Pathol 1999;10:243–9.

269. Luton JP, Mahoudeau JA, Bouchard P, et al. Treatment of Cushing's disease by o,p'-DDD: survey of 62 cases. N Engl J Med 1979;300:459–64.

270. MacKay A. Atlas of human adrenal cortex ultrastructure. In: Symington T, ed. Functional pathology of the human adrenal gland. Edinburgh: Livingstone, 1964:345–489.

271. McArthur RG, Cloutier MD, Hayles AB, Sprague RG. Cushing's disease in children. Findings in 13 cases. Mayo Clin Proc 1972;47:318–26.

272. Muller OA, Von Werder K. Ectopic production of ACTH and corticotropin-releasing hormone (CRH). J Steroid Biochem Molecular Biol 1992;43:403–8.

273. Neville AM, MacKay AM. The structure of the human adrenal cortex in health and disease. Clin Endocrinol Metab 1972;1:361.

274. Neville AM, O'Hare MJ. The human adrenal cortex: pathology and biology, an integrated approach. New York: Springer Verlag, 1982.

275. Neville AM, O'Hare MJ. The human adrenal gland: aspects of structure functional pathology. In: James VH, ed. The adrenal cortex. New York: Raven Press, 1979.

276. Neville AM, Symington T. The pathology of the adrenal gland in Cushing's syndrome. J Pathol Bacteriol 1967;93:19–35.

277. Orth DN, Kovacs WJ. The adrenal cortex. In: Wilson JD, Foster DW, Kronenberg HM, Larsen PR, eds. Williams textbook of endocrinology, 9th ed. Philadelphia: WB Saunders, 1998:517–664.

278. Orth DN, Liddle GW. Results of treatment in 108 patients with Cushing's syndrome. N Engl J Med 1971;285:243–7.

279. Pasqualini RQ, Gurevich N. Spontaneous remission in a case of Cushing's syndrome. J Clin Endocrinol Metab 1956;16:406.

280. Pratt JH, Sawin CT, Melby JC. Remission of Cushing's disease after administration of adrenocorticotropin. Am J Med 1974;57:949–52.

281. Preeyasombat C, Sirikulchayanonta V, Mahachokelertwattana P, Sriphrapradang A, Boonpucknavig S. Cushing's syndrome caused by Ewing's sarcoma secreting corticotrophin releasing factor-like peptide. Am J Dis Child 1992;146:1103–5.

282. Rees LH, Ratcliffe JG. Ectopic hormone production by non-endocrine tumour. Clin Endocrine 1974;3:263–99.

283. Schteingart DE, Lloyd RV, Akil H, et al. Cushing's syndrome secondary to ectopic corticotropin-releasing hormone—adrenocorticotropin secretion. J Clin Endocrinol Metab 1986;63:770–5.

284. Schteingart DE, Tsao HS, Taylor CI, et al. Sustained remission of Cushing's disease with mitotane and pituitary irradiation. Ann Intern Med 1980;92:613–19.

285. Siren J, Valimaki M, Huikuri K, Sivula A, Voutilainen P, Haapiainen R. Adrenalectomy for primary aldosteronism: long-term follow-up study in 29 patients. World J Surg 1998;22:418–21.

286. Symington T. Functional pathology of the human adrenal gland. Edinburgh: Livingstone, 1969.

287. Tannenbaum M. Ultrastructural pathology of the adrenal cortex. Pathol Ann 1973;8:109–56.

288. Thompson GB, Grant CS, van Heerden JA, et al. Laparoscopic versus open posterior adrenalectomy: a case-control study of 100 patients. Surgery 1997;122:1132–6.

289. Zárate A, Kovacs K, Flores M, Moran C, Felix I. ACTH and CRF producing bronchial carcinoid associated with Cushing's syndrome. Clin Endocrinol 1986;24:523–9.

Adrenocortical Macronodular Hyperplasia

290. Aiba M, Hirayama A, Iri H, et al. Adrenocorticotropic hormone-independent bilateral adrenocortical macronodular hyperplasia as a distinct subtype of Cushing's syndrome. Enzyme histochemical and ultrastructural study of four cases with a review of the literature. Am J Clin Pathol 1991;96:334–40.

291. Aiba M, Hirayama A, Iri H, et al. Primary adrenocortical micronodular dysplasia: enzyme histochemical and ultrastructural studies of two cases with a review of the literature. Hum Pathol 1990;21:503-11.

292. Boston BA, Mandel S, LaFranchi S, et al. Activating mutation in the stimulatory guanine nucleotide-binding protein in an infant with Cushing's syndrome and nodular adrenal hyperplasia. J Clin Endocrinol Metab 1994;79:890–3.

293. Doppman JL, Nieman LK, Travis WD, et al. CT and MR imaging of massive macronodular adrenocortical disease: a rare cause of autonomous primary adrenal hypercortisolism. J Computr Assist Tomogr 1991;15:773–9.

294. Hashimoto K, Kawada Y, Murakami K, et al. Cortisol responsiveness to insulin-induced hypoglycemia in Cushing's syndrome with huge nodular adrenocortical hyperplasia. Endocrinol Jpn 1986;33:479–87.

295. Hidai H, Fujii H, Otsuka K, Abe K, Shimizu N. Cushing's syndrome due to huge adrenocortical multinodular hyperplasia. Endocrinol Jpn 1975;22:555–60.

296. Kirschner MA, Powell RD, Lipsett MB. Cushing's syndrome: nodular cortical hyperplasia of adrenal glands with clinical and pathological features suggesting adrenocortical tumor. J Clin Endocr Metab 1964;24:947–55.

297. Lacroix A, Bolte E, Tremblay J, et al. Gastric inhibitory polypeptide-dependent cortisol hypersecretion—a new cause of Cushing's syndrome. N Engl J Med 1992;327:974–80.

298. Lacroix A, Tremblay J, Rousseau G, Bouvier M, Hamet P. Propranolol therapy for ectopic beta-adrenergic receptors in adrenal Cushing's syndrome. N Engl J Med 1997;337:1429–34.

299. Sasano H, Miyazaki S, Sawai T, et al. Primary pigmented nodular adrenocortical disease (PPNAD): immunohistochemical and in situ hybridization analysis of steroidogenic enzymes in eight cases. Mod Pathol 1992;5:23–9.

300. Sasano H, Suzuki T, Nagura H. ACTH-independent macronodular adrenocortical hyperplasia: immunohistochemical and in situ hybridization studies of steroidogenic enzymes. Mod Pathol 1994;7:215–9.

301. Someya T, Koyano H, Ozana V. ACTH-independent macronodular adrenocortical hyperplasia (AIMAH) in two brothers and a sister. Folia Endorinol 1996;72:762.

302. Swain JM, Grant CS, Schlinkert RT, Thompson GB, von Heerden JA, Lloyd RV, Young WF. Corticotropin-independent macronodular adrenal hyperplasia: a clinicopathologic correlation. Arch Surg 1998;133:541–5.

303. Willenberg HS, Stratakis CA, Marx C, Ehrhart-Bornstein M, Chrousos GP, Bornstein SR. Aberrant interleukin-1 receptors in a cortisol-secreting adrenal adenoma causing Cushing's syndrome. N Engl J Med 1998;339:27–31.

Primary Pigmented Nodular Adrenocortical Disease

304. Aiba M, Hirayama A, Iri H, et al. Primary adrenocortical micronodular dysplasia: enzyme histochemical and ultrastructural studies of two cases with a review of the literature. Hum Pathol 1990;21:503–11.

305. Atherton DJ, Pitcher DW, Wells RS, MacDonald DM. A syndrome of various cutaneous pigmented lesions, myxoid neurofibromata and atrial myxoma: the NAME syndrome. Br J Dermatol 1980;103:421–9.

306. Böhm N, Lippmann-Grob B, von Petrykowski W. Familial Cushing's syndrome due to pigmented multinodular adrenocortical dysplasia. Acta Endocrinol 1983;102:428–35.

307. Carney JA, Young WF Jr. Primary pigmented nodular adrenocortical disease and its associated conditions. Endocrinologist 1992;2:6–21.

308. Doppman JL, Travis WD, Nieman L, et al. Cushing syndrome due to primary pigmented nodular adrenocortical disease: findings at CT and MR imaging. Radiology 1989;172:415–20.

309. Grant CS, Carney JA, Carpenter PC, van Heerden JA. Primary pigmented nodular adrenocortical disease: diagnosis and management. Surgery 1986;100:1178–84.

310. Hedinger C. Kombination von Herzmyxomen mit primärer nodulärer Dysplasie der nebennierenrinde, fleckformigen Haut-pigmentierungen und myxomartigen tumoren anderer Lokalisation-ein eigenartiger familiärer symptomenkomplex ("Swiss-syndrome"). Schweiz Med Wschr 1987;117:591–4.

311. Lack EE, Travis WD, Oertel JE. Adrenal cortical nodules, hyperplasia, and hyperfunction. In: Lack EE, ed. Pathology of the adrenal glands. New York: Churchill, Livingstone, 1990:75–113.

312. Larsen JL, Cathey WJ, Odell WD. Primary adrenocortical nodular dysplasia, a distinct subtype of Cushing's syndrome. Case report and review of the literature. Am J Med 1986;80:976–84.

313. Meador CK, Bowdoin B, Owen WC, et al. Primary adrenocortical nodular dysplasia: a rare cause of Cushing's syndrome. J Clin Endocrinol Metab 1967;27:1255–63.

314. Rhodes AR, Silverman RA, Harrist TJ, Perez-Atayde AR. Mucocutaneous lentigines, cardio-mucocutaneous myxomas and multiple blue nevi: the LAMB syndrome. J Am Acad Dermatol 1984;10:72–82.

315. Sarlis NJ, Chrousos GP, Doppman JL, Carney JA, Stratakis CA. Primary pigmented nodular adrenocortical disease: re-evaluation of a patient with Carney complex 27 years after unilateral adrenalectomy. J Clin Endocrinol Metab 1997;82:1274–8.

316. Sasano H, Miyazaki S, Sawai T, et al. Primary pigmented nodular adrenocortical disease (PPNAD): immunohistochemical and in situ hybridization analysis of steroidogenic enzymes in eight cases. Mod Pathol 1992;5:23–9.

317. Shenoy BV, Carpenter PC, Carney JA. Bilateral primary pigmented nodular adrenocortical disease. Rare cause of the Cushing syndrome. Am J Surg Pathol 1984;8:335–44.

318. Stratakis CA, Carney JA, Lin JP, et al. Carney complex, a familial multiple neoplasia and lentiginosis syndrome. Analysis of 11 kindreds and linkage to the short arm of chromosome 2. J Clin Invest 1996;97:699–705.

319. Teding van Berkhout F, Croughs RJ, Kater L, et al. Familial Cushing's syndrome due to nodular adrenocortical dysplasia. A putative receptor-antibody disease? Clin Endocrinol 1986;24:299–310.

320. Travis WD, Tsokos M, Doppman JL, et al. Primary pigmented nodular adrenocortical disease. A light and electron microscopic study of eight cases. Am J Surg Pathol 1989;13:921–30.

321. Young WF Jr, Carney JA, Musa BU, et al. Familial Cushing's syndrome due to primary pigmented nodular adrenocortical disease. Reinvestigation 50 years later. N Engl J Med 1989;321:1659–64.

Aldosterone Excess Due to Adrenocortical Hyperplasia

322. Banks WA, Kastin AJ, Biglieri EG, et al. Primary adrenal hyperplasia: a new subset of primary hyperaldosteronism. J Clin Endocrinol Metab 1984;58:783–5.

323. Bartter FC, Bartter's syndrome. Urol Clin North Am 1977;4:253.

324. Bartter FC, Pronove P, Gill JR Jr, MacCardle RC. Hyperplasia of the juxtaglomerular complex with hyperaldosteronism and hypokalemic alkalosis: a new syndrome. Am J Med 1962;33:811–28.

325. Güllner HG, Gill JR Jr. Beta endorphin selectively stimulates aldosterone secretion in hypophysec-tomized nephrectomized dogs. J Clin Invest 1983;71:124–8.

326. Johnson CM, Sheedy PF, Welch TJ, et al. CT of the adrenal cortex. Semin Ultrastruct CT MR 1985;6:241–60.

327. Neville AM. The nodular adrenal. Invest Cell Pathol 1978;1:99–111.

328. Neville AM, O'Hare MJ. Histopathology of the human adrenal cortex. Clin Endocrinol Metab 1985;14:791–820.

329. Orth DN, Kovacs WJ. The adrenal cortex. In: Wilson JD, Foster DW, Kronenberg HM, Larsen PR, eds. Williams textbook of endocrinology, 9th ed. Philadelphia: WB Saunders, 1998:517–664.

330. Pitcock JA, Hartraft PM. The juxtaglomerular cells in man and their relationship to the level of plasma sodium and to the zona glomerulosa of the adrenal cortex. Am J Pathol 1973;34:863.

331. Rabinowe SL, Taylor T, Dluhy RG, et al. Beta-endorphin stimulates plasma renin and aldosterone release in normal human subjects. J Clin Endocrinol Metab 1985;60:485–9.

332. Young WF Jr. Laparoscopic adrenalectomy. An endocrinologists' perspective. Curr Opin Endocrinol Diabetes 1999;6:199–203.

333. Young WF Jr. Management approaches to adrenal incidentalomas. A view from Rochester, Minnesota. Endocrinol Metabol Clin North Am 2000;29:159–85.

334. Young WF Jr. Primary aldosteronism. A common and curable form of hypertension. Cardiol Rev 1999;7:207–14.

Unilateral Adrenal Cortical Hyperplasia

335. Catania A, Reschini E, Orsatti A, Motta P, Airaghi L, Cantalamessa L. Cushing's syndrome due to unilateral adrenal nodular hyperplasia with incomplete inhibition of the contralateral gland. Hormone Res 1986;23:9–15.

336. Ganguly A, Zager PG, Luetscher JA. Primary aldosteronism due to unilateral adrenal hyperplasia. J Clin Endocrinol Metab 1980;51:1190–4.

337. Josse RG, Bear R, Kovacs K, Higgins HP. Cushing's syndrome due to unilateral nodular adrenal hyperplasia. A new pathophysiological entity? Acta Endocrinol 1980;93:495–504.

338. Neville AM, Symington T. The pathology of the adrenal gland in Cushing's syndrome. J Pathol Bacteriol 1967;93:19–35.

339. Oberfield SE, Levine LS, Firpo A, et al. Primary hyperaldosteronism in childhood due to unilateral macronodular hyperplasia. Case report. Hypertension 1984;6:75–84.

340. Sigman LM, Wallach L. Unilateral adrenal hypertrophy in ectopic ACTH syndrome. Arch Intern Med 1984;144:1869–70.

Congenital Adrenal Hyperplasia

341. Azziz R, Kenney PJ. Magnetic resonance imaging of the adrenal gland in women with late-onset adrenal hyperplasia. Fertil Steril 1991;56:142–4.

342. Biglieri EG, Kater CE. 17-alpha-hydroxylation deficiency. Endocrinol Metab Clin N Am 1991;20:257–68.

343. Blumberg-Tick J, Boudou P, Nahoul K, Schaison G. Testicular tumors in congenital adrenal hyperplasia: steroid measurements from adrenal and spermatic veins. J Clin Endocrinol Metab 1991;73:1129–33.

344. Bongiovanni AM, Root AW. The adrenogenital syndrome. N Engl J Med 1963;268:1391–9.

345. de Crecchio L. Sopra un caso di apparenzi virili in una donna. Morgagni 1865;7:154–88.

346. Johnson RE, Scheithauer B. Massive hyperplasia of testicular adrenal rests in a patient with Nelson's syndrome. Am J Clin Pathol 1982;77:501–7.

347. Kalaitzoglou G, New MI. Congenital adrenal hyperplasia. Molecular insights learned from patients. Receptor 1993;3:211–22.

348. Kim I, Young RH, Scully RE. Leydig cell tumors of the testis. A clinicopathological analysis of 40 cases and review of the literature. Am J Surg Pathol 1985;9:177–92.

349. Kirkland RT, Kirkland JL, Keenan BS, Bongiovanni AM, Rosenberg HS, Clayton GW. Bilateral testicular tumors in congenital adrenal hyperplasia. J Clin Endocrinol Metab 1977;44:369–78.

350. Knudsen JL, Savage A, Mobb GE. The testicular tumour of adrenogenital syndrome—a persistent diagnostic pitfall. Histopathology 1991;19:468–70.

351. Menon PS, Virmani A, Sethi AK, et al. Congenital adrenal hyperplasia: experience at intersex clinic, AIIMS. In J Pediatrics 1992;59:531–5.

352. Migeon CJ, Donohoue PA. Congenital adrenal hyperplasia caused by 21-hydroxylase deficiency. Its molecular basis and its remaining therapeutic problems. Endocrinol Metab Clin N Am 1991;20:277–96.

353. Miller WL. Congenital adrenal hyperplasia. Endocrinol Metab Clin N Am 1991;20:721-49.

354. Neville AM, O'Hare J. The human adrenal cortex. New York: Springer-Verlag, 1982:161–4.

355. New MI. Male pseudohermaphroditism due to 17 alpha-hydroxylase deficiency. J Clin Invest 1970;49:1930–41.

356. New MI. Steroid 21-hydroxylase deficiency (congenital adrenal hyperplasia). Am J Med 1995;98:2S–8S.

357. New MI, White PC. Genetic disorders of steroid hormone synthesis and metabolism. Baillieres Clin Endocrinol Metab 1995;9:525–54.

358. Orth DN, Kovacs WJ. The adrenal cortex. In: Wilson JD, Foster DW, Kronenberg HM, Larsen PR, eds. Williams textbook of endocrinology, 9th ed. Philadelphia: WB Saunders, 1998:517–664.

359. Pang S, Pollack MS, Marshall RN, Immken L. Prenatal treatment of congenital adrenal hyperplasia due to 21-hydroxylase deficiency. N Engl J Med 1990;322:111–5.

360. Speiser PW, Agdere L, Ueshiba H, White PC, New MI. Aldosterone synthesis in salt-wasting congenital adrenal hyperplasia with complete absence of adrenal 21-hydroxylase. N Engl J Med 1991;324:145–9.

361. White PC, New MI, Dupont B. Congenital adrenal hyperplasia. N Engl J Med 1987;316:1519–24.

Beckwith-Wiedemann Syndrome

362. Beckwith JB. Macroglossia, omphalocele, adrenal cytomegaly, gigantism and hyperplastic visceromegaly. Birth defects. Original Article Series 1969;5:188–96.

363. Henry I, Jeanpierre M, Couillin P, et al. Molecular definition of 11p15.5 region involved in Beckwith-Wiedemann syndrome and probably in predisposition to adrenocortical carcinoma. Hum Genet 1989;81:273–7.

364. Lack EE. Tumors of the adrenal gland and extra-adrenal paraganglia. Atlas of Tumor Pathology, 3rd Series, Fascicle 19. Washington, DC: Armed Forces Institute of Pathology, 1997.

365. McCauley RG, Beckwith JB, Elias ER, Faerber EN, Prewitt LH Jr, Berdon WE. Benign hemorrhagic adrenocortical macrocysts in Beckwith-Wiedemann syndrome. Am J Roentgenol 1991;157:549–52.

366. Pettanati MJ, Haines JL, Higgins RR, Wappner RS, Palmer CG, Weaver DD. Wiedemann-Beckwith syndrome: presentation of clinical and cytogenetic data on 22 new cases and review of the literature. Hum Genet 1986;74:143–54.

367. Zhang P, Liegeois NJ, Wong C, et al. Altered cell differentiation and proliferation in mice lacking p57^{kip2} indicates a role in Beckwith-Wiedemann syndrome. Nature 1997;387:151–8.

Adrenal Medullary Hyperplasia

368. Beckwith JB. Extreme cytomegaly of the adrenal fetal cortex, omphalocele, hyperplasia of kidneys and pancreas, and Leydig-cell hyperplasia—another syndrome? Presented at Annual Meeting of Western Society for Pediatric Research, Los Angeles, November 11, 1963.

369. Beckwith JB. Macroglossia, omphalocele, adrenal cytomegaly, gigantism, and hyperplastic visceromegaly. Birth defects: Original Article Series 1969;5:188–96.

370. Bialestock D. Hyperplasia of the adrenal medulla in hypertension of children. Arch Dis Child 1961;36:465–73.

371. Bongiovanni AM, Yakovac WC, Steiker DD. Study of adrenal glands in childhood: hormonal content correlated with morphologic characteristics. Lab Invest 1961;10:956–67.

372. Carlson KM, Bracamontes J, Jackson CE, et al. Parent-of-origin effects in multiple endocrine neoplasia type 2B. Am J Hum Genet 1994;55:1076–82.

373. Carney JA, Sizemore GW, Hayles AB. Multiple endocrine neoplasia, type 2b. Pathol Annu 1978;8:105–53.

374. Carney JA, Sizemore GW, Sheps SG. Adrenal medullary disease in multiple endocrine neoplasia, type 2: pheochromocytoma and its precursors. Am J Clin Pathol 1976;66:279–90.

375. Carney JA, Sizemore GW, Tyce GM. Bilateral adrenal medullary hyperplasia in multiple endocrine neoplasia, type 2: the precursor of bilateral pheochromocytoma. Mayo Clin Proc 1975;50:3–10.

376. Chen SX, Zhou ZQ, Zhao JS, Wang SZ, Sun ND. Catecholamine acute abdomen. A case of adrenal medulla hyperplasia accompanied by acute abdomen. Chin Med J 1989;102:811–3.

377. DeLellis RA, Wolfe HJ, Gagel RT, et al. Adrenal medullary hyperplasia. A morphometric analysis in patients with familial medullary thyroid carcinoma. Am J Pathol 1976;83:177–96.

378. Diaz-Cano SJ. Clonality studies in the analysis of adrenal medullary proliferations: application principles and limitations. Endocr Pathol 1998;9:301–16.

379. Eng C, Smith DP, Mulligan LM, et al. Point mutation within the tyrosine kinase domain of the RET proto-oncogene in multiple endocrine neoplasia type 2b and related sporadic tumours. Hum Mol Genet 1994;3:237–41.

380. Gagel RF. Multiple endocrine neoplasia. In: Wilson JD, Faster DW, Kronenberg HM, Larsen PR, eds. Williams textbook of endocrinology, 9th ed. Philadelphia: WB Saunders, 1998:16, 27–49.

381. Gagel RF, Tashjian AH Jr, Cummings T, et al. The clinical outcome of prospective screening for multiple endocrine neoplasia type 2a. An 18-year experience. N Engl J Med 1988;318:478–84.

382. Keiser HR, Beaven MA, Doppman J, Wells S Jr, Buja LM. Sipple's syndrome: medullary thyroid carcinoma, pheochromocytoma, and parathyroid disease. Studies in a large family. NIH conference. Ann Int Med 1973;78:561–79.

383. Kurihara K, Mizuseki K, Kondo T, Ohoka H, Mannami M, Kawai K. Adrenal medullary hyperplasia. Hyperplasia-pheochromocytoma sequence. Acta Pathol Jap 1990;40:683–6.

384. Lloyd RV. RET proto-oncogene mutations and rearrangements in endocrine diseases. Am J Pathol 1995;147:1539–44.

385. Maki Y, Irie S, Ohashi T, Ohmori H. A case of unilateral adrenal medullary hyperplasia. Acta Medica Okayama 1989;43:311–5.

386. Maurea S, Cuocolo A, Reynolds JC, et al. Iodine-131-metaiodobenzylguanidine scintigraphy in preoperative and postoperative evaluation of paragangliomas: comparison with CT and MRI. J Nucl Med 1993;34:173–9.

387. Mulligan LM, Marsh DJ, Robinson BG, et al. Genotype-phenotype correlation in multiple endocrine neoplasia type 2: report of the Intentional RET Mutation Consortium. J Int Med 1995;238:343–6.

388. Naeye RL. Brain-stem and adrenal abnormalities in the sudden infant death syndrome. Am J Clin Pathol 1976;66:526–30.

389. Norton JA, Froome LC, Farrell RE, Wells SA Jr. Multiple endocrine neoplasia type IIb: the most aggressive form of medullary thyroid carcinoma. Surg Clin N Am 1979;59:109–18.

390. Padberg BC, Garbe E, Achilles E, Dralle H, Bressel M, Schröder S. Adrenomedullary hyperplasia and phaeochromocytoma. DNA cytophotometric findings in 47 cases. Virchows Arch [A] 1990;416:443–6.

391. Schimke RN. Multiple endocrine adenomatosis syndromes. Adv Intern Med 1976;21:249–65.

392. Sipple JH. The association of pheochromocytoma with carcinoma of the thyroid gland. Am J Med 1961;31:163–5.

393. Steiner AL, Goodman AD, Powers SR. Study of a kindred with pheochromocytoma, medullary thyroid carcinoma, hyperparathyroidism and Cushing's disease: multiple endocrine neoplasia, type 2. Medicine 1968;47:371–409.

394. Thomas JE, Rooke ED, Kvale WF. The neurologist's experience with pheochromocytoma. A review of 100 cases. JAMA 1966;197:754–8.

395. Tischler AS. Cell proliferation in the adult adrenal medulla. Chromaffin cells as a model of indirect carcinogenesis. In: Pathology of laboratory animals, endocrine system. ILSI Monograph. New York: Springer-Verlag, 1994.

396. Tischler AS, DeLellis RA. The rat adrenal medulla: II. Proliferative lesions. J Am Coll Toxicol 1988;7:23–44.

397. Tischler AS, DeLellis RA, Perlman RL, et al. Spontaneous proliferative lesions of the adrenal medulla in aging Long-Evans rats. Comparison to PC12 cells, small granule-containing cells, and human adrenal medullary hyperplasia. Lab Invest 1985;53:486–98.

398. Tischler AS, Ruzicka LA, Donahue SR, DeLellis RA. Chromaffin cell proliferation in the adult rat adrenal medulla. Int J Dev Neurosci 1989;7:439–48.

399. Tischler AS, Ruzicka LA, Van Pelt CS, Sandusky GE. Catecholamine-synthesizing enzymes and chromogranin proteins in drug-induced proliferative lesions of the rat adrenal medulla. Lab Invest 1990;63:44–51.

400. Valk TW, Frager MS, Gross MD, et al. Spectrum of pheochromocytoma in multiple endocrine neoplasia. A scintigraphic portrayal using 131I-metaiodobenzylguanidine. Ann Int Med 1981;94:762–7.

401. Verdy M, Weber AM, Roy CC, Morin CL, Cadotte M, Brochu P. Hirschsprung's disease in a family with multiple endocrine neoplasia type 2. J Pediatr Gastroenterol Nutr 1982;1:603–7.

402. Warren S, Grozdev L, Gates O, Chute RN. Radiation-induced adrenal medullary tumors in the rat. Arch Pathol 1966;82:115–8.

403. Williams ED, Pollock DJ. Multiple mucosal neuromata with endocrine tumours: a syndrome allied to von Recklinghausen's disease. J Pathol Bacteriol 1966;91:71–80.

404. Wu CP. Adrenal medullary hyperplasia. Natl Med J Chin 1977;57:331–3.

405. Wu JP, Xu FJ, Zeng ZP. Adrenal medullary hyperplasia. Long-term follow-up of 15 patients. Chin Med J (Engl) 1984;97:653–6.

406. Yobbagy JJ, Levatter R, Sisson JC, Shulkin BL, Polley T. Scintigraphic portrayal of the syndrome of multiple endocrine neoplasia type 2b. Clin Nucl Med 1988;13:433–7.

407. Yoshida A, Hatanaka S, Ohi Y, Umekito Y, Yoshida H. von Recklinghausen's disease associated with somatostatin-rich duodenal carcinoid (somatostatinoma), medullary thyroid carcinoma and diffuse adrenal medullary hyperplasia. Acta Pathol Jap 1991;41:847–56.

408. Zhang ZX, Yu ST. Analysis of 17 cases of adrenal medullary hyperplasia. Natl Med J Chin 1979;59:95–7.

5
DIFFUSE NEUROENDOCRINE SYSTEM

EMBRYOLOGY AND ANATOMY

The expression of specific neuronal and endocrine features by the cells and tissues that make up the diffuse or dispersed neuroendocrine system (DNES) is regulated by many genes. Such features include the presence of cytoplasmic secretory granules, expression of broad-spectrum neuroendocrine markers such as chromogranins and synaptophysin, and expression of specific peptide hormones and amines (2,4–6,12–15). The DNES is comprised of a wide spectrum of cells, located in disparate sites from the skin to the gastrointestinal tract and brain (Table 5-1, fig. 5-1). Specific organs, such as the parathyroid and pituitary glands, are composed mainly of DNES cells, while the adrenal and thyroid glands have a mixture of neuroendocrine cells and non-neuroendocrine cells. The non-neuroendocrine cells of the endocrine system are limited in number and include thyroid follicular cells, adrenal cortical cells, and steroid-producing cells of the ovary and testis. These cells, which form part of the traditional endocrine system, produce thyroxine or steroid hormones. Neuroendocrine cells are found admixed within other tissues and organs such as the prostate, breast, kidney, and larynx.

Development of DNES Concept and Embryology

Feyrter (3) first recognized the pale (neuroendocrine) cells that were widely distributed throughout the body, especially in the gastrointestinal tract. Pearse and colleagues (13,14) observed that many endocrine cells had chemicals in common with neurons, including peptides and amines. The features of these neuroendocrine cells that they observed included amine production and/or amine precursor uptake, production of amino acid decarboxylase, high esterase/cholinesterase levels, high alpha-glycerophosphate dehydrogenase levels, ultrastructurally identifiable endocrine secretory granules, and specific peptide immunohistochemistry. Pearse subsequently proposed that cells of the DNES were of neural crest origin (13). Weston (16) and others showed that a wide spectrum of cells in the body are derived from the

Table 5-1

NEUROENDOCRINE CELLS AND PEPTIDE PRODUCTS

Cell Type	Markers
Adrenal medulla	Catecholamines, somatostatin, S100 protein, VIP,[a] ACTH
Gastrointestinal tract	Gastrin, somatostatin, VIP, secretin, insulin, glucagon, pancreatic polypeptide, cholecystokinins, serotonin
Lung	ACTH, endorphin, calcitonin, gastrin-releasing peptides
Pancreas	Insulin, glucagon, pancreatic polypeptide, somatostatin, VIP, gastrin, serotonin
Parathyroid	Parathyroid hormone, parathyroid hormone-related peptide
Pituitary	ACTH, growth hormone, prolactin, follicle-stimulating hormone, luteinizing hormone, thyroid-stimulating hormone, calcitonin
Thyroid C cell	Calcitonin, somatostatin, ACTH, calcitonin, gene-related peptide
Neuroendocrine cells and tumors of breast, cervix, kidney, larynx, ovary, uterus, paranasal sinus, prostate, testis, and other sites	Chromogranin, synaptophysin, other broad-spectrum neuroendocrine markers

[a]VIP - vasoactive intestinal polypeptide; ACTH - adrenocorticotropic hormone.

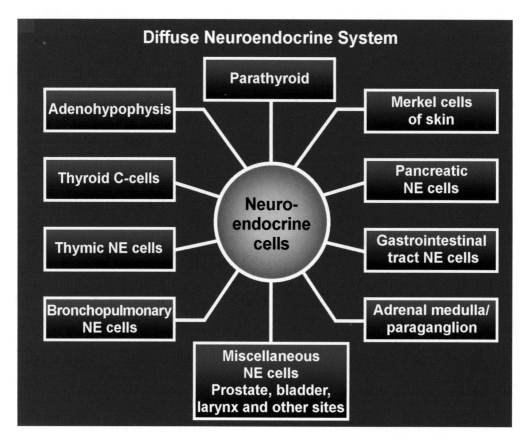

Figure 5-1

DIFFUSE NEUROENDOCRINE SYSTEM

Schematic overview of the diffuse neuroendocrine system which is composed of classic endocrine organs, as well as scattered neuroendocrine cells in various organs and tissues. These cells are characterized by specific peptides such as chromogranin and synaptophysin, and ultrastructural evidence of secretory granules.

neural crest including the sensory and autonomic ganglia; skeletal and supporting tissue components such as mesenchyma in the head and cranial and visceral skeleton; and the pigment cells, indicating the wide diversity of neural crest–derived cells. In developing the amine precursor uptake and decarboxylase (APUD) concept, Pearse presented evidence that a few members of the DNES were derived from the neural crest (13,15). However, the neural crest origin of most of these cells was subsequently disproven by the experiments of LeDourin and colleagues (7–11), by Andrews et al. (1), and by other investigators. The experimental findings showed that only the adrenal medullary cells, paraganglia, thyroid C cells, and a few other cells such as sympathetic ganglia were derived from the neural crest.

In a revision of the original DNES concept, Pearse proposed that 40 individual cell types were members of the DNES, including a central division of the hypothalamic-pituitary axis and pineal gland, and a peripheral division of the gastroenteropancreatic axis, lungs, parathyroid gland, adrenal medulla sympathetic ganglia, skin melanocytes, thyroid C cells, and urogenital tract. Interestingly, the Merkel cell of the skin was not included in the DNES by Pearse, although these cells have DNES properties. In contrast, melanocytes, although derived from the neural crest, do not have immunohistochemical features that fit into the current DNES concept. Other workers have proposed similar unifying concepts analogous to that of the DNES. The paraneuron concept proposed by Fujita (4) stated that receptosecretory cells, which included the typical DNES cells in addition to gustatory cells, olfactory cells, hair cells of the inner ear, and visual cells of the retina, had many common properties including dense core secretory granules, peptides, amines, nucleotides, and acidic carrier proteins including chromogranins which made them similar to the DNES of Pearse. The modified DNES concept, which considers this system to be composed of cells showing a unique genotype and phenotype, provides a unifying approach to explain the various multiple endocrine neoplasia syndromes and tumors commonly involved with ectopic hormone production. The updated DNES theory in use today incorporates the ideas of Pearse et al., the paraneuron concept of Fujita, and observations of other investigators who have contributed to the development and evolution of the DNES concept (2,4,12,13,15).

Pancreas

The endocrine cells of the pancreas are first noted in the 8-week-old fetus as single cells at the base of the primary tubules formed from primitive epithelial cells (17). The insulin (B), glucagon (A), and somatostatin (D) cells are noted first by immunohistochemical staining and the pancreatic polypeptide (PP) cells are detected a few days later. The islet cells continue to develop along the intralobular and intercalated ductules through the rest of gestation until the early postnatal period, but these cells do not develop from the main ducts (18,20). The glucagon and somatostatin cells are more abundant in the fetal than the adult pancreas. They are usually somewhat separate from the insulin cells in some islets. The islets at the posterior inferior part of the pancreatic head, which originates from the ventral pouch, have more pancreatic polypeptide cells, with a few insulin cells, but very few of the two other cell types (20).

In most areas of the neonatal pancreas, the predominant cell is the insulin cell, except in the posterior inferior head where 70 to 80 percent of the cells produce pancreatic polypeptide (19).

Extra-Adrenal Paraganglia

The extra-adrenal paraganglionic cells are derived from the neural crest. They are distributed along the paravertebral and para-aortic axis, paralleling the distribution of the sympathetic nervous system. The head and neck paraganglia are associated with the parasympathetic nervous system and are usually located close to neural and vascular structures in these regions.

Lung

The Kulchitsky or K cells in the lungs are precursor neuroendocrine cells that are present in the bronchial and bronchiolar respiratory epithelium. These cells are numerous in the developing fetus and neonate, and are less common in the adult (21,22).

HISTOLOGY

Pancreas

The pancreatic endocrine cells are mostly present in the islets of Langerhans; a small number are present as single cells or small cell clusters among the ductal cells and paraductal acinar cells (24,25). Pancreatic polypeptide cells are the principal cell type found in the small ducts. Some serotonin and enterochromaffin (EC) cells are present in the epithelium of the large pancreatic duct (23). The islets range from 75 to 225 μm in greatest diameter (26). They are evenly distributed throughout most of the pancreas, and morphometric studies have shown that the body and tail of the pancreas have similar endocrine cell masses (31). The exception is the pancreatic polypeptide–rich islet in the posterior part of the head of the pancreas which may reach 400 to 500 mm in size and show a trabecular architecture suggestive of hyperplasia (27,28).

The islets are composed of compact masses of cells with anastomosing sinusoids. The islet capillaries are lined by endocrine cells that are in direct contact with the blood vessels (26). Innervation is by both sympathetic and parasympathetic nerve fibers which run along the blood vessels. A rich network of peptidergic fibers originating from the autonomic ganglia is present in the islets; the fibers function as neuroregulators in the control of islet cell function.

The most frequent type of islet cell in the body and tail is the insulin or B cell (fig. 5-2), which makes up 60 to 80 percent of cells in these regions and 20 to 30 percent of cells in the posterior head (25). The glucagon or A cell comprises about 15 to 20 percent of the cells in the body and tail of the pancreas and is present largely at the periphery of the islet (fig. 5-3) (25). The somatostatin or D cell comprises about 5 to 10 percent of the body and tail (fig. 5-4).

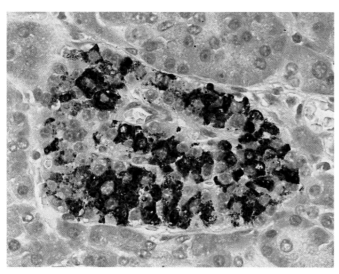
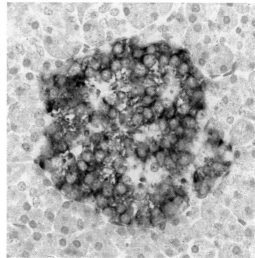

Figure 5-2

NORMAL PANCREATIC ISLET

Left: Normal pancreatic islet immunostained for insulin. Insulin-positive cells constitute 60 to 80 percent of the islet cells (diaminobenzidine chromogen).

Right: Normal pancreatic islet stained for proinsulin messenger RNA by in situ hybridization. Positive cells have dark blue cytoplasmic staining similar to insulin immunostaining (alkaline phosphatase-NBT/BCIP).

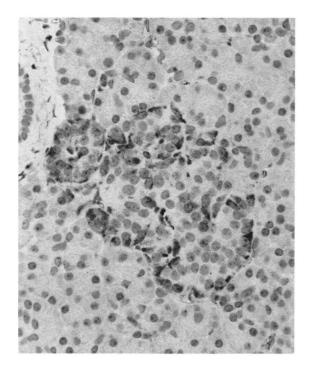

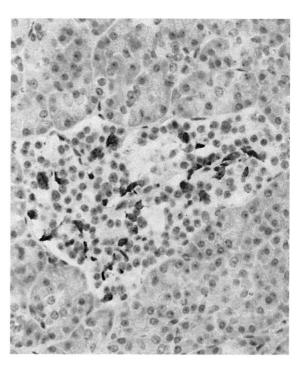

Figure 5-3

NORMAL PANCREATIC ISLET

Glucagon cells are normally at the periphery of the islets and comprise about 15 to 20 percent of the cells.

Figure 5-4

NORMAL PANCREATIC ISLET

Somatostatin-positive cells comprise about 5 to 10 percent of islet cells.

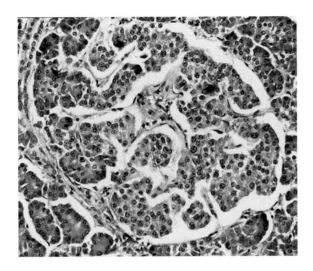
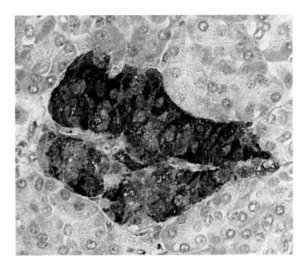

Figure 5-5

NORMAL PANCREATIC ISLET

Left: Pancreatic polypeptide-producing cells in the body of the pancreas comprise about 2 to 5 percent of islet cells.
Right: Pancreatic polypeptide-producing cells in the posterior portion of the head of the pancreas comprise about 70 percent of the islet cells in this region.

Pancreatic polypeptide cells constitute 2 to 5 percent of islet cells in the body and tail, but up to 70 percent of cells in the posterior portion of the head of the pancreas (fig. 5-5) (25). Unique hormones in some islet cells include islet amyloid polypeptide in insulin cells (27) and glicentin-related pancreatic peptide in glucagon cells (30).

Immunohistochemical staining with highly specific antibodies has provided an exact method for quantifying the islet cells as well as for studying other peptides produced by these cells. Broad-spectrum markers such as chromogranin A and B, synaptophysin, proprotein convertases, and neuron-specific enolase are readily identified in islet cells.

Ultrastructural studies have historically been used to identify different types of islet cells by granule morphology (figs. 5-6–5-8). The insulin cells have irregular secretory granules with a crystalline or compact finely granular core (fig. 5-7). The crystalline granules contain mainly insulin, while the compact core granules are less mature and contain proinsulin along with insulin (29). Insulin granules range from 200 to 400 nm in diameter, glucagon granules from 300 to 400 nm and contain a central electron dense core and a pale granular halo (fig. 5-6), and somatostatin granules from 170 to 250 nm and are of uniform density (fig. 5-8). The pancre-

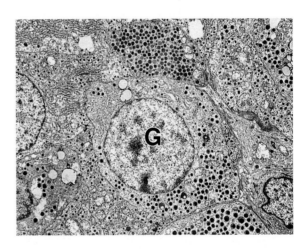

Figure 5-6

NORMAL PANCREATIC ISLET

Ultrastructural features of the normal islet cells show the unique secretory granules. Glucagon cells (G) have granules with a dense core and a less osmophilic peripheral zone. Pancreatic polypeptide cells in the body of the pancreas have small secretory granules ranging from 100 to 200 nm in diameter (X6,500).

atic polypeptide granules from the posterior head of the pancreas are larger (mean diameter, 208 nm) than those in the tail and body which have a mean diameter of 140 nm, and have a dense core and a round shape.

Figure 5-7

NORMAL PANCREATIC ISLET

Ultrastructure of an insulin cell shows distinct crystalline granules with irregular shapes. The more compact secretory granules are less mature and contain more proinsulin along with insulin (X6,500).

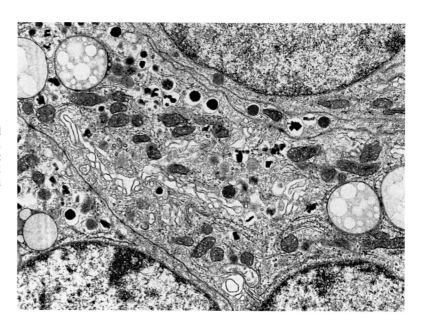

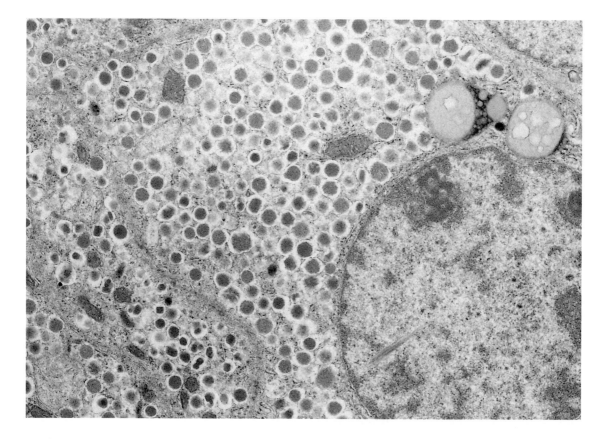

Figure 5-8

NORMAL PANCREATIC ISLET

Ultrastructure of somatostatin cells shows secretory granules of uniform density, which range in size from 170 to 200 nm in a normal islet.

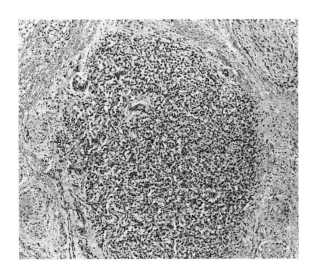

Figure 5-9

NORMAL PARAGANGLIONIC TISSUE

Nests of paraganglionic cells from the organ of Zuckerkandl show uniform cells in an organoid pattern.

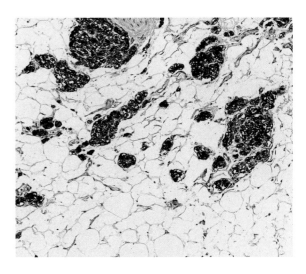

Figure 5-10

NORMAL PARAGANGLIONIC TISSUE

Nest of paraganglionic cells from the organ of Zuckerkandl stains strongly for chromogranin A (diaminobenzidine chromogen).

Extra-Adrenal Paraganglia

The microscopic appearance of the extra-adrenal paraganglia is similar to that of the adrenal medulla discussed in chapter 4. There are paraganglionic chief cells and sustentacular cells (figs. 5-9–5-11). The chief cells are positive for chromogranin A (fig. 5-10) and synaptophysin, and the sustentacular cells stain for S100 protein. A few ganglion cells and myelinated nerve bundles may also be present. Ultrastructural studies show cytoplasmic secretory granules 100 to 200 nm in diameter in the chief cells. The sustentacular cells do not have secretory granules.

Lung

Pulmonary neuroendocrine cells are cylindrical and located in the basal part of the mucosa. They are not ciliated and have cytoplasmic processes that may occasionally reach the airway lumen. The individual cells have clear to eosinophilic cytoplasm, ovoid to round nucleus, and a small nucleolus. The cells are positive for broad-spectrum neuroendocrine markers, including chromogranin (fig. 5-12), synaptophysin, prohormone convertases, and bombesin or gastrin-releasing peptides. Ultrastructural examination shows secretory granules ranging from 100 to 300 nm in diameter (32); microtubules and lipofuscin granules may be present as well.

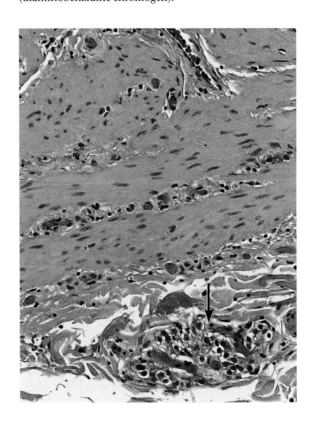

Figure 5-11

NORMAL PARAGANGLIONIC TISSUE

Normal paraganglionic cells present in the wall of the gallbladder (arrow).

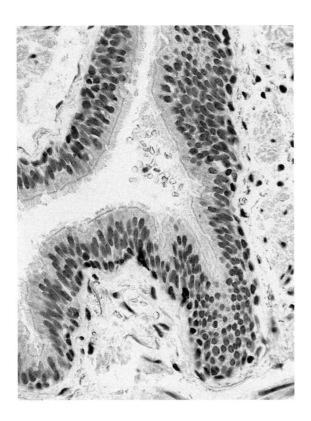 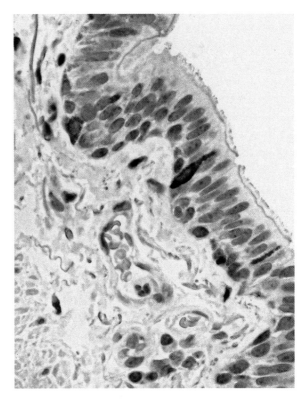

Figure 5-12

NORMAL LUNG ENDOCRINE TISSUE

Left: Neuroendocrine cells (NE) in the normal adult bronchial mucosa stain for chromogranin A (diaminobenzidine chromogen).

Right: Higher magnification of NE cells. These cells are also positive for bombesin and serotonin.

Neuroendocrine bodies are clusters of 4 to 10 neuroendocrine cells which extend from the subepithelial basement membrane to the airway lumen (36). They are positive for neuroendocrine markers (37). Their function is not known, but they may have chemoreceptor or tactile receptor function. Neuroendocrine bodies have been shown to increase in number in experimental animals after treatment with diethylnitrosamine (35). They are increased in number in patients with hypertensive pulmonary disease and in infants with bronchopulmonary dysplasia (33,34), and decreased in patients with hyaline membrane disease (34).

Gastrointestinal Tract

A plethora of cell types in the gastrointestinal tract are members of the DNES, having the typical dense core secretory granules and expressing chromogranin or synaptophysin and other broad-spectrum neuroendocrine markers (Table 5-2). Cholecystokinin (CCK) is present in the I cells of the duodenum and jejunal mucosal glands. There are various forms of the hormone whose principal functions include stimulation of pancreatic enzyme release, stimulation of gallbladder contraction, and relaxation of the sphincter of Oddi (38,44). Gastrin is present in distinct cells of the gastric antrum, duodenum, and jejunum. It stimulates secretion of gastric acid and intrinsic factor.

Gastrin-inhibiting polypeptide (GIP) is present in the Kulchitsky (K) cells of the small intestine. It functions to enhance insulin release after glucose ingestion during hyperglycemic conditions (44). Motilin is present in the M cells of the small intestine and is most abundant in the jejunal mucosa. Motilin stimulates the interdigestive motor activity of the gastric and upper intestinal smooth muscle.

Table 5-2

DISTRIBUTION OF CELLS OF THE DNES IN THE GASTROINTESTINAL TRACT[a]

Hormone/Chemical	Cell Type	Location	Function
Cholecystokinin	I	Small bowel	Stimulate pancreatic enzyme secretion
Gastrin-inhibiting peptide (GIP)	K	Small bowel	Stimulate insulin secretion
Gastrin	G, IG	Antrum and small intestine	Stimulate gastric acid secretion
Gastrin-releasing peptide	—	Digestive system	Stimulate gastrin secretion
Glucagon-like immunoreactivity	L	Small and large intestine	Possible regulation of glucose
Histamine	ECL	Gastric fundus	Stimulate gastric acid secretion
Motilin	M	Small intestine	Intestinal motility
Neurotensin	N	Ileum	Possible vascular regulation
Pancreatic polypeptide	PP	Small intestine	Possible inhibition of pancreatic enzyme
Polypeptide YY	—	Large intestine	Unknown
Secretin	S	Small intestine	Stimulate bicarbonate secretion
Serotonin	EC	Small and large intestine	Motility, possible vascular regulation
Somatostatin	D	Small and large intestine	Inhibition of multiple factors
Substance P	—	Nerves	Possible neurotransmitter
Vasoactive intestinal polypeptide	—	Nerves	Possible neurotransmitter

[a]Modified from Lechago J, Shah IA. The endocrine digestive system. In: Kovacs K, Asa SL, eds. Functional endocrine pathology, 2nd ed. Oxford, UK: Blackwell Science, 1998:488–512.

Neurotensin is present in the N cells of the ileum and jejunal mucosa. It regulates systemic arterial wall relaxation, leading to hypotension, but may also have other functions (40,44). Pancreatic polypeptide inhibits pancreatic exocrine secretion and stimulates gastrointestinal motility. It is present mainly in the posterior head of the pancreas but has also been localized to the large intestine. Peptide YY is present in the ileal and colonic mucosa. It inhibits pancreatic bicarbonate secretion. Secretin is produced by the S cells. It stimulates water and bicarbonate secretion by the pancreas. Somatostatin is produced primarily by the islet cells but also by the stomach and small intestine. It inhibits secretion of gastric acid and release of gastrin. It is also present in nerve fibers in the gastrointestinal tract.

Gastrin-releasing peptide is present in nerve cells of the gastrointestinal tract, in the nerve plexus of Auerbach, in nerve fibers of the musculinus propria, and in the gastric mucosa (39). It is the equivalent of the amphibian peptide bombesin (39) and releases gastrin from the antral G cells. It also has trophic activity in the developing fetal lung. Substance P is present in nerve fibers of the gastrointestinal tract and in enterochromaffin cells (EC) of the small intestine. It is a pain transmitter as well as regulator of smooth muscle contraction in the gastrointestinal tract. Vasoactive intestine polypeptide is present in nerve cells and fibers where it regulates vessel tone to cause vasodilatation, stimulates electrolyte transport across epithelial membranes, and causes smooth muscle relaxation. Serotonin is a biogenic amine and is present throughout the stomach and large and small intestine in the enterochromaffin cells where it regulates gut motility and blood flow (42). Histamine is another amine present in enterochromaffin-like (ECL) cells and stimulates gastric acid secretion.

Immunohistochemical studies of the DNES cells in the gastrointestinal tract have localized broad-spectrum markers such as chromogranin, synaptophysin, and neuron-specific enolase as well as many peptides, in specific cell types (45). Electron microscopic studies have helped to further characterize the various cell types (43).

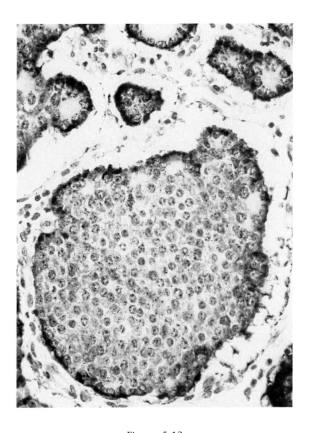

Figure 5-13

FONTANA-MASSON STAIN

Histochemical Fontana-Masson silver stain of a midgut carcinoid shows a dark brown reaction product in the cytoplasm. Positive cells take up silver salt and reduce it to a visible metallic state without an extraneous reducing agent. This staining reaction is highly specific but not very sensitive.

Gastrin-producing cells have round secretory granules 180 to 300 nm in diameter which are located mainly in the basal portion of the cell cytoplasm. In the duodenum, gastrin secretory granules are dark and round and measure 190 ± 30 nm in diameter (43). Somatostatin cells in the stomach have dense core secretory granules measuring 300 to 400 nm in diameter; in the large intestine they have a different appearance (43). Secretin cells have round to slightly irregular granules measuring 180 to 220 nm in diameter and a core of electron dense material with a clear space between this and the limiting membrane. Cholecystokinin-producing cells have dense core granules 250 to 300 nm in diameter. Serotonin-producing cells have pleomorphic secretory granules measuring 200 to 300 nm in diameter, with a dense central core and an ad-

Table 5-3
BROAD-SPECTRUM NEUROENDOCRINE MARKERS

Chromogranin/secretogranin

Synaptophysin

PGP 9.5

Leu-7

Synaptic proteins
    SNAP-25
    Rab3A

Neural cell adhesion nodules (NCAM) (CD57)

Peptidylglycine alpha-amidating monooxygenase

Neuroendocrine-specific protein (NSP) reticulons

jacent limiting membrane. Ultrastructural and immunohistochemical studies have become a more precise way of localizing peptides and other chemicals in secretory granules (41).

METHODS USED TO CHARACTERIZE DNES CELLS

Histochemical Stains

A wide variety of techniques have been used to characterize the cells and tissues of the DNES (55,59). Silver stains such as the argentaffin stain (e.g., Fontana-Masson), are taken up by certain cells that reduce the silver to its visible metallic state without an extraneous reducing agent (fig. 5-13). Midgut DNES cells are typically argentaffin positive. Argyrophilic stains require the addition of a reducing agent to reduce the impregnated silver to a visible metallic end product. The Grimelius and Sevier-Munger argyrophilic stains are more sensitive than argentaffin stains, but less specific (fig. 5-14).

Immunohistochemical Stains

An increasing number of general neuroendocrine markers or immunostains are used to characterize the cells of the DNES (Table 5-3).

Chromogranin-Secretogranin. The chromogranin/secretogranin (Cg/Sg) family is composed of several of the acidic proteins present in the secretory granules of neuroendocrine cells (Table 5-4). The three major Cg/Sg proteins are

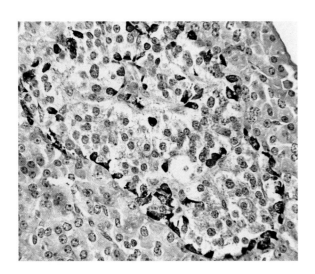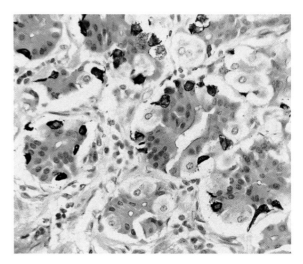

Figure 5-14

ARGYROPHILIC SILVER STAIN

Left: Cells at the periphery of a normal islet, which are associated with glucagon production, stain with Grimelius stain. Argyrophilic stains such as the Grimelius require the addition of a reducing agent to reduce the impregnated silver to a visible metallic end product.

Right: Gastric neuroendocrine cells stain with the Grimelius silver stain. Most of the positive cells are associated with gastrin production.

Table 5-4

CHROMOGRANIN/SECRETOGRANIN MOLECULES

Protein	Molecular Mass (kd)	mRNA (kb)	Chromosome Location	Proteolytic Cleavage Product
Chromogranin A[a]	49	2.1	14	Pancreastatin, chromostatin
Chromogranin B	76	2.5	20	GAWK peptide, CCB peptide
Secretogranin II	68	2.5	—	Secretoneurin
Secretogranin III (1B1075)	57	2.2	9	—
Secretogranin IV (HISL-19)	NA[b]	NA	NA	—
Secretogranin V (7B2)	21	1.35	15	—

[a]Chromogranin A was previously known as bovine secretory protein I; chromogranin B was previously designated as secretogranin I; secretogranin II was previously designated as chromogranin C.

[b]NA = data not available.

currently designated as chromogranin (Cg)A and (Cg)B and secretogranin (Sg)II. Others include SgIII, SgIV, and SgV (or 7B2). The distribution of CgA has been studied extensively in human tumors (61–63,76,88). It is present in most neuroendocrine cells and neoplasms. Because of their widespread distribution and high degree of specificity, Cg/Sg proteins are excellent markers for neuroendocrine cells and neoplasms (fig. 5-15) (87,88).

Most neoplasms with only a few endocrine secretory granules, such as small cell carcinoma of the lung and Merkel's cell carcinoma, do not react strongly with CgA antibodies (88). Although CgA is a highly specific neuroendocrine marker, it may have limited sensitivity in some cells and tumors (47,48). For example, hindgut carcinoid tumors have limited immunoreactivity for CgA, with only 60 percent of cases positive in a recent series (48). Similarly, pituitary

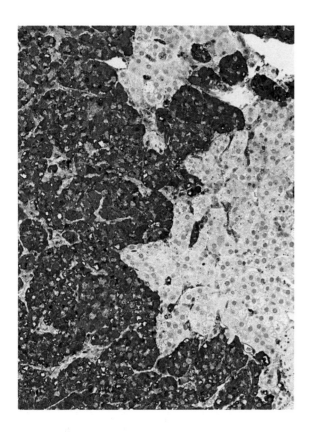 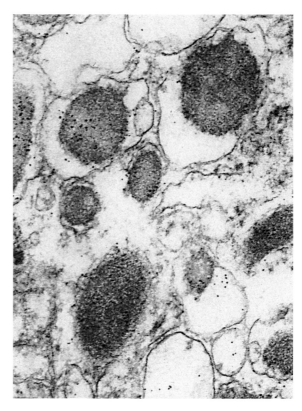

Figure 5-15

CHROMOGRANIN A IMMUNOLOCALIZATION

Left: Chromogranin stains the cells of the adrenal medulla. Adrenocortical cells are negative for chromogranin A (diaminobenzidine chromogen).

Right: Ultrastructural localization of chromogranin A with 5-nm colloidal gold particles in the secretory granules of a pheochromocytoma. This labeling shows the specificity of chromogranin staining in the secretory granules of neuroendocrine cells (X30,000).

prolactinomas are often negative for CgA. Because these tumors often express CgB, the use of antibodies against CgB or a cocktail of CgA and B usually increases the sensitivity for detecting neuroendocrine cells.

Synaptophysin. Synaptophysin, a 38-kd protein molecule, is a component of the membrane of presynaptic vesicles. It is widely distributed in neurons and neuroendocrine cells and their neoplasms, and it is another broad-spectrum neuroendocrine marker (54). Unlike the Cg/Sg proteins that are well preserved in formalin-fixed tissues, ethanol fixation provides optimal preservation of the synaptophysin antigen. However, most of the antisynaptophysin monoclonal antibodies work well in formalin-fixed sections. Synaptophysin is localized to vesicles in the neuroendocrine cells of tumors, but immunostaining is present diffusely in the cytoplasm.

Proconvertases. The proconvertases (PCs) are recently described enzymes that process propeptides into active peptides within cells (61,78). Some of these, including PC1/PC3 and PC2, are highly specific for neuroendocrine cells and tumors, and can be used as specific neuroendocrine markers (fig. 5-16). Others, such as PC4, are present in the testis, whereas PC5/6 is more prevalent in the gastrointestinal tract and adrenal gland.

Neuron-Specific Enolase (NSE). The enzyme, also known as gamma-enolase, is a very sensitive, but not too specific, marker for neuroendocrine cells and tumors. It is commonly found in neurons, peripheral nerves, and neuroendocrine cells (64,75). Some non-neuroendocrine

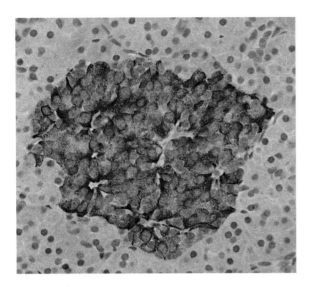 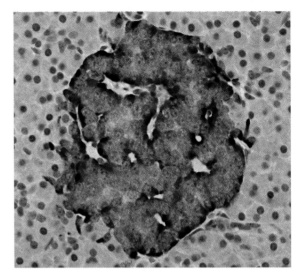

Figure 5-16

BROAD-SPECTRUM NEUROENDOCRINE MARKERS

Left: Immunohistochemical staining of an islet for the proconvertase PC1/3 shows diffuse brown staining in most of the islet cells (diaminobenzidine chromogen).

Right: Immunohistochemical staining of an islet for the proconvertase PC2 shows diffuse staining, with stronger staining in the peripheral glucagon-producing cells (diaminobenzidine chromogen).

cells and neoplasms also react with antisera against NSE. NSE should be used only with other broad-spectrum markers of neuroendocrine cells in the diagnosis of neuroendocrine tumors because of its relative lack of specificity.

Bombesin/Gastrin-Releasing Peptide and Leu-7 (HNK-1). Bombesin is a tetradecapeptide originally isolated from amphibian skin. It is present in many endocrine cells as well as in central and peripheral neurons (86). Gastrin-releasing peptide, the proposed mammalian analogue of bombesin, has been found in many lung and gastrointestinal endocrine cells and tumors, and can be used as a broad-spectrum marker for many endocrine neoplasms (49).

Leu-7 (HNK-1), a monoclonal antibody that was produced against a T-cell leukemia cell line, recognizes natural killer cells in blood and lymphoid tissue. It also reacts with small cell carcinomas of the lung as well as with pheochromocytomas and other neuroendocrine neoplasms (50,84).

PGP 9.5. PGP 9.5 is a soluble protein that was originally isolated from brain. It is a good general marker for neuronal and neuroendocrine tissues (71,83). Interestingly, about half of mela-

nomas stain for PGP 9.5, whereas these melanocytic tumors are usually negative for Cg/Sg and synaptophysin. PGP is a cytoplasmic soluble protein that frequently co-localizes in normal and neoplastic neuroendocrine tissues.

Neural Cell Adhesion Molecule (NCAM). NCAM is a member of the family of membrane-bound glycoproteins present mainly in brain and muscle (51,57). It is involved in neuron-neuron and nerve-muscle interactions. The distribution of NCAM in neuroendocrine tissues and tumors was first reported by Jin et al. (57), who found it in widespread distribution. NCAM is present in about 20 percent of nonsmall cell lung carcinomas and is often associated with a poor prognosis (69). Small cell lung carcinomas also frequently stain with NCAM antibodies (56,58,73).

Peptidylglycine Alpha-Amidating Monooxygene (PAM). Amidation is an important step in the maturation of some neuropeptides (52,55,56,60,82). The enzyme PAM catalyzes the post-translational modification of many neuropeptides. It consists of two enzymes that convert peptidylglycine substrates into alpha-amidating products and glyoxylate. The PAM proteins are usually released along with their peptide products

271

during exocytosis, whereas membrane-bound PAM remains associated with the cell (52). Several studies have examined PAM expression in neuroendocrine cells (53,67,70,78). A recent study by Scopsi et al. (78) found PAM in all neuroendocrine cell types. They found a close correlation between PAM expression and at least one of the three principal granin proteins (CgA, CgB, or SgII) (78).

Synaptic Proteins. A series of proteins involved in neurotransmitter secretion has also been associated with neuroendocrine cells and tumors. These synaptic proteins include SNAP-25 and Rab3A (46,72,74,81). SNAP-25 was originally identified as a neuron-specific protein associated with the plasma membrane of the presynaptic nerve terminal. It was shown to be part of the putative docking complex that is implicated in membrane fusion. A homologous protein, SNAP-23, is expressed ubiquitously in human non-neuronal tissues, including endocrine organs.

Rab3A is a small guanosine 5'-triphosphate-binding protein of the Rab family that is expressed mainly in neurons and neuroendocrine cells (65,66,68). Rab3A is thought to be important in the control of exocytosis in neuron and neuroendocrine cells. A recent study showed increased SNAP-25 immunoreactivity in most prolactin (PRL) and growth hormone (GH) cell adenomas, suggesting that this protein is involved in the mechanism of exocytosis in neoplasms derived from these cell types (65).

Neuroendocrine-Specific Protein (NSP) Reticulons. NSP reticulons are endoplasmic reticulum–associated protein complexes consisting of two closely related protein constituents: NSP-A and NSP-C (79–81,85). In a recent report (81), the expression of these NSP reticulons was examined in lung carcinomas. NSP-A and NSP-C were reactive with most carcinoid tumors and small cell lung carcinomas. There was a high concordance between expression of NSP-A and NSP-C in neuroendocrine tumors. The investigators noted that NSP-A was more sensitive than synaptophysin, chromogranin A, Leu-7, and neurofilament proteins in detecting neuroendocrine differentiation in nonsmall cell lung carcinomas. NSP-A expression also showed a stronger correlation with conventional neuroendocrine markers than did NCAM.

Molecular Biology

Molecular approaches have provided new insight into the analysis of the DNES cells and tumors. In situ hybridization has been applied to examine gene expression of such broad-spectrum neuroendocrine markers as chromogranins and secretogranins (98,100,104,110, 111). The cloning of most members of the chromogranin family (Tables 5-3, 5-4) has provided the tools for the examination of the function and expression of members of the chromogranin/secretogranin family (98,111). Molecular analysis of chromogranin A gene expression has been used to detect neuroendocrine phenotype even in tumors that do not appear to be neuroendocrine (89).

The genes responsible for multiple endocrine neoplasia (MEN) types 1, 2a, and 2b have been cloned and characterized. Abnormalities of these genes lead to hyperplasia and neoplasia of multiple endocrine tissues, most of which are members of the DNES. MEN 1 is associated with a tumor suppressor gene located on chromosome 11q which produces the protein product menin (92,96,112). An abnormality of this suppressor gene is associated with hyperplasia and neoplasia of the pituitary gland, pancreas, and parathyroid gland. Some patients develop the Zollinger-Ellison syndrome. The genetic abnormality of MEN 2a and 2b is an activating mutation of tyrosine kinase of the RET proto-oncogene located on chromosome 10q (95,101–103). Abnormalities associated with these syndromes include hyperplasias and neoplasias of the thyroid C cells, adrenal medulla, and parathyroid gland in patients with MEN 2a and hyperplasias and neoplasias of the thyroid C cells and adrenal medulla, as well as mucosal neuromas and gastrointestinal tract ganglioneuromas in patients with MEN 2b (101–103). Patients and other family members affected with these inherited diseases can now be diagnosed by screening for the abnormal gene (95).

Molecular clonality analyses have provided insight into the proliferative activity of hyperplastic lesions of the DNES. Studies of primary and secondary parathyroid hyperplasia by Arnold et al. (90) showed that most secondary hyperplasias were monoclonal, suggesting that they had become true neoplasias, while the primary hyperplasias were polyclonal. Clonal analysis of pancreatic endocrine tumors showed that most benign tumors were polyclonal while the malignant tumors were monoclonal or oligoclonal (108).

Most recent molecular studies have focused on neoplasms rather than hyperplasias or inflammatory lesions involving members of the DNES. However, these studies can serve as models to explore nonneoplastic disorders of the DNES in the future, so a few of these will be cited here. The molecular technique of comparative genomic hybridization has been used to study many tumors of the DNES. With this cytogenetic technique the entire tumor genome is screened simultaneously for chromosomal gains or losses. With this approach, various new chromosomal abnormalities have been identified in various benign DNES tumors (93,105), for example, gains and losses of various chromosomes not previously detected in parathyroid and pituitary tumors have been reported. These new findings should help to focus future investigations on specific chromosomal abnormalities.

The p53 gene is most commonly altered in human tumors. Some tumors derived from the DNES, such as neuroendocrine tumors of lung, show point mutations and overexpression of the p53 protein in high-grade tumors, such as small cell carcinomas, but not in atypical or typical carcinoid tumors, emphasizing the role of these genes in tumor progression (109). p53 wild-type overexpression is more common in olfactory neuroblastomas that are likely to show local aggressive behavior and to recur (106). Similar findings of p53 overexpression have been reported in pituitary carcinomas as opposed to pituitary adenomas (107).

Recent studies of cell cycle proteins, such as cyclin-dependent kinase inhibitors including p27^{kip1}, cyclins such as cyclin D1, and other markers such as Ki67, have shown that they may have important roles in separating some hyperplastic from neoplastic lesions of the DNES, as well as adenomas from carcinomas (91,94,97,99). For example, high levels of p27^{kip1} protein are present in normal endocrine cells, with decreased levels in some hyperplastic endocrine tissues, such as with parathyroid hyperplasia (99). Even lower levels of this nuclear protein are present in many neuroen-

docrine adenomas and carcinomas (97). These findings indicate that these molecular markers can be used to analyze the hyperplastic and/or neoplastic status of DNES members and may be potentially useful in diagnostic pathology.

HYPOFUNCTION IN CELLS AND TISSUES OF THE DNES

Hypofunction of the DNES cells affects some tissues more than others. While many cells and tissues of the endocrine system, such as those of the adrenal glands, are affected by both types I and II polyglandular autoimmune syndrome (PGA), the cells of the parathyroid gland and pancreatic islets are affected the most (Table 5-5). Autoimmune parathyroid insufficiency has been discussed in chapter 2; autoimmune involvement of the pancreatic islets in types I and II diabetes mellitus is discussed here.

Polyglandular Autoimmune Syndrome

These autoimmune diseases involve several endocrine as well as nonendocrine tissues. The two principal types of PGA are type I and type II (Table 5-5); PGA type II is more common. There is usually a female predominance as with other autoimmune diseases. PGA usually develops in adulthood and there is a familial aggregation. Adrenal cortical insufficiency, autoimmune thyroid disease, and type I diabetes mellitus are the most common manifestations (117).

Polyglandular Autoimmune Syndrome Type II (PGA II). PGA II is recognized by the occurrence in the same individual of two or more of the following diseases: adrenal insufficiency, Graves' disease, autoimmune thyroiditis, type I diabetes mellitus, primary hypogonadism, myasthenia gravis, and celiac diseases (115). Thyroid peroxidase autoantibodies are present in 10 percent of children with type I diabetes mellitus (126), and 2 to 3 percent of patients with type I diabetes mellitus have celiac disease (123). Although hypoparathyroidism is rare in patients with PGA II, it may occur (117). In patients with type I diabetes mellitus and Addison's disease associated with PGA II, the high risk of developing PGA II is associated with heterozygosity for human leukocyte antigen (HLA)-DR3 and HLA-DR4 haplotypes (124).

Organ-specific autoantibodies are useful in the diagnosis of PGA. Most endocrine autoantigens

Table 5-5

POLYGLANDULAR AUTOIMMUNE
SYNDROMES ASSOCIATED WITH THE
DIFFUSE NEUROENDOCRINE SYSTEM
AND OTHER ENDOCRINE TISSUES[a]

Disorder[b]	Prevalence (%)
Type I	
Hypoparathyroidism	89
Chronic mucocutaneous candidiasis	75
Adrenal insufficiency	60
Gonadal failure	45
Hypothyroidism	12
Insulin-dependent diabetes mellitus	1
Hypopituitarism	<1
Diabetes insipidus	<1
Type II	
Adrenal insufficiency	100
Autoimmune thyroid disease	70
Insulin-dependent diabetes mellitus	50
Gonadal failure	5-50
Diabetes insipidus	<1

[a]Compiled from references 115 and 118.

[b]Other conditions involving nonendocrine tissue include: malabsorption syndrome, alopecia totalis or areata, pernicious anemia, chronic active hepatitis, and vitiligo in type I; vitiligo, alopecia, pernicious anemia, myasthenia gravis, immune thrombocytopenia purpura, Sjögren's syndrome, and rheumatoid arthritis in type II.

are hormones, such as insulin, or enzymes associated with specific endocrine function, such as thyroid peroxidase (117). In type I diabetes mellitus, several autoantibodies that react with insulin, including glutamic acid decarboxylase, are useful in the diagnosis. The mode of inheritance of PGA II is uncertain.

Polyglandular Autoimmune Syndrome Type I (PGA I). PGA I is characterized by autoimmune hypoparathyroidism, adrenal insufficiency, and mucocutaneous candidiasis. This is an uncommon disease with a little more than 140 patients reported. The largest series studied included 68 patients (114). The syndrome is usually detected in early childhood in contrast to type II which is commonly seen between ages 20 and 40. The presence of chronic mucocutaneous candidiasis suggests a T-cell function defect in the pathogenesis of the syndrome. Patients usually have antiparathyroid and antiadrenal anti-

bodies. Most patients have autoantibodies to glutamic acid decarboxylase (GAD65) which is similar to PGA II. This autoantibody may be detected up to 8 years before the development of diabetes mellitus (125).

PGA I is not associated with specific class II HLA alleles. It is inherited as an autosomal recessive disorder (115). The genetic locus is on the short arm of chromosome 21 (113).

Other Autoimmune Disorders Associated with Diabetes Mellitus

A few other autoimmune disorders associated with type I diabetes mellitus have been reported.

Trisomy 21. Down's syndrome is associated with type I diabetes mellitus and thyroiditis. Affected individuals have a T-cell abnormality that may be involved in the pathogenesis of some of these disorders (121).

Congenital Rubella. Patients with this viral infection have a 20 percent risk of acquiring diabetes mellitus, which is usually associated with expression of HLA-DR3 and HLA-DR4. There is also an increased risk of thyroiditis and hypothyroidism, which may be related to damage to the immune system by the rubella virus (116,120).

Wolfram's Syndrome. This rare autosomal recessive syndrome is associated with diabetes mellitus, diabetes insipidus, bilateral optic atrophy, and sensorineural deafness. This is a slowly progressive neurodegenerative process that has been localized to the short arm of chromosome 4 (119). The selective destruction of the islet insulin-producing cells starts in early childhood (122).

Diabetes Mellitus

Definition. Diabetes mellitus is a chronic disease in which there is sustained hyperglycemia due to relative or absolute insulin deficiency.

General Remarks. There are two principal types of diabetes mellitus (136,146,163). Type I or insulin-dependent diabetes mellitus used to be designated as juvenile onset diabetes mellitus, a disease associated with an absolute loss of insulin-producing beta cells (Table 5-6). Type II or noninsulin-dependent diabetes mellitus is associated with a relative lack of insulin due to defective secretion of hormones.

These two types of diabetes account for greater than 95 percent of all cases. Rare causes of diabetes may be due to chronic pancreatitis, cystic fibrosis, hemachromatosis, and conditions associated with other diseases, such as acromegaly and Cushing's syndrome.

Type I, Insulin-Dependent Diabetes Mellitus (IDDM). Type I diabetes mellitus is most common in whites and rare in Japanese, Chinese, African blacks, Filipinos, and Asiatic Indians (163). The prevalence in the United States is 260 per 100,000 people (0.26 percent) by age 20 years and an equal number develop the disease after age 20. The incidence is 3.7 to 20.0 per 100,000 (148).

Both class I and class II HLA molecules may be important in the development of type I diabetes: HLA-DR3 or HLA-DR4 antigens are present in 95 percent of these patients (154). The mode of inheritance of type I diabetes mellitus is unknown; a dominant mode of inheritance has been suggested, but this may be affected by complex environmental-genetic interactions. A viral contribution to the etiology of type I diabetes is supported by indirect evidence linking its onset to viral infections from rubella, mumps, cytomegalovirus, polio virus, or Epstein-Barr virus. Coxsackie virus B has been implicated as a possible significant etiologic agent, but viruses have not been isolated from the tissues of patients with beta cell destruction due to postinfectious diabetes (168). Molecular mimicry, in which another protein cross-reacting with a beta cell protein induces an antiviral CD8 lymphocyte response to beta cells, has been proposed as an etiologic agent. This theory is based mainly on experimental work with autoimmune diabetes in mice (155).

Another autoantibody involved in type I diabetes mellitus is the islet cell antibody which is present in the serum of 60 to 90 percent of newly diagnosed patients with type I diabetes mellitus (163). These antibodies react not only with insulin (B) cells but also with glucagon (A), somatostatin (D), and pancreatic polypeptide (PP) cells (134). Most of the islet cell antibodies disappear within 2 to 3 years of the onset of type I diabetes (163). Glutamic acid decarboxylase antibody is a major autoantigen in type I diabetes (128) and insulin antibodies may be present in up to 50 percent of patients with new onset type I diabetes, especially proinsulin autoantibodies (131).

Table 5-6

PRINCIPAL TYPES OF DIABETES MELLITUS

Feature	Type I (IDDM)[a]	Type II (NIDDM)
Loss of beta cell mass	+	-
Defective release of insulin	-	+
Anti-islet cell antibody	+	-
Associated with PGA I and II[b]	+	-
Obesity associated	-	+
HLA-D[c] linked	+	-
Young age onset	+	-
Ketoacidosis common	+	-
Concordance in twins	+	+

[a]IDDM – Insulin-dependent diabetes mellitus; NIDDM – Noninsulin-dependent diabetes mellitus.
[b]PGA - Polyglandular autoimmune syndrome.
[c]HLA - Human leukocyte antigen.

Type II Noninsulin-Dependent Diabetes Mellitus (NIDDM). Type II diabetes is present in all populations. While the Pima Indians of Arizona have rates that approach 40 percent (129), the prevalence is about 10 percent in the older population of the United States (163). In 1990 to 1992, 625,000 cases were diagnosed in the U.S. each year (163). With type II diabetes concordance in identical twins can approach 100 percent compared to 50 percent or less for type I diabetes (163). There is no association between HLA and type II diabetes (163). The major defects in type II NIDDM are insulin resistance and hyperinsulinemia, followed by failure to secrete enough insulin to compensate for the insulin resistance. The failure of insulin secretion correlates with glucose tolerance and is thought to be its cause (163).

Many factors affect the inheritance of type II NIDDM. The maturity onset diabetes of the young (MODY), a form of NIDDM, is inherited as an autosomal dominant defect (141). Molecular defects have been identified in type II NIDDM. The genes for the MODY type of type II diabetes have been linked to specific chromosomes, including MODY 1 to chromosome 20q, MODY 2 to 7p13-15 at the glucokinase enzyme, and MODY 3 to chromosome 12q. Specific mutations

Table 5-7

NORMAL VALUES FOR SOME NEUROENDOCRINE HORMONES[a]

Hormone	SI[b]	Conventional
Gastrin, plasma	<120 ng/L	<120 pg/mL
Glucagon, plasma	50-100 ng/L	50-100 pg/mL
Glucose, plasma		
Overnight fast, normal	4.2–6.4 mmol/L	75–115 mg/dL
Overnight fast, diabetes mellitus		
National Diabetes Data Group	>7–8 mmol/L	>140 mg/dL
American Diabetes Association	>7.0 mmol/L	>126 mg/dL
72 hr fast, normal men	>2.8 mmol/L	>50 mg/dL
72 hr fast, normal women	>2.2 mmol/L	>40 mg/dL
Glucose Tolerance Test		
2-hr postprandial plasma glucose		
Normal	<7.8 mmol/L	<140 mg/dL
Impaired glucose tolerance	7.8–11.1 mmol/L	140-200 mg/dL
Diabetes mellitus	>11.1 mmol/L	>200 mg/dL
Insulin, plasma		
Fasting	35–145 pmol/L	5–20 µU/mL
During hypoglycemia (plasma glucose <2.8 nmol/L <50 ng/mL)	<35 pmol/L	<5 µU/mL
Insulin C peptide, plasma	0.5–2.0 µg/L	0.5-2.0 pg/mL

[a]Wilson JD, Foster DW, Kronenberg DW, Larsen PR, eds. Williams textbook of endocrinology, 9th ed. Philadelphia: WB Saunders, 1998: back cover.

[b]SI - System of international units.

have been identified in the insulin receptor gene, but these mutations are not thought to cause the insulin resistance in the usual type II NIDDM (162). Other possible genetic defects affect the GLUT-2 glucose transporter, glucokinase gene, sulfonylurea receptor, and a mitochondrial gene associated with type II diabetes and deafness. Leptin and leptin receptor genes have been found to be abnormal due to genetic defects in some cases of type II NIDDM, but more of these have been shown to be candidate genetic defects in type II diabetes mellitus (163).

Clinical Features. Type I IDDM is associated with hyperglycemia, polyuria, polydipsia, and polyphagia, with weight loss due to the severe catabolic state. In children symptoms develop over a relatively short period, although the destruction of the insulin-producing cells probably occurs over a 3-year period on average (163). Patients may present with diabetic ketoacidosis precipitated by stress or another illness.

Patients with type II NIDDM may present with hyperglycemia which usually develops gradually or with glycosuria detected on routine urinalysis. Occasionally the presenting symptoms may be diabetic complications, such as peripheral neuropathy, gangrene, or a vascular insult (163). Presentation with symptoms of an acute illness from stress as in type I diabetes mellitus is very rare.

Laboratory Findings. Hyperglycemia is the most common initial finding in type I disease (Table 5-7). Patients presenting with diabetic ketoacidosis usually have hyperglycemia, hyponatremia, hyperkalemia, metabolic acidosis, and hypertriglyceridemia.

Hyperglycemia and/or glycosuria is the common initial finding with type II disease. Patients presenting with hyperosmolar nonketotic coma have marked hyperglycemia and increased osmolarity lactic acidosis, elevated blood urea nitrogen, and elevated creatinine.

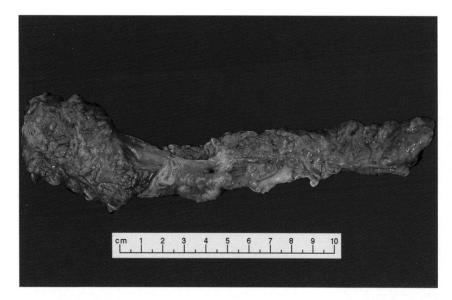

Figure 5-17

TYPE I INSULIN-DEPENDENT
DIABETES MELLITUS

Pancreas from a patient with
longstanding type I insulin-
dependent diabetes mellitus
(IDDM). The pancreas is
decreased in size with atrophy of
the acinar cells.

Measurement of glycosylated hemoglobulin can provide information about the control of the diabetes mellitus (163).

Macroscopic Findings. In type I IDDM, the pancreas is normal in size and weight if the disease develops during the first year of life. With longstanding disease, the pancreas is decreased in weight and size with atrophy of acinar cells (130,148–150). The atrophy is secondary to the lack of insulin, which has a trophic effect on the acinar cells (fig. 5-17).

There are no specific gross abnormalities in the pancreas in patients with type II NIDDM.

Microscopic Findings. In type II IDDM the microscopic findings depend on the duration of the disease. Insulitis or infiltration of lymphocytes, which are primarily T cells, is present during the initial weeks to months (139). Most of the infiltrate consists of CD8 suppressor cells with a few B cells and macrophages (133). Insulitis is most common in type I IDDM patients who are less than 5 years of age and is rarely seen after age 15 (146); it is also rare 12 months after the onset of diabetes mellitus.

With chronic type I IDDM (after one or more years), there is marked acinar cell atrophy. The islets contain very few insulin B cells, but glucagon, somatostatin, and pancreatic polypeptide cells are prominent (fig. 5-18) (140, 142,144). Islet amyloidosis, which is common in type II NIDDM, is rarely seen in type I IDDM.

The histologic features of type II NIDDM can vary from normal-appearing islets to islets with marked deposition of amyloid (fig. 5-19). Islet amyloidosis only affects insulin-producing islet cells, since amyloid is produced by these cells. The amyloid is deposited between the islet capillaries and the insulin-producing cells, and is made up of the islet amyloid polypeptide or amylin, a 37-amino acid product which has been shown by in situ hybridization to be produced by the insulin cells (165). Studies have shown islet cell amyloid in 80 to 90 percent of pancreases from patients with type II NIDDM (137, 166) compared to 2 to 3 percent of individuals without a history of overt diabetes mellitus.

Differential Diagnosis. A variety of conditions affecting the pancreas may lead to diabetes mellitus. If a history of type I IDDM or type II NIDDM is not available, morphologic examination of the pancreas should allow distinction between some of these diseases.

About 25 percent of patients with chronic pancreatitis develop diabetes mellitus (145,158). The exocrine pancreas is quite fibrotic and calcification may be present. Immunohistochemical staining for islet cell hormone shows increased numbers of glucagon cells and decreased numbers of insulin cells.

Individuals with carcinoma of the pancreas can develop diabetes mellitus secondary to obstructive disease if the tumor involves the

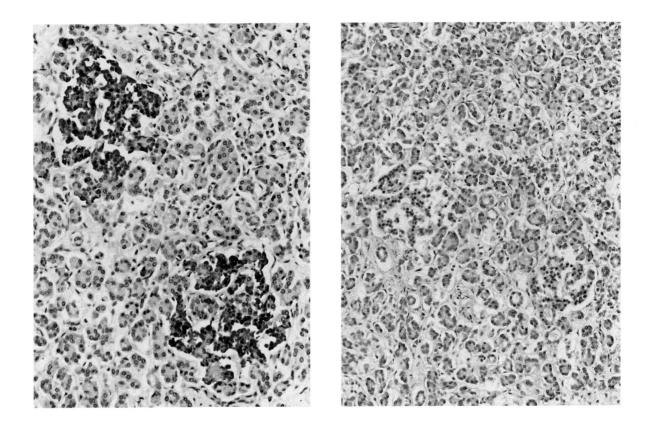

Figure 5-18

TYPE I INSULIN-DEPENDENT DIABETES MELLITUS

Left: In patients with type I IDDM, there is an increase in the number of glucagon-positive cells in the islet after immunostaining (diaminobenzidine chromogen).

Right: Immunostaining for insulin in an adjacent section from the same patient shows complete absence of insulin-producing cells.

pancreatic duct, leads to chronic pancreatitis, and infiltrates other areas of the pancreas (135). Recognition of the malignant infiltrating cells allows diagnosis even in small biopsy specimens.

Hemochromatosis due to iron overload, with iron deposition in the islet cells as well as in the exocrine pancreas, can lead to diabetes mellitus (157). The detection of iron overload in the serum and special stains for iron in pancreatic biopsy secretions are diagnostic.

Patients with cystic fibrosis may develop overt diabetes mellitus. The histologic features of cystically dilated ducts with inspissated secretions as well as extensive fibrosis and atrophy are helpful diagnostically (148). Specific chemicals, such as streptozotocin and alloxan which have been used therapeutically in patients with hyperinsulinemic hypoglycemia sec-

ondary to insulin-producing tumors or islet cell hyperplasia, may also lead to diabetes mellitus (163). These chemicals have produced diabetes in experimental animals (163). Alloxan and streptozotocin can lead to death of insulin cells in humans within a few hours (132,167).

Treatment. Insulin therapy is used for patients with type I IDDM. The goal is to achieve a normal plasma glucose level (138) and thus prevent many of the severe complications of diabetes mellitus that are discussed below. Various methods of treatment including meticulous control with daily subcutaneous insulin, continuous subcutaneous insulin infusion, and implantable intraperitoneal pumps have been used but are beyond the scope of this chapter.

The treatment of type II NIDDM is more individualized because of the older age of the

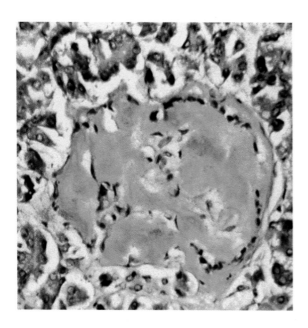

Figure 5-19

TYPE II NONINSULIN-DEPENDENT
DIABETES MELLITUS

Islet from a patient with type II NIDDM shows deposition of amyloid, which is made up of amylin or islet amyloid polypeptide. Amyloid is present in 80 to 90 percent of pancreases of patients with type II NIDDM.

patients and the greater frequency of clinical problems (163). Diet therapy and oral anti-hyperglycemic drugs such as sulfonylureas or metformin are used before resorting to insulin therapy. Insulin is used only for patients who do not respond to these measures (163).

More recent forms of treatment include pancreas transplantation which does not reverse the established complications of chronic diabetes mellitus. Since pancreas transplantation requires ongoing immunosuppression, it is usually done with kidney transplantation at the time of renal failure (161). Islet cell transplantation has also been used therapeutically (164). Porcine fetal islet cell transplants have been recently attempted, but the results are still too preliminary to assess (143).

Complications of Diabetes Mellitus. The major complications of diabetes mellitus are macrovascular disease, which includes atherosclerosis and its sequelae, and microvascular disease, including nephropathy, neuropathy, and retinopathy. The relationship between the

strict control of blood glucose and diabetic complications has been established by the Diabetes Control and Complications Trial (138). There are several mechanisms involved in the tissue changes that lead to diabetic complications. Overglycosylation of proteins occurs with elevated glucose levels because there is an increase in advanced glycation end products. Overglycosylation of basement membrane proteins, collagen, hemoglobin, and others results in advanced glycation end products. These glycation end products represent nonenzymatic cross-linked protein adducts. Advanced glycation end products cause tissue damage. It is not known whether the glycation of collagen in basement membrane contributes to the basement membrane thickening that is present in diabetes mellitus. However, studies have shown that glycated collagen is more resistant to collagenase digestion and more insoluble (159).

The polyol pathway is another possible cause of diabetic complications. When glucose is reduced to sorbitol, this sugar can be oxidized to fructose by sorbitol dehydrogenase. The accumulation of polyols has been implicated in the development of many of the diseases associated with chronic diabetes mellitus, including atherosclerosis, neuropathy, and retinopathy (142,153). The polyol pathway may also contribute to nonenzymatic glycation of proteins, since fructose can bind to various proteins nonenzymatically.

An altered hemodynamic pathway may also contribute to the complications of diabetes. According to this hypothesis, there is a decrease in blood flow and arteriolar resistance along with an increase in hydrostatic pressure in the capillary bed. This leads to leaking of proteins and other macromolecules, especially in diabetic nephropathy (127).

Atherosclerosis. Atherosclerosis probably accounts for 80 percent of deaths in patients with type II diabetes (160). Multiple vessels including the coronary, central, and peripheral vessels develop atherosclerosis, resulting in an increased incidence of myocardial infarction, stroke, and gangrene of the feet. These complications account for up to 75 percent of all deaths in diabetic patients (151). Peripheral atherosclerosis can develop rapidly in diabetic patients, leading to leg and foot amputations.

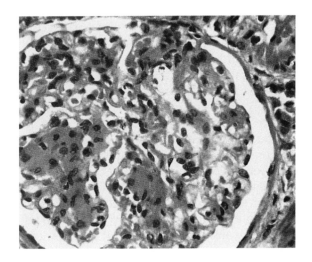
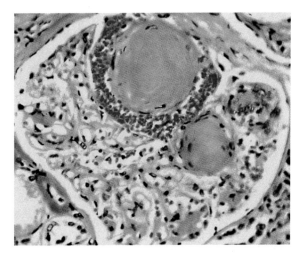

Figure 5-20

DIABETIC NEPHROPATHY

Left: Patient with diabetic nephropathy in which the kidney shows diffuse and nodular glomerulosclerosis with mesangial thickening. (Left and right figures courtesy of Dr. J. P. Grande, Rocheser, MN.)

Right: Kidney with a nodular glomerulosclerosis (Kimmelsteil-Wilson nodules) in a patient with chronic type I diabetes mellitus.

Figure 5-21

DIABETIC NEPHROPATHY

Electron micrograph of diabetic glomerulosclerosis. There is an increase in the mesangial matrix and thickening of the basement membrane of the capillary lumen (X 6,000). (Courtesy of Dr. J.P. Grande, Rochester, MN.)

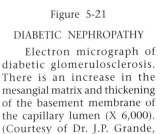
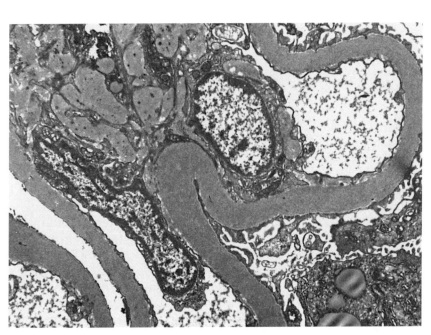

Nephropathy. Nephropathy is present in up to 50 percent of patients with type I diabetes that started in childhood (figs. 5-20, 5-21) (152). The histopathologic features include diffuse and nodular glomerulosclerosis with mesangial thickening and Kimmelstiel-Wilson nodules consisting of periodic acid–Schiff (PAS)-positive material of collagen, basement membrane, mes-enchymal matrix, and others. Diabetic nephropathy accounts for about 9 percent of deaths in diabetics (151).

Retinopathy. Retinopathy and other eye diseases are also related to the severity and duration of the diabetes mellitus (fig. 5-22). An early nonproliferative stage with microaneurysms, lipid exudates, hemorrhage, and microinfarcts

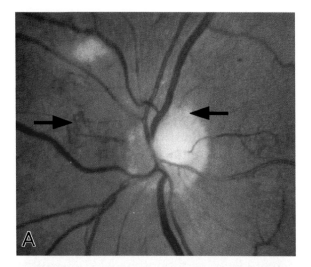

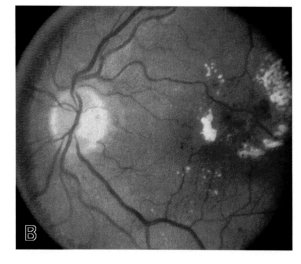

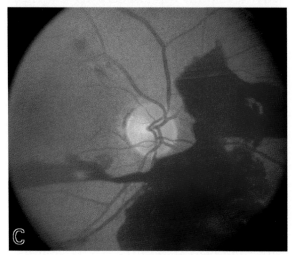

Figure 5-22

DIABETIC EYE DISEASE

A: Simple or background retinopathy with microaneurysms (arrows) in a patient with type I IDDM.

B: Simple retinopathy in a patient with type I IDDM showing cotton-wool exudates representing microinfarctions.

C: Diabetic proliferative retinopathy with retinal hemorrhage probably secondary to traction caused by glial proliferation.

(fig. 5-22) is followed by a proliferative stage with new vessels and fibrous tissues. Adhesions between the newly formed fibrovascular tissue on the retina and the vitreous body lead to hemorrhage and retinal detachment (fig. 5-22C). Ninety-nine percent of patients with type I diabetes have retinopathy after 15 years of disease and 67 percent have proliferative retinopathy after 35 years (144).

Neuropathy. About 50 percent of patients with type II diabetes have neuropathy after 25 years of disease (156). This can involve mononeuropathy affecting a major nerve such as the sciatic, median, or ulnar nerve; symmetrical peripheral polyneuropathy with sensory loss in the distal lower extremities; and autonomic neuropathy with motility disturbances of the gastrointestinal tract, genitourinary dysfunction, and erectile dysfunction.

Prognosis. The prognosis in patients with diabetes mellitus depends on the extent of glucose control, the duration of the disease, and many other factors (163). The most serious complication is macrovascular disease, which accounts for 80 percent of the deaths of patients with NIDDM, 60 percent of which are secondary to ischemic heart disease. The atherosclerotic risk is greatest in poorly controlled patients. The morbidity associated with diabetic complications including eye disease, renal disease, and peripheral nerve diseases, is also devastating (163).

DNES CELL HYPERPLASIA

Increased function and/or mass of the cells and tissues of the DNES caused by hyperplasia is uncommon. Only a limited number of disease conditions, including those involving the pancreas and the gastric G, gastric enterochromaffin-like (ECL), and enterochromaffin (EC) cells of the small intestine are well documented. Hyperplasia of the paraganglionic cells and the pulmonary endocrine cells is rare.

Pancreas: Hyperplasia in Infants of Diabetic Mothers

Definition. This islet cell hyperplasia is associated with macrosomia in infants of mothers with uncontrolled diabetes.

General Remarks. The most common finding in such infants is macrosomia or oversized fetuses. They also have hypoglycemia, hypocalcemia, respiratory distress syndrome, and congenital defects. Because insulin does not cross the placenta, the metabolism of maternal substrates by the fetus is dependent on endogenous insulin produced by the fetus. With poorly controlled maternal diabetes, the maternal hyperglycemia leads to fetal hyperinsulinemia and hyperplasia of the beta cells in the fetal pancreas (189). The increased insulin levels stimulate fetal growth, so the fetus is much larger at birth. There is delay in lung maturation from the hyperglycemia leading to respiratory distress syndrome. There is also an increase in the incidence of organ system malformations (171,173,193). The caudal regression syndrome with hypoplasia of the lower segment of the body is more common in these infants (192).

Macroscopic Findings. The gross appearance and weight of the pancreas are normal.

Microscopic Findings. The islets are increased in diameter and volume, with hypertrophy and hyperplasia of the insulin cells (178, 188). There is pleomorphism of the insulin cell nuclei within the islets. Lymphocytic infiltrates and eosinophils are present around the islets and in the islet interstitium, and fibrosis forms around the islets (196).

Islet Cell Hyperplasia (Nesidioblastosis) in Children

Definition. This is a proliferation of islet cells in focal and/or diffuse areas, and includes ductuloinsular complex formation. Synonyms include *multifocal ductuloinsular proliferation, islet cell adenomatosis, endocrine cell dysplasia,* and *nesidiodysplasia.*

General Remarks. A variety of descriptions have been used for the process of persistent hypoglycemia in childhood (175–177,181,185,186,194, 195,200). The studies of Klöppel and Heitz (177, 181,182) provide a systematic way of examining these abnormalities, with distinction between focal and diffuse nesidioblastosis.

Patients with nesidioblastosis have an inappropriately high level of insulin secretion. There may be a genetic component in some patients with an association or linkage to chromosome 11p (174). Mutations in the sulfonylurea receptor on chromosome 11p15.1 has also been associated with hypoglycemia (172). These mutated insulin-producing cells have inactive adenosine triphosphate (ATP)-sensitive potassium channels and are permanently depolarized, which could lead to inappropriate insulin release (182).

The hypertrophy of the insulin cells in nesidioblastosis is associated with increased insulin secretion. There may also be abnormalities in the mechanisms controlling the differentiation of the islet cells (182). This hypothesis is based on the fact that some of the features of the fetal pancreas are seen in the pancreas of patients with nesidioblastosis, such as clusters of endocrine cells throughout the acinar tissue and formation of ductuloinsular complexes (182).

Clinical Features. Patients present with hyperinsulinemia and hypoglycemia associated with somnolence, seizures, ataxia, and possible loss of consciousness. In most cases the signs and symptoms occur during the first 3 months of life and almost always during the first year of life (183,184). Macrosomia and early obesity are common findings. If the condition is not recognized and treated early, neurological damage, including severe mental retardation from the neuroglycopenia, can develop.

Laboratory Findings. These include hyperinsulinemia and hypoglycemia, with a high insulin-glucose ratio in the blood. Leucine sensitivity is sometimes present (190).

Macroscopic Findings. A small pancreatic nodule, from a few millimeters up to 1 cm in size, may be present with focal nesidioblastosis (fig. 5-23). The nodule may protrude from the surface of the gland on occasion (182). In diffuse nesidioblastosis, there are usually no gross abnormalities in the pancreas.

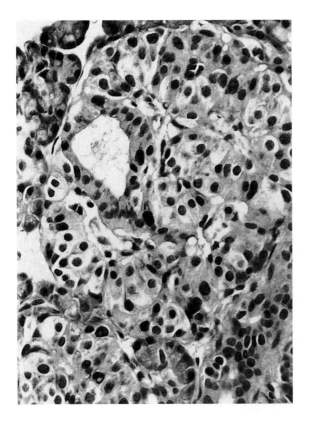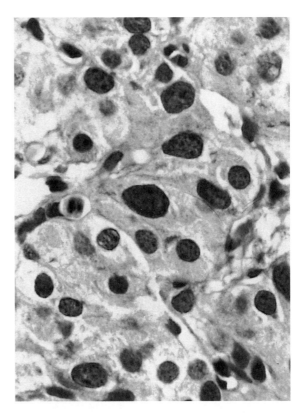

Figure 5-23

FOCAL NESIDIOBLASTOSIS IN PERSISTENT NEONATAL HYPERINSULINEMIC HYPOGLYCEMIA

Left: Clusters of proliferating islet cells associated with a ductuloinsular complex. (Figure 8-5 left, Fascicle 20, 3rd Series.)
Right: Higher magnification shows proliferating islet cells with pleomorphic nuclei. (Figure 8-5 right, Fascicle 20, 3rd Series.)

Microscopic Findings. There is usually one distinct focus in one area of the pancreas with focal nesidioblastosis, but multifocal lesions may be present in some cases (194). The lesions are composed of markedly enlarged islets and endocrine cell clusters with ductuloinsular complexes. The clusters of islet cells are often admixed with acinar tissue. The endocrine cells are enlarged and have large nuclei, some of which may be up to 1.5 times the normal size. The discrete nodules may look like small tumors, but there is usually fibrous stroma separating them from the adjacent exocrine pancreas.

In the diffuse pattern there is islet cell hypertrophy with enlarged, bizarre-appearing nuclei. The islet clusters are of variable sizes and irregular contours (fig. 5-24). Small clusters of islet cells are scattered among the acinar parenchyma. Islet cells budding off small ducts are common (ductuloinsular complexes) (figs. 5-25–5-27).

Immunohistochemical Findings. In focal nesidioblastosis immunohistochemical staining for pancreatic hormones shows insulin, glucagon, somatostatin, and pancreatic polypeptide cells with an increase in the number of insulin cells (178,181,186,191). These adenoma-type lesions contain a mixture of cell types, a difference from true islet cell adenoma, which consists of only one predominant cell type. The islets outside the focal areas contain endocrine cells of normal size, appearance, and distribution.

Immunohistochemical staining in diffuse nesidioblastosis shows all four major types of islet cells: insulin, glucagon, somatostatin, and pancreatic polypeptide. The hypertrophied islet cells are predominately insulin-producing (fig. 5-26). Some studies have suggested that there is a decrease in the volume density of somatostatin cells (191), although this observation has not been confirmed by other investigators.

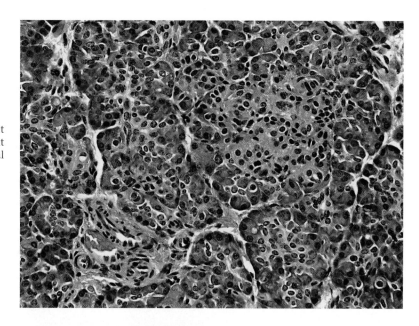

Figure 5-24

DIFFUSE NESIDIOBLASTOSIS

Proliferating small nests of islet cells shown here as pale cells are present in a patient with persistent neonatal hyperinsulinemic hypoglycemia.

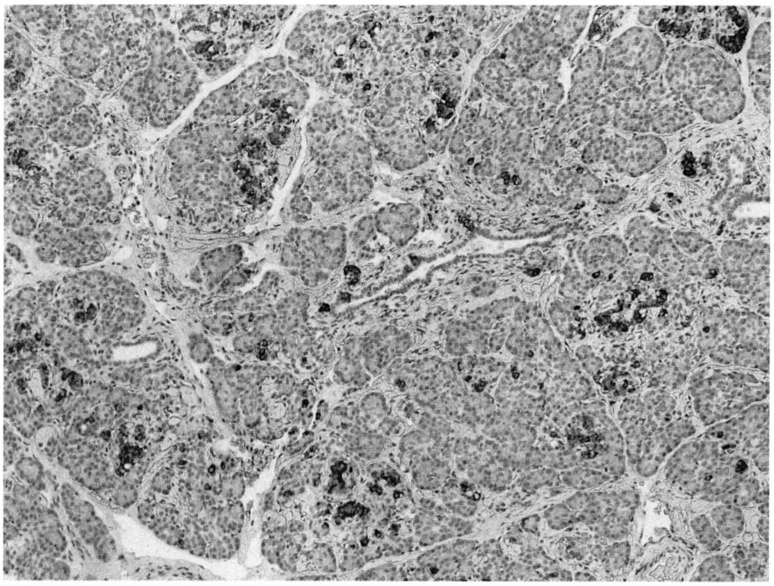

Figure 5-25

DIFFUSE NESIDIOBLASTOSIS

Immunohistochemical staining for insulin accentuates the small clusters of proliferating islet cells in the pancreas (diaminobenzidine chromogen).

Ultrastructural Findings. Electron microscopic studies of diffuse nesidioblastosis show islet cells with ultrastructural features similar to normal islet cells. An unusual finding observed by several investigators is the presence of large zymogen-type granules in insulin and glucagon cells, suggesting dual differentiation of abnormal endocrine-exocrine cell mixtures (175,179,187).

Differential Diagnosis. Morphologically similar lesions are islet cell hyperplasia in infants of diabetic mothers and the Beckwith-Wiedemann syndrome. In islet cell hyperplasia associated with neonates of diabetic mothers, the islets are markedly enlarged with an increased islet cell volume, but ductuloinsular complexes are not as prominent. The lymphocytic and eosinophilic infiltrates in this condition are more prominent than in nesidioblastosis.

Patients with the Beckwith-Wiedemann syndrome (which is associated with macroglossia, gigantism, visceromegaly, renal dysplasia, omphalocele, adrenal cortical hyperplasia, cytomegaly, and Leydig cell hyperplasia) often

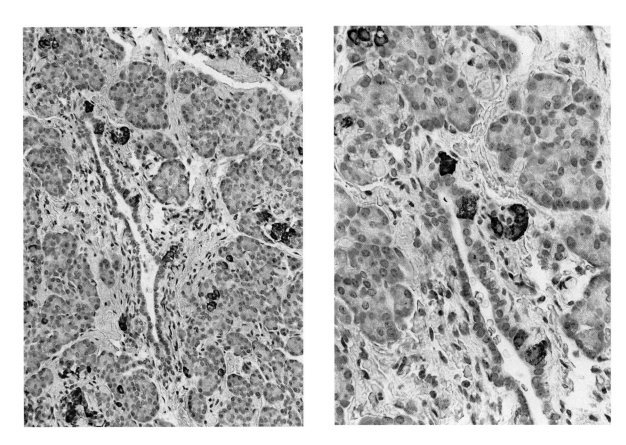

Figure 5-26

DIFFUSE NESIDIOBLASTOSIS

Left: Several ductuloinsular complexes, present in a small duct, are demonstrated by insulin staining (diaminobenzidine chromogen).

Right: Higher magnification shows the ductuloinsular complexes budding off the pancreatic duct (diaminobenzidine chromogen).

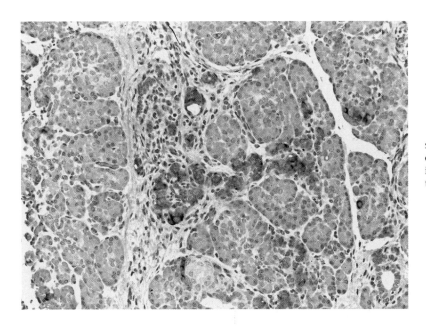

Figure 5-27

DIFFUSE NESIDIOBLASTOSIS

Proinsulin mRNA staining by in situ hybridization shows small cell clusters and single cells expressing the insulin gene product (alkaline phosphatase-NBT/BCIP).

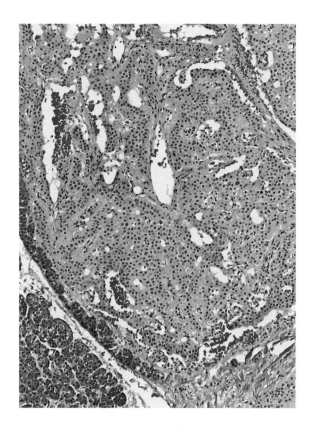

Figure 5-28

INSULINOMA

A solitary islet cell tumor in a sporadic insulinoma.

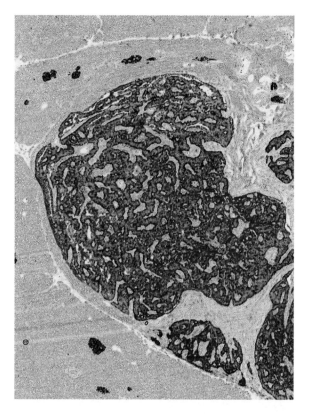

Figure 5-29

INSULINOMA

Immunostaining for insulin shows diffuse reactivity in the tumor and in the adjacent normal islets (diaminobenzidine chromogen).

have hyperinsulinemia and hypoglycemia (169, 198). In this condition the islets are enlarged, but their distribution in the pancreas is normal. There is an increase in all cell types, especially insulin and glucagon cells. Ductuloinsular complexes are not as prominent as in nesidioblastosis.

Although chronic pancreatitis is often associated with diabetes mellitus, islet cell hyperplasia is also seen in chronic pancreatitis (180). The presence of extensive fibrosis with loss of the acinar cells allows distinction between this condition and nesidioblastosis. Anecdotal reports of islet cell hypertrophy and hyperplasia have been reported in infants with congenital cardiac malfunctions and alpha-1-antitrypsin deficiency, but these cases are not well documented by morphometric studies (186,192).

Focal nesidioblastosis may be confused with an adenoma, especially when only one focus of nesidioblastosis is present. However, im-

munohistochemical staining shows an admixture of all four major pancreatic hormone cell types in focal nesidioblastosis along with prominent ductuloinsular complexes which are usually not present in adenomas (figs. 5-28, 5-29).

Treatment and Prognosis. Surgery is the usual treatment for patients with nesidioblastosis. In focal nesidioblastosis, a solitary nodule is relatively easy to remove surgically. With diffuse nesidioblastosis, a 75 to 95 percent pancreatectomy is often done (197,199). Response to subtotal pancreatectomy is quite variable, with many patients becoming normoglycemic (197) while others develop recurrent hypoglycemia (181). In a recent study of 52 neonates with hyperinsulinemia, 13 of the 30 patients with diffuse hyperfunction had persistent hypoglycemia after near-total pancreatectomy (170). Hypoglycemia developed in 7, diabetes mellitus in 8, and only 2 patients were normoglycemic 1 year after surgery.

Nesidioblastosis in Adults

Definition. Nesidioblastosis in adults is persistent hyperinsulinemic hypoglycemia caused by islet cell abnormalities in the absence of an insulinoma.

General Remarks. Insulinoma is the most common cause of hyperinsulinemic hypoglycemia in adults; islet cell hypertrophy and nesidioblastosis are rarer causes (201,202,204,205,208, 211,213). The morphologic evidence of this disorder has been challenged by some investigators who failed to show a correlation between the anatomic changes and the hypoglycemia (203).

Although mutations in the sulfonylurea receptor (SURI) gene and the inwardly rectifying potassium channel (Kir 6.2) gene have been found in some patients with pediatric familial persistent hyperinsulinemic hypoglycemia (207,210), such mutations have not been detected in the small numbers of adults with nonfamilial nesidioblastosis in which this has been investigated (208).

Macroscopic Findings. Gross examination of the pancreas sectioned at 1 mm intervals is usually unremarkable.

Microscopic Findings. Histologic findings consist of hypertrophic islets, some of which have pleomorphic nuclei, and increased numbers of islet cells budding off ducts (ductuloinsular complexes) or neoformation of islets from ducts (figs. 5-30–5-33). In one recent study, the mean diameter of the hypertrophied islets ranged from 228 to 262 μm, while normal islets were 75 to 225 μm (208). Individual islets contain cells with enlarged pleomorphic nuclei that are 1.5- to 2-fold larger than the normal islet cell nucleus. Peliosis or a type of vascular ectasia of the islet with prominently dilated vascular sinusoids may be observed. This finding has been previously reported in the pancreas of a patient with multiple endocrine neoplasia type 1 (206).

Immunohistochemical Findings. The hypertrophied islets contain all major islet cell types: insulin, glucagon, somatostatin, and pancreatic polypeptide. Insulin-positive cells are present in the ductuloinsular complexes (fig. 5-33). In one study the peripheral ring of glucagon cells present in normal islets was reported to be absent (213).

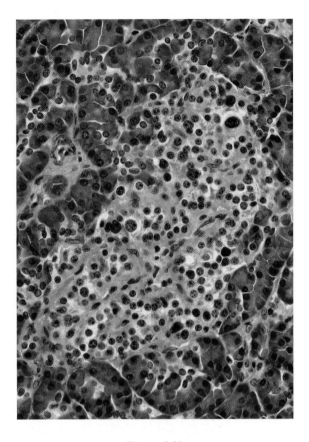

Figure 5-30

ADULT NESIDIOBLASTOSIS

Islet shows hypertrophy and hyperplasia in an adult with hyperinsulinemic hypoglycemia. Some of the enlarged islet cells have pleomorphic nuclei.

Ultrastructural Findings. Prominent insulin-producing cells, identified by the irregular crystalline structure of the secretory granules, are present (213). These insulin-producing cells may be present at the periphery of the islets, which is usually occupied by glucagon cells. Some acinar cells show degranulation and evidence of increased secretory activity, with dilated cisterns of rough endoplasmic reticulum and only occasional acinar zymogen granules (213).

Differential Diagnosis. Since insulinomas are the cause of endogenous hypoglycemia in more than 99 percent of patients with hyperinsulinemic hypoglycemia, the gross specimen must be carefully examined for minute insulinomas. This is done by microscopic examination of 1 mm sections of the pancreas. The differential diagnosis includes small adenomas.

Figure 5-31

ADULT NESIDIOBLASTOSIS

Islet from an adult with hyperin-sulinemic hypoglycemia showing peliosis-type vascular ectasia. These changes are seen in less than 1 percent of islet cells, but are usually a consistent finding.

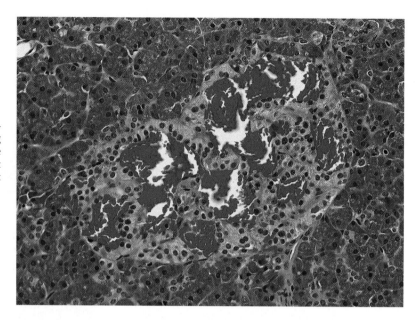

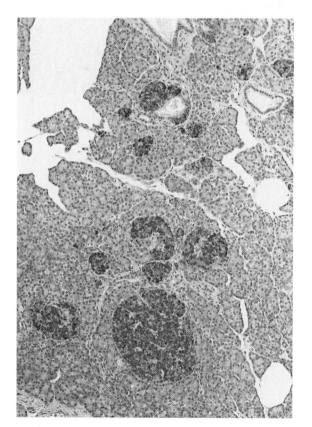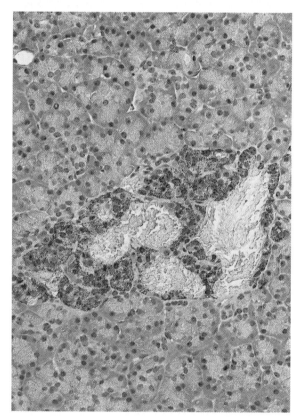

Figure 5-32

ADULT NESIDIOBLASTOSIS

Left: Insulin immunostaining shows a range of sizes of islets expressing insulin, from small clusters to hypertrophied islets (diaminobenzidine chromogen).

Right: Insulin immunostaining of an islet with peliosis-type vascular ectasia (diaminobenzidine chromogen).

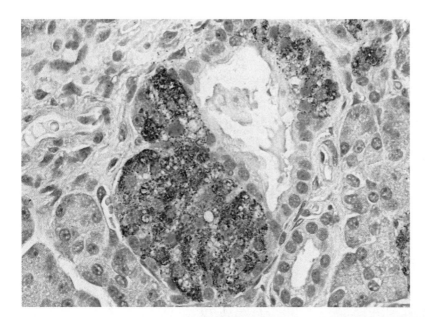

Figure 5-33

ADULT NESIDIOBLASTOSIS

Ductuloinsular complex in an adult with hyperinsulinemic hypoglycemia (diaminobenzidine chromogen).

Figure 5-34

MULTIPLE ENDOCRINE NEOPLASIA TYPE 1

An intraoperative ultrasound shows multiple hypoechoic masses (arrows) in the pancreas indicating many islet cell nodules in a patient with MEN 1.

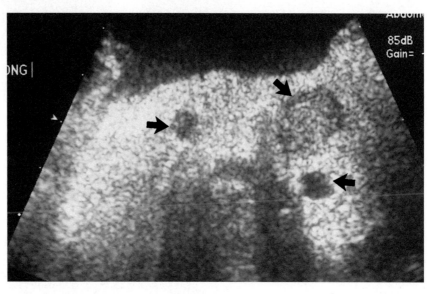

Immunostaining shows that adenomas consist of one predominant cell population, while hypertrophied islets with nesidioblastosis have an admixture of different cell types. Patients with multiple endocrine neoplasia type 1 (MEN 1) may have insulinomas associated with hypoglycemia. These patients have multifocal disease that is difficult to cure by surgery (212). The pancreas in MEN 1 patients usually has multiple nodules ranging from less than 1 mm to several centimeters in diameter (figs. 5-34, 5-35). Most of these nodules are chromogranin A positive, but many are negative for pancreatic hormones and are nonfunctional.

In the evaluation of islet cell hypertrophy and hyperplasia in adults, hyperplastic islets in areas of fibrosis is a common finding (fig. 5-36) and should not be misinterpreted as a primary islet cell abnormality. The pancreas in chronic pancreatitis may also show islet cell hypertrophy and hyperplasia (fig. 5-37). The presence of extensive fibrosis with loss of acinar cells allows distinction between this condition and adult nesidioblastosis.

Treatment and Prognosis. Partial pancreatectomy with resection of up to 75 percent or more of the pancreas is the usual treatment

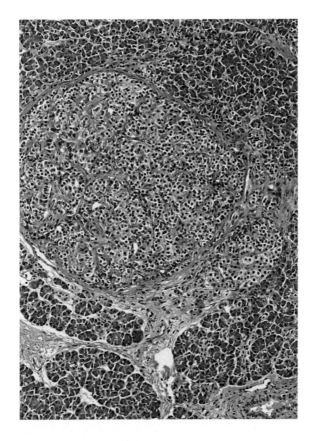

Figure 5-35

MULTIPLE ENDOCRINE NEOPLASIA TYPE 1

This hyperplastic nodule represents one of several nodules of proliferating islet cells in a patient with MEN 1.

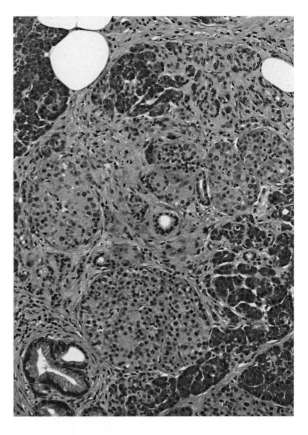

Figure 5-36

FOCAL ISLET CELL PROLIFERATION WITH FIBROSIS

Focal islet cell proliferation in a background of fibrosis. This is a common finding in the pancreas of adults and is not associated with hyperinsulinemic hypoglycemia.

Figure 5-37

CHRONIC PANCREATITIS WITH ISLET CELL HYPERPLASIA

There is diffuse and nodular proliferation of islet cells in a patient with chronic pancreatitis.

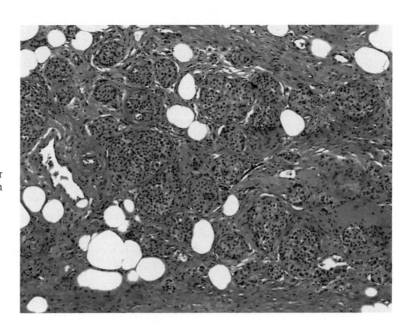

for this uncommon disorder. The prognosis is quite variable, with resolution of signs and symptoms in some patients and continued hypoglycemia or seizures in others (208,209). In a Mayo Clinic series of five patients, four were free of hypoglycemic symptoms up to 3 years after surgery (208). One patient who had a limited distal pancreatectomy had a brief recurrence of symptoms.

Gastric Endocrine Cell Hyperplasia: Gastrin (G)-Cell Hyperplasia

Definition. G-cell hyperplasia is an absolute increase in the number of gastrin-immunoreactive cells in the gastric mucosa.

General Remarks. G-cell hyperplasia has been divided into primary and secondary types, depending on the etiology. Primary G-cell hyperplasia in which the G-cell mass increases without an antecedent stimulus is uncommon (220, 224). After a test meal patients have moderate basal hypergastrinemia and exaggerated gastrin release. Antrectomy usually leads to the return of gastrin levels in gastric acid output to normal (224). It has been postulated that the peptic ulcers seen in patients with primary hypergastrinemia may be related to infection with *Helicobacter pylori* via inhibition of somatostatin secretion and increased gastrin release (218).

Secondary G-cell hyperplasia, the most common type observed, develops when the G cells are no longer regulated by the feedback inhibition normally provided by gastric acid. Pathologic conditions associated with secondary G-cell hyperplasia include atrophic gastritis associated with hypochlorhydria or achlorhydria (223), gastric atrophy associated with pernicious anemia (225), surgical procedures in which the gastric antrum is separated from the rest of the stomach and from the acid secreted by the parietal cells (215), and surgical excision of the vagus nerve branches leading to hypochlorhydria (214, 216). Patients with atrophic gastritis, pernicious anemia, and hypergastrinemia do not appear to have any clinical manifestations from the elevated gastrin levels, since their gastric mucosa can no longer secrete acid. However, in patients with a surgically excluded antrum, the hypergastrinemia is associated with gastric acid hypersecretion and peptic ulceration.

Clinical Features. Primary G-cell hyperplasia is characterized by peptic ulcers and hypergastrinemia. Patients have acid hypersecretion, fasting hypergastrinemia, and an exaggerated gastrin response to a protein meal (224). Symptoms associated with peptic ulcers include epigastric pain, intractable nausea, and vomiting.

Patients with secondary G-cell hyperplasia with gastric atrophy and pernicious anemia (type A gastritis) have elevated serum gastrin levels which are in the same range as those of patients with Zollinger-Ellison syndrome. The latter is largely an autoimmune disease in which patients have antibodies to parietal cells that are cytotoxic to gastric mucosal cells. Antibodies to parietal cells are found in about 90 percent of patients with pernicious anemia, 50 percent of whom also have antibodies to thyroid antigens. Serum antibodies to intrinsic factor are more specific for type A gastritis than are parietal cell antibodies, and are present in 40 percent of patients with pernicious anemia (217).

Macroscopic Findings. Peptic ulcers involving the gastric mucosa and duodenum are often present. Microcarcinoid tumors related to enterochromaffin-like hyperplasia may also be present as nodules or polyps in the stomach.

Microscopic Findings. There is an increase in the number of antral G cells, atrophic changes in the body of the stomach, and decreased or absent parietal cells (figs. 5-38–5-40).

Morphometric studies are needed to document G-cell hyperplasia, especially in biopsy specimens. The criteria for G-cell hyperplasia include (217,221–223): 1) an increase in the number of G cells from a normal of 41–93 per linear mm to 192–259 per linear mm; 2) extension of the G cells upward and inward within the gastric glands and expansion of their normal compartment; and 3) appearance of clusters of G-cell clones in the antral mucosa.

In the studies of Lewin et al. (219), the control patients had mean G-cell numbers of 19 ± 9.5 per linear mm with a range of 6 to 41, while patients with primary G-cell hyperplasia had a mean of 48 ± 8.9 per linear mm, with a range of 39 to 63. Other investigators have quantified G-cell hyperplasia by endoscopic biopsy (221,225).

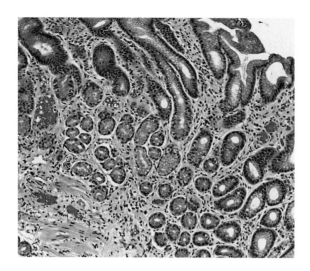

Figure 5-38

GASTRIN CELL HYPERPLASIA

Atrophic gastritis and endocrine cell hyperplasia in the gastric antrum of a patient with secondary G-cell hyperplasia.

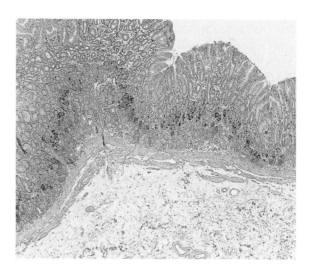

Figure 5-39

SECONDARY GASTRIN CELL HYPERPLASIA

Secondary G-cell hyperplasia showing an increase in the number of gastrin-positive cells (diaminobenzidine chromogen).

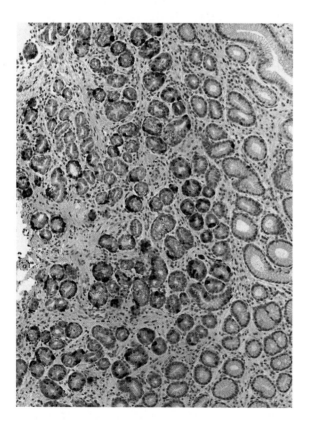

Figure 5-40

SECONDARY GASTRIN CELL HYPERPLASIA

G-cell hyperplasia showing increased numbers of gastrin-positive cells (diaminobenzidine chromogen).

Differential Diagnosis. The differential diagnosis includes enterochromaffin-like (ECL) cell hyperplasia secondary to hypergastrinemia, Zollinger-Ellison syndrome associated with a gastrinoma, or hypergastrinemia in the setting of type A atrophic gastritis. Adequate sampling of the stomach can determine the state of the parietal cells in the antrum; these are hyperplastic in Zollinger-Ellison syndrome. Distinction between G cells and ECL-like cells can be made by immunostaining. Both cell types are positive for chromogranin A, but only the G cells are positive for gastrin.

Treatment. Patients with primary G-cell hyperplasia and ulcers have been treated with antrectomy and vagotomy for the ulcer disease, although medical treatment is used more commonly. No specific treatment is required for patients with type A gastritis and pernicious anemia but they require lifelong regular parenteral administration of vitamin B12 (216).

Enterochromaffin-Like Cell Hyperplasia

Definition. This is an increase in the number of argyrophil cells with a characteristic ultrastructure in the glands of the gastric oxyntic mucosa.

General Remarks. Hyperplasia of the ECL cells is usually seen in patients with type A gastritis and pernicious anemia (226,231) or with Zollinger-Ellison syndrome (227,233,236). Gastrin is a potent trophic factor for the ECL cells, so elevated gastrin levels lead to ECL hyperplasia and gastric carcinoid formation (233).

In patients with longstanding pernicious anemia, ECL hyperplasia may progress to dysplastic and neoplastic microcarcinoid and invasive carcinoid tumors (228,229,235). Bordi et al. (228) classified the hyperplastic lesions into various groups: simple hyperplasia, linear hyperplasia, micronodular hyperplasia, and adenomatoid hyperplasia which may be single or multiple. Dysplastic lesions are classified into several groups as well: enlarging micronodules, fusing micronodules, microinvasive micronodules, and nodules with newly formed stroma (233). These changes are all noted adjacent to carcinoid tumors in patients with chronic atrophic gastritis.

Patients with Zollinger-Ellison syndrome (ZES) have peptic ulcers, increased gastric acid secretion, and gastrin-producing tumors of the pancreas and/or small intestine. The hypergastrinemia leads to hyperplasia of the ECL cells in the stomach. Islet cell hyperplasia has been reported in some patients with ZES, probably in association with multiple endocrine neoplasia (MEN) type 1. Approximately 20 to 60 percent of patients with ZES have MEN 1 associated with abnormalities of the menin gene on chromosome 11. In such patients the parietal cell mass is expanded three to six times normal due to the trophic effects of circulatory gastrin.

Microscopic Findings. Patients with ECL hyperplasia, ZES, and MEN 1 have diffuse and micronodular hyperplasia of the antral gastrin cells (234). In ZES there is diffuse and linear hyperplasia of argyrophil endocrine cells, which are positive for chromogranin, synaptophysin, and serotonin, but negative for gastrin (figs. 5-41, 5-42). Argyrophilic microcarcinoid tumors are closely linked to ZES with MEN 1 and may develop in 10 to 20 percent of patients (232). The carcinoid tumors are multiple and very small, and most develop in the mucosa and submucosa. They are sessile polypoid lesions with the characteristic histologic features of carci-

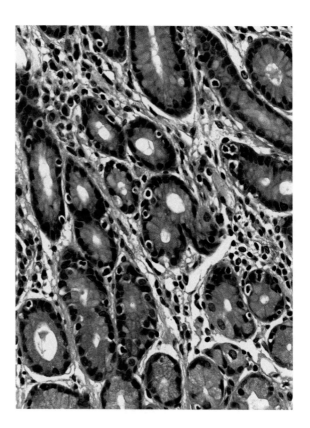

Figure 5-41

ENTEROCHROMAFFIN-LIKE CELL HYPERPLASIA

There is a proliferation of ECL cells in a patient with hypergastrinemia.

noid tumors: uniform cells in a vascular stroma with few mitotic figures. Immunostaining for broad-spectrum neuroendocrine markers (chromogranin and synaptophysin) is positive, while some cells also react with antibodies to gastrin, serotonin, and somatostatin. Ultrastructural studies show the characteristic ECL-type secretory granules, vesicular granules, and solid granules with cerebroid punctate morphology.

Treatment. Patients with ZES are usually resistant to the medical and surgical therapies that are effective for the patients with usual peptic ulcers. Drugs such as H2-receptor antagonists are effective in reducing gastric acid secretion and may heal the ulcers (230). Surgical resection of the gastrinomas and temporary treatment with omeprazole are done while the diagnosis are being established (230).

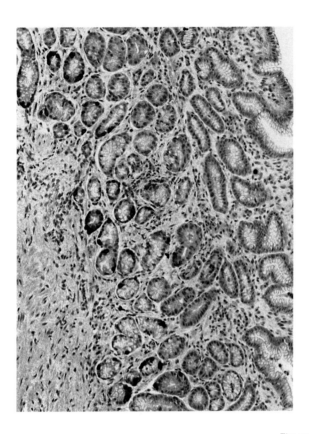 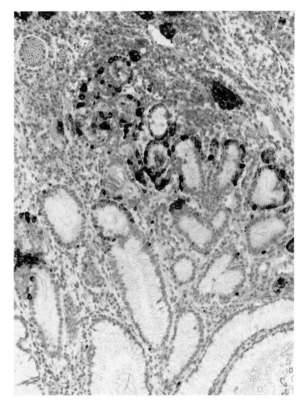

Figure 5-42

ENTEROCHROMAFFIN-LIKE CELL HYPERPLASIA

Left: Serotonin stain reveals the proliferating ECL cells in a patient with Zollinger-Ellison syndrome (diaminobenzidine chromogen).

Right: Chromogranin stain highlights the hyperplastic ECL cells and a few nests of dysplastic micronodules present in the stroma (diaminobenzidine chromogen).

Enterochromaffin Cell Hyperplasia

Hyperplasia of the enterochromaffin (EC) cells in the small intestine is an uncommon pathologic finding. It has been reported in association with specific disorders, such as celiac sprue (238,239,242), in which it is thought to be a nonspecific response to the chronic inflammatory changes. This hyperplasia regresses when a gluten-free diet is used to treat the celiac sprue. Other inflammatory conditions such as appendicitis and chronic gastritis have also been associated with EC cell hyperplasia (243). EC cell hyperplasia has been reported in the duodenum of patients with familial adenomatous polyposis (241) in which there is hyperplasia of other endocrine cells as well. A single case report of megacolon associated with focal EC hyperplasia has been reported (240). Patients with Crohn's ile-itis have increased numbers of endocrine cells including EC cells in the small intestine. EC cell hyperplasia has not been reported to progress to microcarcinoid or invasive carcinoid tumors as has been reported with ECL cells in patients with type A chronic atrophic gastritis (237).

Hyperplasia of Extra-Adrenal Paraganglia

Definition. This hyperplasia consists of an increase in the chief cells and sustentacular cells, especially in the carotid body paraganglia.

General Remarks. Hyperplasia and hypertrophy of paraganglionic tissues have been studied more often in the carotid body paraganglia (245,249,250,251,254,255,259), but can also affect vagal and other paraganglia (252). Chronic hypoxemia has been associated with carotid body enlargement in bovines (244) and in humans living at higher elevations

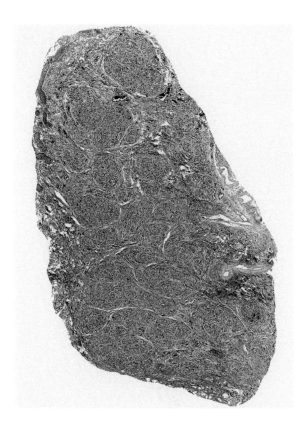

Figure 5-43

HYPERPLASTIC CAROTID BODY PARAGANGLION

Hyperplastic carotid body from a 21-year-old woman with cystic fibrosis, showing increased numbers of lobules. Some of the lobules appear to have become confluent. (Figure 15-12 from Fascicle 19, 3rd Series.)

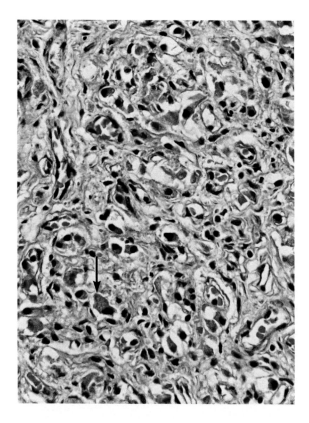

Figure 5-44

HYPERPLASTIC CAROTID BODY

Enlarged hyperplastic carotid body from a young adult with cystic fibrosis. Lobules are increased in size and appear to merge. Most chief cell nuclei are hyperchromatic and some are slightly enlarged. Some chief cells have small cytoplasmic vacuoles (arrow). (Figure 15-13 from Fascicle 19, 3rd Series.)

(247,256–258). Some of these hyperplastic carotid bodies have been considered as tumors or chemodectomas (258). Other diseases such as chronic obstructive pulmonary disease and systemic hypertension have also be associated with enlarged non-neoplastic carotid bodies (252,255–257). Patients with chronic hypoxemia secondary to cyanotic heart disease and cystic fibrosis can develop hyperplasia of the carotid bodies as well as of the vagal and aorticopulmonary paraganglia (252,253,255).

Macroscopic Findings. Hyperplastic carotid bodies have combined weights of over 30 mg, mean diameters greater than 565 μm, and greater than a 47 percent increase in the differential count of elongated cells over chief cells (figs. 5-43, 5-44) (248). It is recommended that the combined weight of the carotid bodies should always be correlated with a control population to correct for age-related variations before making a diagnosis of hyperplasia (254).

Microscopic Findings. There is usually variable hyperplasia of the lobule with an increase in both the chief cells and sustentacular cells. There may be a decrease in chromogranin A immunoreactivity and argyrophilia with hyperplastic carotid bodies developing at high altitudes (253). A prominent spindle cell component with elongated sustentacular cells may be present (259).

Immunohistochemical Findings. The hyperplastic chief cells are positive for chromogranin A, synaptophysin, and neuron-specific enolase while the hyperplastic sustentacular cells are positive for S100 protein.

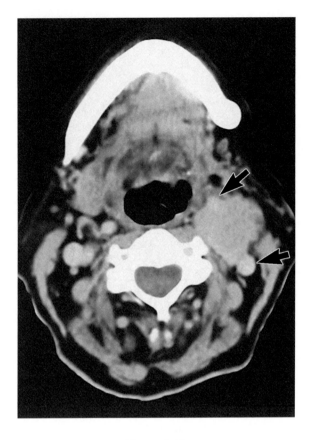

Figure 5-45

CAROTID BODY TUMOR

Contrast-enhanced CT of the neck at the level of the mandible shows an enhancing mass just above the left carotid bifurcation, which displaces the internal and external carotid arteries (arrows).

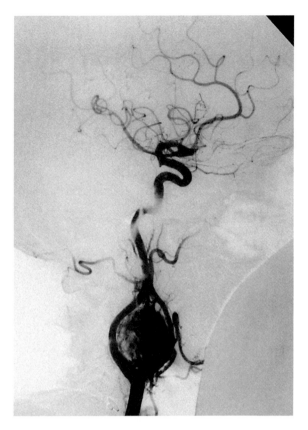

Figure 5-46

CAROTID BODY TUMOR

Left carotid angiogram confirms a vascular mass consistent with a carotid body tumor.

Ultrastructural Findings. A decrease in the number of secretory granules in hyperplastic carotid bodies from patients with cystic fibrosis has been reported (250). There may be proliferation of the S100-positive sustentacular cells as well as nerve axons (251). The myelin sheaths formed by Schwann cells are well developed, but the ones in the sustentacular cells are rudimentary. The hyperplasia does not involve fibrosis or pericytes in the carotid body (251).

Hyperplasia of the vagal paraganglia has been reported in patients with chronic obstructive pulmonary disease and chronic hypoxemia, cystic fibrosis, and cyanotic heart disease (252). The changes are similar to those seen in other forms of carotid body hyperplasia (247).

Differential Diagnosis. The principal differential diagnosis is between hyperplasia and benign paraganglioma. Paragangliomas of the carotid body (figs. 5-45–5-48) are usually larger than 300 mg while hyperplastic carotid bodies are less than 100 mg (254). There is also a higher density of chief cells in carotid body tumors compared to normal and hyperplastic paraganglionic tissues.

Pulmonary Endocrine Cell Hyperplasia

Hyperplasias of neuroendocrine cells in the lungs have been reported in humans living at high altitudes and in patients with cystic fibrosis (fig. 5-49) and chronic pulmonary diseases such as emphysema and chronic bronchitis (260–264,266–271). The studies of Gould

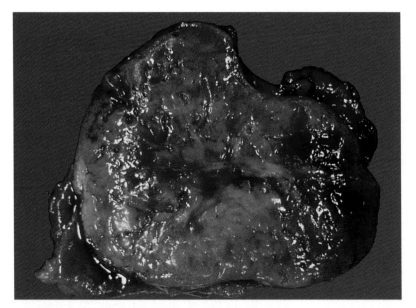

Figure 5-47

CAROTID BODY TUMOR

Gross photograph showing a tan carotid body tumor. The tumor is highly vascular and has focal areas of hemorrhage.

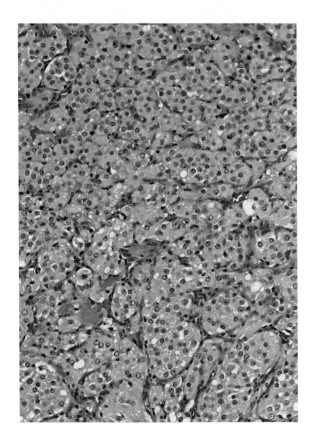 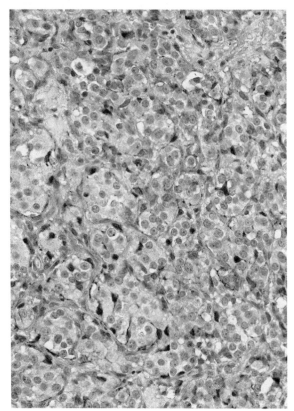

Figure 5-48

CAROTID BODY TUMOR

Left: A prominent zellballen (organoid) pattern is present in this carotid body tumor.

Right: Immunostaining for S100 protein accentuates the organoid pattern, with positively stained sustentacular cells surrounding the nests of neoplastic chief cells (diaminobenzidine chromogen).

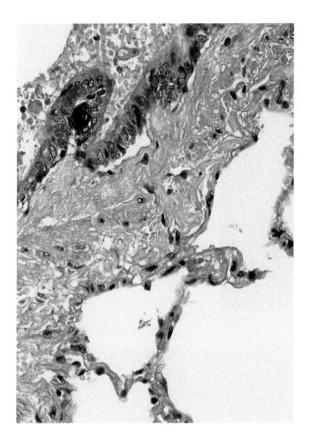 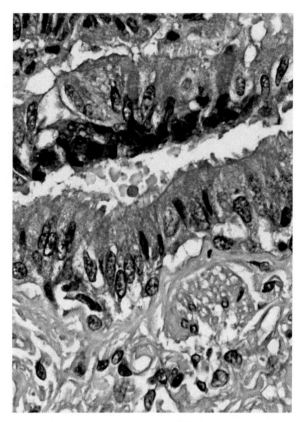

Figure 5-49

PULMONARY NEUROENDOCRINE BODY

Left: The bronchial respiratory epithelium from a patient with cystic fibrosis contains a cluster of neuroendocrine cells or a neuroendocrine body (NEB) revealed by staining for chromogranin A (diaminobenzidine chromogen).

Right: Neuroendocrine cell hyperplasia from a patient with cystic fibrosis detected by chromogranin A immunostaining. These cells are usually positive for bombesin and serotonin. Severely hyperplastic and dysplastic NEBs produce other hormones ectopically such as adrenocorticotropic hormone and vasoactive intestinal polypeptide (diaminobenzidine chromogen).

and colleagues (261) have shown that with severe hyperplasia and dysplasia, peptides generally regarded as ectopic, such as ACTH and vasoactive intestinal polypeptide, can be detected in the neuroendocrine bodies. Tsutsumi et al. (270) found immunoreactivity for ACTH and gastrin-releasing peptide in hyperplastic neuroendocrine cells in adults under pathologic conditions. This is reminiscent of the increase in the numbers of neuroen-

docrine bodies, which are also immunoreactive for bombesin present in the fetal lungs (261, 263,268). Hyperplasia of pulmonary neuroendocrine cells can be seen in experimental animals (261,262, 264,265), where chemicals such as diethylnitrosamine can lead to hyperplasia of the neuroepithelial bodies. The relationship between pulmonary neuroendocrine cell hyperplasia and the development of neuroendocrine tumors in the lung is still unclear.

REFERENCES

Embryology and Anatomy

1. Andrew A. Further evidence that enterochromaffin cells are not derived from the neural crest. J Embryol Exp Morphol 1974;31:589–98.
2. DeLellis RA, Wolfe HJ. The polypeptide hormone-producing neuroendocrine cells and their tumors: an immunohistochemical analysis. Methods Achiev Exp Pathol 1981;10:190–220.
3. Feyrter F. Die Peripheren endokrinen (parakriken) Drusen. In: Kauffman-Staemler, eds. Lehrbuch der speziellen pathologischen anatomie. vols 11-12. Berlin: De Guyrter, 1969.
4. Fujita T. Present status of paraneuron concept. [Review] Arch Histol Cytol 1989;52(Suppl):1–8.
5. Klöppel G, Heitz PU. Classification of normal and neoplastic neuroendocrine cells. Ann NY Acad Sci 1994;733:19–23.
6. Langley K. The neuroendocrine concept today. Ann NY Acad Sci 1994;733:1–17.
7. Le Douarin NM. The neural crest. Cambridge, England: Cambridge University Press, 1982.
8. Le Douarin NM. On the origin of pancreatic endocrine cells. Cell 1988;53:169–71.
9. Le Douarin NM. The ontogeny of the neural crest in avian embryo chimaeras. Nature 1980;286:663–9.
10. Le Douarin NM, Fontaine J, Le Lievre C. New studies on the neural crest origin of the avian ultimobronchial glandular cells. Interspecific combinations and cytochemical characterization of C cells based on the uptake of biogenic amine precursors. Histochemistry 1974;38:297–305.
11. Le Douarin NM, Teillet MA. The migration of neural crest cells to the wall of the digestive tract in avian embryo. J Embryol Exp Morpol 1973;30:31–48.
12. Lloyd RV. Overview of neuroendocrine cells and tumors. Endocr Pathol 1996;7:323–8.
13. Pearse AG. The APUD cell concept and its implications in pathology. Pathol Annu 1974;9:27–41.
14. Pearse AG. The diffuse neuroendocrine system: peptide, amines, placodes and the APUD theory. Prog Brain Res 1986;68:25–31.
15. Pearse AG, Takor T. Embryology of the diffuse neuroendocrine system and its relationship to the common peptides. Fed Proc 1979;38:2288–94.
16. Weston JA. The migration and differentiation of neural crest cells. Adv Morphog 1970;8:41–114.

Pancreas

17. Githens S. Development of duct cells. In: Lebenthal E, ed. Human gastrointestinal development. New York: Raven Press, 1989:669–83.

18. Rahier J, Falt K, Munterfering H, Becker K, Gepts W, Falkmer S. The basic structural lesion of persistent neonatal hypoglycemia with hyperinsulinism: deficiency of pancreatic D cells or hyperactivity of B cells? Diabetalogia 1984; 26:282–9.
19. Rahier J, Wallon J, Henquin JC. Cell populations in the endocrine pancreas of human neonates and infants. Diabetologia 1981;20:540–6.
20. Solcia E, Capella C, Klöppel G. Tumors of the pancreas. Atlas of Tumor Pathology, 3rd Series. Fascicle 20. Washington, DC: Armed Forces Institute of Pathology, 1997.

Lungs

21. Hage E. Electron microscopic identification of several types of endocrine cells in the bronchial epithelium of human foetuses. Z Zellforsch Mikrosk Anat 1973;141:401–12.
22. McDowell EM, Barrett LA, Trump BF. Observations on small granule cells in adult human bronchial epithelium and in carcinoid and oat cell tumors. Lab Invest 1976;34:202–6.

Histology–Pancreas

23. Capella C, Solcia E, Frigerio B, Buffa R, Usellini L, Fontana P. The endocrine cells of the pancreas and related tumours. Ultrastructural study and classification. Virchows Arch [A] 1977;373:327–52.
24. Chen J, Baithun SI, Pollock DJ, Berry CK. Argyrophilic and hormone immunoreactive cells in normal and hyperplastic pancreatic ducts and exocrine pancreatic carcinoma. Virchows Arch [A] 1988;413:399–405.
25. Goossens A, Heitz P, Klöppel G. Pancreatic endocrine cells and their non-neoplastic proliferations. In: Dayal Y, ed. Endocrine pathology of the gut and pancreas. Boca Raton: CRC Press, 1991:69–104.
26. Grube D, Bohn R. The microanatomy of human islets of Langerhans with special reference to somatostatin (D) cells. Arch Histol Jap 1983;46:327–53.
27. Johnson KH, O'Brien TD, Hayden DW, et al. Immunolocalization of islet amyloid polypeptide (IAPP) in pancreatic beta cells by means of peroxidase in antiperoxidase (PAP) and protein A-gold techniques. Am J Pathol 1988;130:1–8.
28. Malaisse-Lagae F, Stefan Y, Cox J, Perrelet A, Orci L. Identification of a lobe in the adult human pancreas rich in pancreatic polypeptide. Diabetologia 1979;17:361–5.

29. Orci L, Ravazzola M, Storch MJ, Anderson RG, Vassalli JD, Perrelet A. Proteolytic maturation of insulin is a post-Golgi event which occurs in acidifying Clathrin-coated secretory vesicles. Cell 1987;49:865–8.

30. Ravazzola M, Orci L. Glucagon and glicentin immunoreactivity are topologically segregated in the alpha granules of the human pancreatic A cell. Nature 1980;284:66–7.

31. Solcia E, Capella C, Klöppel G. Tumors of the pancreas. Atlas of Tumor Pathology, 3rd Series, Fascicle 20. Washington, DC: Armed Forces Institute of Pathology, 1997.

Lungs

32. Bensch KG, Gordon GB, Miller LR. Studies on the bronchial counterpart of the Kultchitzky (argentaffin) cell and innervation of bronchial glands. J Ultrastruct Res 1965;12:668–86.

33. Heath D, Yacoub M, Gosney JR, Madden B, Caslin AW, Smith P. Pulmonary endocrine cells in hypertensive pulmonary vascular disease. Histopathology 1990;16:21–8.

34. Johnson DE, Kulik TJ, Lock JE, Elde RP, Thompson TR. Bombesin, calcitonin and serotonin—immunoreactive pulmonary neuroendocrine cells in acute and chronic neonatal lung disease. Pediatr Pulmonol 1985;1(3 Suppl):S13–20.

35. Kleinerman J, Marchevsky A. Quantitative studies of argyrophilic APUD cells in airways: II. The effects of transplacental diethylnitrosamine. Am Rev Respir Dis 1982;126:152–5.

36. Lauweryns JM, Peuskens JC. Neuroepithelial bodies (neuroreceptor and secretory organs?) in human infant bronchial and bronchiolar epithelium. Anat Rec 1972;172:471–81.

37. Tsutsumi Y, Osamura RY, Watanabe K, Yonaihara N. Immunohistochemical studies on gastrin-releasing peptide and adrenocorticotropic hormone-containing cells in the human lung. Lab Invest 1983;48:623–32.

Gastrointestinal Tract

38. Buffa R, Solcia E, Go VL. Immunohistochemical identification of the cholecystokinin cell in the intestinal mucosa. Gastroenterology 1976;70:528–32.

39. Buffa R, Solovieva I, Fiocca R, et al. Localization of bombesin and GRP (gastrin releasing peptide) sequences in gut nerves or endocrine cells. Histochemistry 1982;76:457–67.

40. Carraway R, Leeman SE. The isolation of a new hypotensive peptide, neurotensin, from bovine hypothalamus. J Biol Chem 1973;248:6854–61.

41. Crawford BG, Lechago J. Electron immunohistochemistry of gut peptides in tissue processed for routine electron microscopy. In: Grossman

MI, Brazier MA, Lechago J, eds. UCLA Forum in Medical Sciences #23. Cellular basis of chemical messengers in the digestive system. New York: Academic Press, 1981:73–82.

42. Forsberg EJ, Miller RJ. Cholinergic agonists induce vectorial release of serotonin from duodenal enterochromaffin cells. Science 1982;217:355–6.

43. Lechago J. The endocrine cells of the gastrointestinal tract. In: Lechago J, Gould VE, eds. Bloodworth's endocrine pathology, 3rd ed. Baltimore: Williams & Wilkins, 1997:463–93.

44. Lechago J, Shah IA. The endocrine cells of the gastrointestinal tract. In: Kovacs K, Asa SL, eds. Functional endocrine pathology, 2nd ed. Malden, MA: Blackwell Science, 1998:488–512.

45. Lloyd RV. Morphologic methods. In: Kovacs K, Asa SL, eds. Functional endocrine pathology, 2nd ed. Malden, MA: Blackwell Science, 1998:100–17.

Neuroendocrine Markers

46. Aguado F, Majó G, Ruiz-Montasell B, et al. Expression of synaptosomal-associated protein SNAP-25 in endocrine anterior pituitary cells. Eur J Cell Biol 1996;69:351–9.

47. Al-Khafaji B, Noffsinger AE, Miller MA, et al. Immunohistologic analysis of gastrointestinal and pulmonary carcinoid tumors. Hum Pathol 1998;29:992–9.

48. Bostwick DG, Roth KA, Evans CJ, et al. Gastrin-releasing peptide, a mammalian analog of bombesin, is present in human neuroendocrine lung tumors. Am J Pathol 1984;117:195–200.

49. Bunn PA Jr, Linnoila I, Minna JD, et al. Small cell lung cancer endocrine cells of the fetal bronchus and other neuroendocrine cells express the Leu-7 antigenic determinant present on natural killer-cells. Blood 1985;65:764–8.

50. Cunningham BA, Hemperly JJ, Murray BA, et al. Neural cell adhesion molecule: structure, immunoglobulin-like domains, cell surface modulation, and alternative RNA splicing. Science 1987;236:799–806.

51. Eipper BA, Stoffers DA, Mains RE. The biosynthesis of neuropeptides: peptide alpha amidation. Annu Rev Neurosci 1992;15:57–85.

52. Fischer von Mollard G, Mignery GA, Baumert M, et al. Rab3 is a small GTP-binding protein exclusively localized to synaptic vesicles. Proc Natl Acad Sci USA 1990;87:1988–92.

53. Gether U, Aakerlund L, Schwartz TW. Comparison of peptidylglycine alpha-amidation activity in medullary thyroid carcinoma cells, pheochromocytomas, and serum. Mol Cell Endocrinol 1991;79:53–63.

54. Gould VE, Lee I, Wiedenmann B, et al. Synaptophysin: a novel marker for neurons, certain neuroendocrine cells and their neoplasms. Hum Pathol 1986;17:979–83.

55. Grimmelikhuijzen CJ, Leviev I, Carstensen K. Peptides in the nervous systems of cnidarians: structure function and biosynthesis. Int Rev Cytol 1996;167:37–89.

56. Jin L, Hemperly JJ, Lloyd RV. Expression of neural cell adhesion molecule in normal and neoplastic human neuroendocrine tissues. Am J Pathol 1991;138:961–9.

57. Johannes L, Lledo PM, Roa M, et al. The GPTase Rab3a negatively controls calcium-dependent exocytosis in neuroendocrine cells. EMBO J 1994;13:2029–37.

58. Kibbelaar RE, Moolenaar KE, Michalides RJ, et al. Neural cell adhesion molecule expression, neuroendocrine differentiation and prognosis in lung carcinoma. Eur J Cancer 1991;27:431–5.

59. Lloyd RV. Morphologic methods. In: Kovacs K, Asa SL, eds. Functional endocrine pathology, 2nd ed. Malden, MA: Blackwell Science, 1998:100–117.

60. Lloyd RV, D'amato CJ, Thiny MT, et al. Corticotroph (basophil) invasion of the pars nervosa in the human pituitary: localization of proopiomelanocortin peptides, galanin and peptidylglycine alpha-amidating monoxygenase-like immunoreactivities. Endocr Pathol 1993;4:86–94.

61. Lloyd RV, Jin L, Qian X, et al. Analysis of the chromogranin A post-translational cleavage product pancreastatin and the prohormone convertases PC2 and PC3 in normal and neoplastic human pituitaries. Am J Pathol 1995;146:1188–98.

62. Lloyd RV, Mervak T, Schmidt K, et al. Immunohistochemical detection of chromogranin and neuron-specific enolase in pancreatic endocrine neoplasms. Am J Surg Pathol 1984;8:607–14.

63. Lloyd RV, Sisson JC, Shapiro B, Verhofstad AA. Immunohistochemical localization of epinephrine, norepinephrine, catecholamine-synthesizing enzymes, and chromogranin neuroendocrine cells and tumors. Am J Pathol 1986;125:45–54.

64. Lloyd RV, Warner TF. Immunohistochemistry of neuron-specific enolase. In: DeLellis RA, ed. Advances in immunochemistry. New York: Masson, 1984:127–40.

65. Majo G, Ferrer I, Marsal J, et al. Immunocytochemical analysis of the synaptic proteins SNAP-25 and Rab3A in human pituitary adenomas. Overexpression of SNAP-25 in the mammosomatotroph lineages. J Pathol 1997;183:440–6.

66. Martelli AM, Bareggi R, Baldini G, Scherer PE, Lodish HF, Baldini G. Diffuse vesicular distribution of Rab3D in the polarized neuroendocrine cell line AtT-20. FEBS Lett 1995;368:271–5.

67. Martinez A, Montuenga LM, Springall DR, Trston A, Cuttitta F, Polak JM. Immunocytochemical localization of peptidylglycine, alpha-amidating monooxygenase enzymes (PAM) in human endocrine pancreas. J Histochem Cytochem 1993;41:375–80.

68. Oyler GA, Higgins GA, Hart RA, et al. The identification of a novel synaptosomal-associated protein. SNAP-25, differentially expressed by neuronal subpopulations. J Cell Biol 1989;109:3039–52.

69. Patel K, Moore SE, Dickson G, et al. Neural cell adhesion molecule (NCAM) is the antigen recognized by monoclonal antibodies of similar specificity in small-cell lung carcinoma and neuroblastoma. Int J Cancer 1989;44:573–8.

70. Quinn KA, Treston AM, Scott FM, et al. Alpha-amidation of peptide hormones in lung cancer. Cancer Cells 1991;3:504–10.

71. Rode J, Dhillon AP, Doran JF, et al. PGP9.5, a new marker for human neuroendocrine tumours. Histopathology 1985;9:147–58.

72. Roth D, Burgoyne RD. SNAP-25 is present in a SNARE complex in adrenal chromaffin cells. FEBS Lett 1994; 351:207–10.

73. Rygaard K, Moller C, Bock E, Spang-Thomsen M. Expression of cadherin and NCAM in human small cell lung cancer cell lines and xenografts. Br J Cancer 1992;65:573–7.

74. Sadoul K, Lang J, Montecucco C, et al. SNAP-25 is expressed in islets of Langerhans and is involved in insulin release. J Cell Biol 1995;128:1019–28.

75. Schmechel D, Marangos PJ, Brightman M. Neurone-specific enolase is a molecular marker for peripheral and central neuroendocrine cells. Nature 1978;276;834–6.

76. Schmid KW, Kross M, Hittmair A, et al. Chromogranin A and B in adenomas of the pituitary. An immunohistochemical study of 42 cases. Am J Surg Pathol 1991;15:1072–77.

77. Scopsi L, Gullo M, Rilke F, Martin S, Steiner DF. Proprotein convertases (PC1/PC3 and PC2) in normal and neoplastic human tissues: their use as markers of neuroendocrine differentiation. J Clin Endocrinol Metab 1995;80:294–301.

78. Scopsi L, Lee R, Gullo M, et al. Peptidylglycine a-amidating monooxygenase in neuroendocrine tumors. Its identification, characterization, quantification and relation to the grade of morphologic differentiation, amidated peptide content and granin immunocytochemistry. Appl Immunohistochem 1998;6:120–32.

79. Senden NH, Timmer ED, Boers JE, et al. Neuro-endocrine-specific protein C (NSP-C): subcellular localization and differential expression in relation to NSP-A. Eur J Cell Biol 1996;69:197–213.

80. Senden NH, Timmer ED, deBruine A, et al. A comparison of NSP-reticulons with conventional neuroendocrine markers in immunophenotyping of lung cancers. J Pathol 1997;182:13–21.

81. Senden NH, Van de Velde HJ, Broers JL, et al. Cluster 10 lung cancer antibodies recognize NSPs. Novel neuroendocrine proteins associated with membranes of the endoplasmic reticulum. Int J Cancer Suppl 1994;8:84–8.

82. Steel JH, Martinez A, Springall DR, et al. Peptidylglycine alpha-amidating monooxygenase (PAM) immunoreactivity and messenger RNA in human pituitary and increased expression in pituitary tumours. Cell Tissue Res 1994;276:197–207.

83. Thompson RJ, Doran JF, Jackson P, et al. PGP9.5—a new marker for vertebrate neurons and neuroendocrine cells. Brain Res 1983;278:224–8.

84. Tischler AS, Mobtaker H, Mann K, et al. Anti-lymphocyte antibody Leu-7 (HNK-1) recognizes a constituent of neuroendocrine granule matrix. J Histochem Cytochem 1986;34:1213–6.

85. Van de Velde HJ, Senden NH, Roskams TA, et al. NSP-encoded reticulons are neuroendocrine markers of a novel category in human lung cancer diagnosis. Cancer Res 1994;54:4769–76.

86. Wharton J, Polak JM, Bloom SR, et al. Bombesin-like immunoreactivity in the lung. Nature 1978;273:769–70.

87. Wiedenmann B, Huttner WB. Synaptophysin and chromogranins/secretogranins—widespread constituents of distinct types of neuroendocrine vesicles and new tools in tumor diagnosis. Virchows Arch [Cell Pathol] 1989;58:95–121.

88. Wilson BS, Lloyd RV. Detection of chromogranin in neuroendocrine cells with a monoclonal antibody. Am J Pathol 1984;115:458–68.

Molecular Biology

89. Abbona G, Papotti M, Viberti L, Macri L, Stella A, Bussolati G. Chromogranin A gene expression in nonsmall cell lung carcinomas. J Pathol 1998;186:151–6.

90. Arnold A, Brown MF, Urena P, Gaz RD, Sarfati E, Drueke TB. Monoclonality of parathyroid tumors in chronic renal failure and in primary parathyroid hyperplasia. J Clin Invest 1995;95:2047–53.

91. Arnold A, Kim HG, Gaz RD, et al. Molecular cloning and chromosomal mapping of DNA rearranged with the parathyroid hormone gene in a parathyroid adenoma. J Clin Invest 1989;83:2034–40.

92. Chandrasekharappa SC, Guru SC, Manickam P, et al. Positional cloning of the gene for multiple endocrine neopalsia-type 1. Science 1997;276:404–7.

93. Daniely M, Aviram A, Adams EF, Buchfelder M. Comparative genomic hybridization analysis of nonfunctioning pituitary tumors. J Clin Endocrinol Metab 1998;83:1801–5.

94. Erickson LA, Jin L, Wollan PC, Thompson, GB, van Heerden JA, Lloyd RV. Parathyroid hyperplasia, adenomas, and carcinomas: differential expression of p27kip1 protein. Am J Surg Pathol 1999;23:288–95.

95. Gagel RF. Multiple endocrine neoplasia. In: Wilson JD, Foster DW, Kronenberg HM, Larsen PR, eds. Williams textbook of endocrinology, 9th ed. Philadelphia: WB Saunders, 1998:1627–49.

96. Guru SC, Goldsmith PK, Burns AL, et al. Menin, the product of the MEN1 gene, is a nuclear protein. Proc Natl Acad Sci USA 1998;95:1630–4.

97. Lloyd RV, Erickson LA, Jin L, et al. p27kip1: a multifunctional cyclin-dependent kinase inhibitor with prognostic significance in human cancers. Am J Pathol 1999;154:313–23.

98. Lloyd RV, Jin L, Kulig E, Fields K. Molecular approaches for the analysis of chromogranin and secretogranins. Diagn Mol Pathol 1992;1:2–15.

99. Lloyd RV, Jin L, Qian X, Kulig E. Abberant p27kip1 expression in endocrine and other tumors. Am J Pathol 1997;150:401–7.

100. Mouland AJ, Bevan S, White JH, Hendy GN. Human chromogranin A gene. Molecular cloning, structural analysis, and neuroendocrine cell-specific expression. J Biol Chem 1994;269:6918–26.

101. Mulligan LM, Marsh DJ, Robinson BG, et al. Genotype-phenotype correlation in multiple endocrine neoplasia type 2: report of the international RET mutation consortium. J Int Med 1995;238:343–6.

102. Mulligan LM, Ponder BA. Genetic basis of endocrine disease: multiple endocrine neoplasia type 2. J Clin Endocrinl Metab 1995;80:1989–95.

103. Nakamura T, Ishizaka Y, Nagao M, Hara M, Ishikawa T. Expression of the ret proto-oncogene product in human normal and neoplastic tissue of neural crest origin. J Pathol 1994;172:255–60.

104. Pagani A, Forni M, Tonini GP, Papotti M, Bussolati G. Expression of members of the chromogranin family in primary neuroblastomas. Diagn Mol Pathol 1992;1:16–24.

105. Palanisamy N, Imanishi Y, Rao PH, Tahara H, Chaganti RS, Arnold A. Novel chromosomal abnormalities identified by comparative genomic hybridization in parathyroid adenomas. J Clin Endocrinol Metab 1988;83:1766–70.

106. Papadaki H, Kounelis S, Kapadia SB, Bakker A, Swalsky PA, Finkelstein SD. Relationship of p53 gene alterations with tumor progression and recurrence in olfactory neuroblastoma. Am J Surg Pathol 1996;20:715–21.

107. Pernicone PJ, Scheithauer BW, Sebo TJ, et al. Pituitary carcinoma: a clinicopathologic study of 15 cases. Cancer 1997;79:804–12.

108. Perren A, Roth J, Muletta-Feunrer S, et al. Clonal analysis of sporadic pancreatic endocrine tumors. J Pathol 1998;186:363–71.

109. Przygodzki RM, Finkelstein SD, Langer JC, et al. Analysis of p53, K-ras-2 and c-raf-1 in pulmonary neuroendocrine tumors. Correlation with histological subtype and clinical outcome. Am J Pathol 1996;148:1531–41.

110. Winkler H, Fischer-Colbrie R. The chromogranin A and B: the first 25 years and future perspectives. Neuroscience 1992;49:497–528.

111. Wu H, Rozansky DJ, Webster NJ, O'Connor DT. Cell type-specific gene expression in the neuroendocrine system. A neuroendocrine-specific regulatory element in the promotor of chromogranin A, a ubiquitous secretory granule core protein. J Clin Invest 1994;94:118–29.

112. Zhuang Z, Vertneyer AO, Pack S, et al. Somatic mutations of the MEN1 tumor suppressor gene in sporadic gastrinomas and insulinomas. Cancer Res 1997;57:4682–6.

Hypofunction

113. Aaltonen J, Bjorses P, Sandkuijl L, Perhcentupa J, Pettonen L. An autosomal locus causing autoimmune disease: autoimmune polyglandular disease type I assigned to chromosone 21. Nat Genet 1994;8:83–7.

114. Ahonen P, Myllarniemi S, Sipila I, et al. Clinical variation of autoimmune polyendocrinopathy—candidiasis-ectodermal dystrophy (APECED) in a series of 68 patients. N Engl J Med 1990;322:1829–36.

115. Eisenbarth GS, Verge CF. Immunoendocrinopathy syndromes. In: Wilson JD, Foster DW, Kronenberg HM, Larsen PR, eds. Williams textbook of endocrinology, 9th ed. Philadelphia: WB Saunders, 1998:1651–62.

116. Menser MA, Forrest JM, Bransby RD. Rubella infection and diabetes mellitus. Lancet 1978;1:57–60.

117. Neufeld M, Maclaren NK, Blizzard RM. Two types of autoimmune Addison's disease associated with different polyglandular autoimmune (PGA) syndromes. Medicine 1981;60:355–62.

118. Orth DN, Kovacs WJ. The adrenal cortex. In: Wilson JD, Foster DW, Kronenberg HM, Larsen PR, eds. Williams textbook of endocrinology, 9th ed. Philadelphia: WB Saunders, 1998:517–664.

119. Polymeropoulos MH, Swift RG, Swift M. Linkage of the gene for Wolfram syndrome to markers on the short arm of chromosome 4. Nat Genet 1994;8:95–7.

120. Rabinowe SL, George KL, Loughlin R, et al. Congenital rubella. Monoclonal antibody defined T cell abnormalities in young adults. Am J Med 1986;81:779–82.

121. Rabinowe SL, Rubin IL, George KL, Adri MN, Eisenbarth GS. Trisomy 21 (Down's syndrome): autoimmunity, aging and monoclonal antibody defined T cell abnormalities. J Autoimmun 1989;2:25–30.

122. Rando TA, Horton JC, Layzer RB. Wolfram syndrome: evidence of a diffuse neurodegenerative disease by magnetic resonance imaging. Neurology 1992;42:1220–4.

123. Savilahti E, Simell O, Koskimies S, Rilva A, Akerblom HK. Celiac disease in insulin-dependent diabetes mellitus. J Pediatr 1986;108:690–3.

124. Thompson G, Robinson WP, Kuhner MK, et al. Genetic heterogeneity, modes of inheritance and risk estimates for a joint study of Caucasians with insulin-dependent diabetes mellitus. Am J Hum Genet 1988;43:799–816.

125. Tuomi T, Bjorses P, Falorri A, et al. Antibodies to glutamic acid decarboxylase and insulin-dependent diabetes in patients with autoimmune polyendocrine syndrome type I. J Clin Endocrinol Metab 1996;81:1488–94.

126. Verge CF, Howard NJ, Rouley MJ, et al. Antiglutamate decarboxylase and other antibodies at the onset of childhood IDDM: a population-based study. Diabetologia 1994;37:1113-20.

Diabetes Mellitus

127. Anderson S, Brenner BM. Pathogenesis of diabetic glomeruloscleropathy: hemodynamic consideration. Diabetes Metab Res 1988;4:163–77.

128. Baekkeskov S, Nielsen JH, Marner B, Bilde T, Ludvigsson J, Lernmark A. Autoantibodies in newly diagnosed diabetic children immunoprecipitate human pancreatic islet cell proteins. Nature 1982;298:167–9.

129. Bennett PH, Rushforth NB, Miller M, et al. Epidemiologic studies of diabetes in the Pima Indians. Recent Prog Horm Res 1976;32: 333–76.

130. Bloodworth JM Jr. The endocrine pancreas. In: Lechago J, Gould VE, eds. Bloodworth's endocrine pathology, 3rd ed. Baltimore: Williams & Wilkins, 1997:519–57.

131. Böhmer K, Keilacker H, Kuglin B, et al. Proinsulin autoantibodies are more closely associated with type I (insulin-dependent) diabetes mellitus than insulin antibodies. Diabetologia 1991;34:830–4.

132. Boquist L. The endocrine pancreas in early alloxin diabetes. Acta Pathol Microbiol Scand Sect A 1977;85A:219–29.

133. Bottazzo GF, Dean BM, McNally JM, McKay EH, Swift PG, Gamble DR. In situ characterization of autoimmune phenomena in diabetic insulitis. N Engl J Med 1985;313:353–60.

134. Bottazzo GF, Lendrum R. Separate autoantibodies to human pancreatic glucagon and somatostatin cells. Lancet 1976;2:873–6.

135. Cersosimo E, Pisters PW, Pesola G, McDermott K, Bajorunas D, Brennan MF. Insulin secretion and action in patients with pancreatic cancer. Cancer 1991;67:486–93.

136. Cryer PE, Polonsky KS. Glucose homeostasis and hypoglycemia. In: Wilson JD, Foster DW, Kronenberg HM, Larsen PR, eds. Williams textbook of endocrinology, 9th ed. Philadelphia: WB Saunders, 1998:939–71.

137. DeKoning EJ, Fleming KA, Gray DW, Clark A. High prevalence of pancreatic islet amyloid in patients with end-stage renal failure on dialysis treatment. J Pathol 1995;175:253–8.

138. The Diabetes Control and Complications Trial Research Group. The effect of intensive treatment of diabetes on the development and progression of long-term complications in insulin-dependent diabetes mellitus. N Engl J Med 1993;329:977–86.

139. Gepts W. Pathologic anatomy of the pancreas in juvenile diabetes mellitus. Diabetes 1965;14:619–33.

140. Gepts W, DeMey J. Islet cell survival determined by morphology. An immunocytochemical study of the islets of Langerhans in juvenile diabetes mellitus. Diabetes 1978;27(Suppl 1):251–61.

141. Goto Y, Kakizaki M, Toyota T. Hereditary diabetes mellitus. In: Melish JS, Hanna J, Baba S, eds. Genetic-environmental interaction in diabetes mellitus. Amsterdam: Excerpta Medica, 1982:18–29.

142. Greene DA, Lattimer SA, Sima AA. Are disturbances of sorbitol phosphoinositide and Na+-K+-ATPase one regulation involved in pathogenesis of diabetic neuropathy? Diabetes 1988;37:688–93.

143. Groth CG, Korsgren O, Tibell A, et al. Transplantation of porcine fetal pancreas to diabetic patients. Lancet 1994;344:1402–4.

144. Klein R, Klein BE, Moss SE, et al. The Wisconsin Epidemiologic Study of Diabetic Retinopathy II. Prevalence and risk of diabetic retinopathy when age at diagnosis is less than 30 years. Arch Ophthalmol 1984;102:520–6.

145. Klöppel G, Bommer G, Commandeur G, Heitz P. The endocrine pancreas in chronic pancreatitis. Immunocytochemical and ultrastructural studies. Virchows Arch [A] 1978;377:157–74.

146. Klöppel G, Int Veld PA, Komminoth P, Heitz PU. The endocrine pancreas. In: Kovacs K, Asa SL, eds. Functional endocrine pathology, 2nd ed. Oxford: Blackwell Sciences, 1998:415–87.

147. La Porte RE, Fishbein HA, Drash AL, et al. The Pittsburgh insulin-dependent diabetes mellitus (IDDM) registry: the incidence of insulin-dependent diabetes mellitus in Allegheny County, Pennsylvania (1965-1976). Diabetes 1981;30:279–84.

148. Löhr M, Goertchen P, Nizze H, et al. Cystic fibrosis associated islet changes may provide a basis for diabetes. An immunocytochemical and morphometrical study. Virchows Arch [A] 1989;414:179–85.

149. Löhr M, Klöppel G. Residual insulin positivity and pancreatic atrophy in relation to duration of chronic type I (insulin-dependent) diabetes mellitus and microangiopathy. Diabetologia 1987;30:757–62.

150. MacLean N, Ogilvie RF. Observations on the pancreatic islet tissue of young diabetic subjects. Diabetes 1959;8:83–91.

151. Marble A. Late complications of diabetes. A continuing challenge. The Elliot P Joslin Memorial Lecture of the German Diabetes Federation. Diabetologia 1976;12:193–9.

152. Marks HH. Longevity and mortality of diabetics. Am J Public Health 1965;55:416–23.

153. Morrison AD, Clements RS Jr, Winegrad AI. Effects of elevated glucose concentrations on the metabolism of the aortic wall. J Clin Invest 1972;51:3114–23.

154. Nerup J, Mandrup-Poulsen T, Molvig J. The HLA-IDDM association: implications for etiology and pathogenesis of IDDM. Diabetes Metab Rev 1987;3:779–802.

155. Oldstone MB, Nenenberg M, Southern P, Price J, Lewicki H. Virus infection triggers insulin-dependent diabetes mellitus in a transgenic model: role of anti-self (virus) immune response. Cell 1991;65:319–31.

156. Partanen J, Niskanen L, Lehtinen J, Mervaala E, Siitonen O, Usitupa M. Natural history of peripheral neuropathy in patients with non-insulin-dependent diabetes mellitus. N Engl J Med 1995;333:89–94.

157. Rahier J, Loozen S, Goebbels RM, Abrahem M. The haemochromatotic human pancreas: a quantitative immunohistochemical and ultrastructural study. Diabetologia 1987;30:5–12.

158. Rao RH. Diabetes in the undernourished: coincidence or consequence? Endocrine Rev 1988;9:67–87.

159. Schnider SL, Kohn RR. Effects of age and diabetes mellitus on the solubility and nonenzymatic glucosylation of human skin collagen. J Clin Invest 1981;67:1630–5.

160. Soler NG, Bennett MA, Pentecost BL, Fitzgerald MG, Malins JM. Myocardial infarction in diabetics. Q J Med 1975;44:125–32.

161. Sutherland DE. Who should get a pancreas transplant? Diabetes Care 1988;11:681–5.

162. Taylor SI, Werthheimer E, Accili D, et al. Mutations in the insulin-receptor gene: update. Endocr Rev 1994;2:58–65.

163. Unger RH, Foster DW. Diabetes mellitus. In: Wilson JD, Foster DW, Kronenberg HM, Larsen PR, eds. Williams textbook of endocrinology, 9th ed. Philadelphia: WB Saunders, 1998:973–1059.

164. Warnock GL, Knetemen NM, Ryan EA, Rabinovitch A, Rajotte RV. Long-term follow-up after transplantation of insulin-producing pancreatic islets into patients with type I (insulin-dependent) diabetes mellitus. Diabetologia 1992;35:89–95.

165. Westermark GT, Christmanson L, Terenghi G, et al. Islet amyloid polypeptide: demonstration of mRNA in human pancreatic islets by in situ hybridization in islets with and without amyloid deposits. Diabetologia 1993;36:323–8.

166. Westermark P, Wilander E, Westermark GT, Johnson KH. Islet amyloid polypeptide-like immunoreactivity in the islet B cells of type II (non-insulin-dependent) diabetic and non-diabetic individuals. Diabetologia 1987;30:887–92.

167. Wilander E, Boquist L. Streptozotocin-diabetes in the Chinese hamster. Blood glucose and structural changes during the first 24 hours. Horm Metab Res 1972;4:426–33.

168. Yoon-JW, Austin M, Onodera T, Notkins AL. Virus-induced diabetes mellitus: isolation of a virus from the pancreas of a child with diabetic ketoacidosis. N Engl J Med 1979;300:1173–9.

Hyperplasia-Pancreas in Children

169. Dahms BB, Landing BH, Blaskovics M, Roe TF. Nesidioblastosis and other islet cell abnormalities in hyperinsulinemic hypoglycemia of childhood. Hum Pathol 1980;11:641–9.

170. deLonlay-Dobony P, Poggi-Travert F, Fournet JC, et al. Clinical features of 52 neonates with hyperinsulinism. N Engl J Med 1999;340:1169–75.

171. deMarais CF, Lopes EA, Bisi H, Alves, de Macedo Santos RT. Nesidioblastosis associated with congenital malformations of the heart—morphological and immunohistochemical study of 5 necropsy cases. Pathol Res Pract 1986;181:175–9.

172. Dunne MJ, Kane C, Shepherd RM, et al. Familial persistent hyperinsulinemic hypoglycemia of infancy and mutations of the sulfanylurea receptor. N Engl J Med 1997;336:703–6.

173. Gabbe SG. Diabetes mellitus in pregnancy: have all the problems been solved? Am J Med 1981;70:613–8.

174. Glaser B, Chiu KC, Anker R, et al. Familial hyperinsulinism maps to chromosome 11p 14-15.1, 30 cM centromeric to the insulin gene. Nat Genet 1994;7:185–8.

175. Gould VE, Memoli VA, Dardi LE, Gould NS. Nesidiodysplasia and nesidioblastosis of infancy: structural and functional correlations with the syndrome of hyperinsulinemic hypoglycemia. Pediatr Pathol 1983;1:7–31.

176. Hansson G, Redin B. Familial neonatal hypoglycemia. A syndrome resembling foetopathia diabetica. Acta Paediatr 1963;52:145–52.

177. Heitz PU, Klöppel G, Häcki WH, Polak JM, Pearse AG. Nesidioblastosis: the pathologic basis of persistent hyperinsulinemic hypoglycemia in infants. Morphologic and quanitative analysis of seven cases based on specific immunostaining and electron microscopy. Diabetes 1977;26:632–42.

178. Hultquist GT, Olding LB. Endocrine pathology of infants of diabetic mothers. A quantitative morphological analysis including a comparison with infants of iso-immunized and non-diabetic mothers. Acta Endocrinol 1981;(Suppl 241):1–202.

179. Jaffe R, Hashida Y, Yunis EJ. Pancreatic pathology in hyperinsulinemic hypoglycemia of infancy. Lab Invest 1980;42:356–65.

180. Klöppel G, Bommer G, Commandeur G, Heitz P. The endocrine pancreas in chronic pancreatitis. Immunocytochemical and ultrastructural studies. Virchows Arch [A] 1978;377:157–74.

181. Klöppel G, Heitz PhV. Nesidioblastosis: a clinical entity with heterogenesis lesions of the pancreas. In: Folkner S, Hakanson R, Sundler F, eds. Evolution and tumor pathology of the neuroendocrine system. New York: Elsevier, 1984:349–70.

182. Klöppel G, Int Veld PA, Komminoth P, Heitz PU. The endocrine pancreas. In: Kovacs K, Asa SL, eds. Functional endocrine pathology, 2nd ed. Malden, MA: Blackwell Science, 1998:415–87.

183. Kogut MD, Blaskovics M, Donnell GN. Idiopathic hypoglycemia: a study of 26 children. J Pediatr 1969;74:853–71.

184. Kramer JL, Bell MJ, DeSchyver K, Bower RJ, Ternberg JL, White NH. Clinical and histologic indications for extensive pancreatic resection in nesidioblastosis. Am J Surg 1982;143:116–9.

185. Laidlaw GF. Nesidioblastoma, the islet tumor of the pancreas. Am J Pathol 1938;14:125–34.

186. Lloyd RV, Caceres V, Warner TF, Gilbert EF. Islet cell adenomatosis: a report of two cases and review of the literature. Arch Pathol Lab Med 1981;105:198–202.

187. Misugi K, Misugi N, Sotos J, Smith B. The pancreatic islets of infants with severe hypoglycemia. Arch Pathol 1970;89:208–20.

188. Naeye RL. Infants of diabetic mothers: a quantitative morphologic study. Pediatrics 1965;35:980–9.

189. Obenshau SS, Adam PA, King KC, et al. Human fetal insulin response to sustained maternal hyperglycemia. N Engl J Med 1970;283:566–70.

190. Pagliara AS, Karl IE, Haymond M, Kipni DM. Hypoglycemia in infancy (Part 1). J Pediatr 1973;82:365–79.

191. Rahier J, Falt K, Munterfering H, Becker K, Gepts W, Falkmer S. The basic structural lesion of persistent neonatal hypoglycemia with hyperinsulinism: deficiency of pancreatic D cells or hyperactivity of B cells? Diabetologia 1984;26:282–9.

192. Ray MB, Zumwalt R. Islet cell hyperplasia in genetic deficiency of alpha-1-proteinase inhibitor. Am J Clin Pathol 1986;85:681–7.

193. Rusnak SL, Driscoll SG. Congenital spinal anomalies in infants of diabetic mothers. Pediatrics 1965;35:989–95.

194. Schwartz JF, Zwiren GT. Islet cell adenomatosis and adenoma in an infant. J Pediatr 1971;79:232–8.

195. Schwartz SS, Rich BH, Lucky AW, et al. Familial nesidioblastosis: severe neonatal hypoglycemia in two families. J Pediatr 1979;95:44–53.

196. Silverman JL. Eosinophile infiltration in the pancreas of infants of diabetic mothers. A clinicopathologic study. Diabetes 1963;12:528–37.

197. Spitz L, Buick RG, Grant DB, et al. Surgical treatment of nesidioblastosis. Pediatr Surg Int 1986;1:26–9.

198. Stefan Y, Bordi C, Grasso S, Orci L. Beckwith-Wiedemann syndrome: a quantitative immunohistochemical study of pancreatic islet cell population. Diabetalogia 1985;28:914–9.

199. Thomas CG Jr, Underwood LE, Carney CN, et al. Neonatal and infantile hypoglycemia due to insulin excess: new aspects of diagnosis and surgical management. Ann Surg 1977;185:505–17.

200. Yakovac WC, Baker L, Hummeler K. Beta cell nesidioblastosis in idiopathic hypoglycemia of infancy. J Pediatr 1971;79:226–31.

Nesidioblastosis in Adults

201. Albers N, Löhr M, Bogner U, Loy V, Kloppel G. Nesidioblastosis of the pancreas in an adult with persistent hyperinsulinemic hypoglycemia. Am J Clin Pathol 1989;91:336–40.

202. Carlson T, Eckhauser ML, DeBaz B, et al. Nesidioblastosis in an adult: an illustrative case and collective review. Am J Gastroenterol 1987;82:566–71.

203. Goudswaard WB, Houthoff HJ, Koudstal J, Zwierstra RP. Nesidioblastosis and endocrine hyperplasia of the pancreas: a secondary phenomenon. Hum Pathol 1986;17:46–54.

204. Gould VE, Chejfec G, Shah K, Paloyan E, Lawrence AM. Adult nesidiodysplasia. Semin Diag Pathol 1984;1:43–53.

205. Harness JK, Geelhoed GW, Thompson NW, et al. Nesidioblastosis in adults. A surgical dilemma. Arch Surg 1981;116:575–80.

206. Kovacs K, Horvath E, Asa SL, Murray D, Singer W, Reddy SS. Microscopic peliosis of pancreatic islets in a woman with MEN-1 syndrome. Arch Pathol Lab Med 1986;110:607–10.

207. Nestorowicz A, Inagaki N, Gonoi T, et al. A nonsense mutation is the inward rectifier potassium channel gene, Kir 6.2, is associated with a familial hyperinsulinism. Diabetes 1997;46:1743–8.

208. Service FJ, Natt N, Thompson GB, et al. Noninsulinoma pancreatogenous hypoglycemia: a novel syndrome of hyperinsulinemic hypoglycemia in adults independent of mutations in Kir6.2 and SUR1 genes. J Clin Endocrinol Metab 1999;84:1582–9.

209. Spitz L, Buick RG, Grant DB, Leonard JV, Pincott JR. Surgical treatment of nesidioblastosis. Pediatr Surg Int 1986;1:26–9.

210. Thomas PM, Cote GJ, Wohllk N, et al. Mutations in the sulfonylurea receptor gene in familial hyperinsulinemic hypoglycemia of infancy. Science 1995;268:426–9.

211. Tibaldi JM, Lorber D, Lomansky S, Steinberg JJ, Reisman R, Shamoon H. Postprandial hypoglycemia in islet beta cell hyperplasia with adenomatosis of the pancreas. J Surg Oncol 1992;50:53–7.

212. Van Heerden JA, Edis AJ, Service FJ. The surgical aspects of insulinomas. Ann Surg 1979;189:677–82.

213. Weidenheim KM, Hinchey WW, Campbell WG Jr. Hyperinsulinemic hypoglycemia in adults with islet cell hyperplasia and degranulation of exocrine cells of the pancreas. Am J Clin Pathol 1983;79:14–24.

Gastrin Cell Hyperplasia

214. Creutzfeldt W, Arnold R. Endocrinology of duodenal ulcer. World J Surg 1979;3:605–13.

215. Dayal Y, DeLellis RA, Wolfe HJ. Hyperplastic lesions of the gastrointestinal endocrine cells. Am J Surg Pathol 1987;11(Suppl 1):87–101.

216. Friedman LS, Peterson WL. Peptic ulcer and related disorders. In: Fauci AS, Braunwald E, Isselbacher KJ, et al, eds. Harrison's principles of internal medicine, 14th ed. New York: McGraw-Hill, 1998:1596–616.

217. Lechago J. The endocrine cells of the gastrointestinal tract. In: Lechago J, Gould VE, eds. Bloodworth's endocrine pathology, 3rd ed. Baltimore: Williams & Wilkins, 1997:463–93.

218. Lechago J. Gastrointestinal neuroendocrine cell proliferations. Hum Pathol 1994;25:1114–22.
219. Lewin KJ, Yang K, Ulich T, Elashoff JD, Walsh J. Primary gastrin cell hyperplasia. Report of five cases with a review of the literature. Am J Surg Pathol 1984;8:821–32.
220. McHenry L Jr, Vuyyuru L, Schubert ML. Helicobacter pylori and duodenal ulcer disease: the somatostatin link. Gastroenterology 1993;104:1573–5.
221. McIntyne RL, Piris J. A method for the qualification of human gastric G-cell density in endoscopic biopsy specimens. J Clin Pathol 1981;34:514–8.
222. Nielsen HO, Halken S, Lorentzen M. Quantitative studies of the gastrin-producing cells of the human antrum. A methodological study. Acta Pathol Microbiol Scand 1980;88:255–61.
223. Polak JM, Hoffbrand AV, Reed PI, Bloom SR, Pearse AG. Qualitative and quantitative studies of antral and fundic G cells in pernicious anemia. Scand J Gastroenterol 1973;8:361–7.
224. Polak JM, Stagg B, Pearse AG. Two types of Zollinger-Ellison syndrome: immunofluorescent, cytochemical and ultrastructural studies of the antral and pancreatic gastrin cells in different clinical states. Gut 1972;13:501–12.
225. Solcia E, Vassallo G, Capella C. Cytology and cytochemistry of hormone producing cells of the upper gastrointestinal tract. In: Creutzfeldt W, ed. Origin, chemistry, pathology and pathophysiology of the gastrointestinal hormones. Stuttgart: Schattaner-Verlag, 1970:3–29.

Enterochromaffin-Like Cell Hyperplasia

226. Borch K, Renvall H, Kullman E, Wilander E. Gastric carcinoid associated with the syndrome of hypergastrinemic atrophic gastritis. A prospective analysis of 11 cases. Am J Surg Pathol 1987;11:435–44.
227. Bordi C, Cocconi G, Togni R, et al. Gastric endocrine cell proliferation. Association with Zollinger-Ellison syndrome. Arch Pathol 1974;98:274–8.
228. Bordi C, Yu JY, Baggi MT, Moore SB, Alport EC, Nora FE. Gastric carcinoids and their precursor lesions. A histologic and immunohistochemical study of 23 cases. Cancer 1991;67:663–72.
229. Carney JA, Go VL, Fairbanks VF, et al. The syndrome of gastric argyrophil carcinoid tumors and non-antral gastric atrophy. Ann Intern Med 1983;99:761–6.
230. Friedman LS, Peterson WL. Peptic ulcer and related disorders. In: Fauci AS, Braunwald E, Isselbacher KJ, et al, eds. Harrison's principles of internal medicine, 14th ed. New York: McGraw Hill, 1998:1596–616.
231. Hodges JR, Isaacson P, Wright R. Diffuse enterochromaffin-like (ECL) cell hyperplasia and multiple gastric carcinoids. A complication of pernicious anaemia. Gut 1981;22:237–41.
232. Lehy T, Cadiot G, Mignon M, Ruszniewski P, Bonfils S. Influence of multiple endocrine neoplasia type 1 on gastric endocrine cells in patients with the Zollinger-Ellison syndrome. Gut 1992;33:1275–9.
233. Rindi G. Clinicopathologic aspects of gastric neuroendocrine tumors. Am J Surg Pathol 1995;19(Suppl 1):S20–9.
234. Solica E, Capella C, Buffa R, Frigerio B, Fiocca R. Pathology of the Zollinger-Ellison syndrome. Prog Surg Pathol 1980;1:119–33.
235. Solcia E, Capella C, Sessa F, et al. Gastric carcinoids and related endocrine growth. Digestion 1986;35(Suppl 1):3–22.
236. Solcia E, Capella C, Vassallo G, et al. Endocrine cells of the gastric mucosa. Int Rev Cytol 1975;42:223–86.

Enterochromaffin Cell Hyperplasia

237. Bishop AE, Pietroleltti R, Taat CW, Brummelkamp WH, Polak JM. Increased population of endocrine cells in Crohn's ileitis. Virchows Arch [A] 1987;410:391–6.
238. Challacombe DN, Robertson K. Enterochromaffin cells in the duodenal mucosa of children with coeliac disease. Gut 1977;18:373–6.
239. Lechago J. Gastrointestinal neuroendocrine cell proliferations. Hum Pathol 1994;25:1114–22.
240. Lindop GB. Enterochromaffin cell hyperplasia and megacolon: report of a case. Gut 1983;24:575–8.
241. Mogensen AM, Hage E, Bulow S. Electron microscopic studies of endocrine hyperplasia in duodenal adenomas in familial adenomatous polyposis. Virchows Arch [A] 1989;414:321–4.
242. Sjolund K, Aluments J, Berg NO, H kanson R, Sundler F. Enteropathy of coeliac disease in adults: increased number of enterochromaffin cells in the duodenal mucosa. Gut 1982;23:42–8.
243. Solcia E, Vassallo G, Capella C. Cytology and cytochemistry of hormone producing cells of the upper gastrointestinal tract. In: Creutzfeldt W, ed. Origin, chemistry, pathology and pathophysiology of the gastrointestinal hormones. Stuttgart: Schattauer-Verlag, 1970:3–29.

Hyperplasia of Extra-Adrenal Paraganglia

244. Arias-Stella J, Bustos F. Chronic hypoaxia chemodectomas in bovine at high altitudes. Arch Pathol Lab Med 1976;100:636–9.

245. Arias-Stella J, Valcarcel J. Chief cell hyperplasia in the human carotid body at high altitudes: physiologic and pathologic significance. Hum Pathol 1976;7:361–73.

246. Edwards C, Heath D, Harris P. The carotid body in emphysema and left ventricular hypertrophy. J Pathol 1971;104:1–13.

247. Gaylis H, Davidge-Pitts K, Pantanowitz D. Carotid body tumours. A review of 52 cases. S Afn Med J 1987;72:493–6.

248. Habeck JO. Morphological findings at the carotid bodies of humans suffering from different types of systemic hypertension or severe lung diseases. Anat Ariz 1986;162:17–27.

249. Heath D, Smith P, Jago R. Hyperplasia of the carotid body. J Pathol 1982;138:115–27.

250. Jago R, Smith P, Heath D. Electron microscopy of carotid body hyperplasia. Arch Pathol Lab Med 1984;108:717–22.

251. Karasov RS, Sheps SG, Carney JA, van Heerden JA, DeQuattro V. Paragangliomatosis with numerous catecholamine-producing tumors. Mayo Clin Proc 1982;57:590–5.

252. Lack EE. Hyperplasia of vagal and carotid body paraganglia in patients with chronic hypoxemia. Am J Pathol 1978;91:497–516.

253. Lack EE. Pathology of adrenal and extra-adrenal paraganglia. Major problems in pathology, vol. 29. Philadelphia: WB Saunders, 1994.

254. Lack EE. Tumors of the adrenal gland and extra-adrenal paraganglia. Atlas of Tumor Pathology, 3rd Series, Fascicle 19. Washington, DC: Armed Forces Institute of Pathology, 1997.

255. Lack EE, Perez-Atayde AR, Young JB. Carotid body hyperplasia in cystic fibrosis and cyanotic heart disease. A combined morphometric, ultrastructural and biochemical study. Am J Pathol 1985;119:301–14.

256. Pacheco-Ojeda L, Durango E, Rodriquez C, Vivar N. Carotid body tumors at high altitudes. Quito, Ecuador, 1987. World J Surg 1988;12:856–60.

257. Rodriguez-Cuevas H, Lau I, Rodriguez HP. High altitude paragangliomas, diagnostic and therapeutic considerations. Cancer 1986;57:672–6.

258. Saldana MJ, Salem LE, Travezan R. High altitude hypoxia and chemodectomas. Hum Pathol 1973;4:251–63.

259. Smith P, Jago R, Heath D. Anatomical variation and quantitative histology of the normal and enlarged carotid body. J Pathol 1982;137:287–304.

Pulmonary Neuroendocrine Hyperplasia

260. Gosney JR, Sisson MC, Alliborne RO, Blakey AF. Pulmonary endocrine cells in chronic bronchitis and emphysema. J Pathol 1989;157:127–33.

261. Gould VE, Warren WH. The bronchopulmonary tract. In: Lechago J, Gould VE, eds. Bloodworth's endocrine pathology, 3rd ed. Baltimore: Williams & Wilkins, 1997:495–518.

262. Huntrakoon M, Menon CD, Hung KS. Diethylnitrosoamine-induced pulmonary endocrine cell hyperplasia and its association with adenomatosis and adenocarcinoma in rabbits. Am J Pathol 1989;135:1119–28.

263. Kamey T, Yamaguchi K. The endocrine lung. In: Kovacs K, Asa SL. Functional endodrine pathology, 2nd ed. Malden, MA: Blackwell Science, 1998:513–28.

264. Lauweryns JM, Cokelaere M, Theunynck P. Neuroepithelial bodies in the respiratory mucosa of various mammals. A light optical histochemical and ultrastructural investigation. Z Zellforsch Mikrosk Anat 1972;135:569–92.

265. Linnoila RI, Becker KL, Silva OL, Snider RH, Moore CF. Calcitonin as a marker for diethylnitrosamine-induced pulmonary endocrine cell hyperplasia in hamsters. Lab Invest 1984;51:39–45.

266. Memoli VA, Linnoila I, Warren WH, Rios-Dalenz J, Gould VE. Hyperplasia of pulmonary neuroendocrine cells and neuroepithelial bodies [Abstract]. Lab Invest 1983;48:57A.

267. Sorokin SP, Hayt RF Jr. Workshop on pulmonary neuroendocrine cells in health and disease. Anat Rec 1993;236:1–256.

268. Sunday ME. Pulmonary neuroendocrine cells and lung development. Endocr Pathol 1996;7:173–201.

269. Taylor W. Pulmonary argyrophil cells at high altitude. J Pathol 1977;122:137–44.

270. Tsutsumi Y, Osamura RY, Watanabe K, Yanaihara N. Immunohistochemical studies on gastrin-releasing peptide and adrenocorticotropic hormone containing cells in human lung. Lab Invest 1983;48:623–32.

271. Williams D, Heath D, Gosney J, Rios-Dalenz J. Pulmonary endocrine cells of Aymara Indians from the Bolivian Andes. Thorax 1993;48:52–6.

Index*

---

*Numbers in boldface indicate table and figure pages.